PROCEDURES IN RECONSTRUCTIVE SURGERY

DVD Contents

Series Editor: Gregory RD Evans

Cosmetic and Reconstructive
Breast Surgery

Approx run time 150 mins

D1710313

Cosmetic and
Reconstructive
Breast Surgery

PROCEDURES IN RECONSTRUCTIVE SURGERY

Series Editor: Gregory R.D. Evans MD FACS

General Reconstructive Surgery
Gregory R.D. Evans MD FACS and Garret A. Wirth MD
ISBN: 978-0-7020-2925-7

Head and Neck Reconstruction
Charles E. Butler MD FACS
ISBN: 978-0-7020-2926-4

Hand and Upper Extremity Reconstruction
Kevin C. Chung MD MS
ISBN: 978-0-7020-2916-5

Cosmetic and Reconstructive Breast Surgery
Maurice Y. Nahabedian MD FACS
ISBN: 978-0-7020-2915-8

Cosmetic and Reconstructive Breast Surgery

Edited by

Maurice Y. Nahabedian, MD FACS
Associate Professor of Plastic Surgery
Georgetown University
Washington, DC, USA

Series Editor

Gregory R.D. Evans MD FACS
Professor of Surgery and Biomedical Engineering
Chief, Aesthetic and Plastic Surgery Institute
University of California, Irvine
Orange, CA, USA

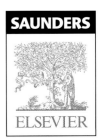

Edinburgh London New York Oxford Philadelphia St Louis Sydney Toronto 2009

SAUNDERS
ELSEVIER

An imprint of Elsevier Limited

© 2009, Elsevier Limited. All rights reserved.

First published 2009

ISBN: 978-0-7020-2915-8

British Library Cataloguing in Publication Data
A catalogue record for this book is available from the British Library
Cosmetic and reconstructive breast surgery. – (Procedures in reconstructive surgery series)
  1. Mammaplasty
  I. Nahabedian, Maurice
  618.1'9059

  ISBN-13: 9780702029158

Library of Congress Cataloging in Publication Data
A catalog record for this book is available from the Library of Congress

Notice

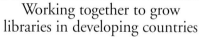

Working together to grow
libraries in developing countries

www.elsevier.com | www.bookaid.org | www.sabre.org

ELSEVIER   BOOK AID International   Sabre Foundation

your source for books,
journals and multimedia
in the health sciences
www.elsevierhealth.com

The
publisher's
policy is to use
**paper manufactured
from sustainable forests**

Printed in China

Commissioning Editor: Sue Hodgson
Development Editor: Claire Bonnett
Project Manager: Kathryn Mason
Cover designer: Jayne Jones
Designer: Sarah Russell
Illustration Manager: Kirsteen Wright
Illustrator: EPS, Inc.

TABLE OF CONTENTS

SERIES PREFACE

When I was studying for my Plastic Surgery Oral Boards and during my training, I was struck by the lack of a book that would explain common procedures in plastic surgery for specific problems. This is probably due to the unique and creative drive of our specialty and its emphasis on multiple approaches. Spurred by this seeming lack of a one volume book to carry to the operating room or utilize for studying, we produced an atlas for plastic surgery that would focus of common approaches to commonly seen problems. Now eight years later, the continued interest in such a book has produced this four volume set. The purpose of these volumes is to allow the student, resident or plastic surgeon to read and absorb common approaches to plastic surgery problems seen routinely. It is our hope that the procedures discussed in these volumes will allow quick in depth approaches, proposing common indications, surgical techniques, postoperative care and avoidance of pitfalls for common surgical problems. The student, resident or plastic surgeon should be able to utilize each of these volumes as a quick and easy access to treatment options for their patients. It is our desire that these volumes will become as popular as our first volume eight years ago and that a new generation of plastic surgeons will use, benefit and enjoy the books for years to come.

G.R.D.E.

VOLUME PREFACE

Cosmetic and Reconstructive Breast Surgery represents a novel approach in the preparation of a learning tool for plastic surgeons. The text is structured in a 'how-to' approach with a basic template that has been applied to all chapters. It has been highly illustrated with clinical pearls that should be useful to those who perform these operations. Many of the chapters have an audiovisual component that is intended to take the reader step-by-step through an operation. We feel that the combination of written and audiovisual material sets it apart from all previously published textbooks on cosmetic and reconstructive breast surgery and should facilitate one's ability to perform these operations at a higher level of understanding and ability.

The book is intended for all surgeons interested in breast surgery to review many of the essential principles, concepts, and techniques associated with cosmetic and reconstructive breast surgery and to provide some insight and clinical pearls that will facilitate one's ability to better master these procedures. There is a mix of reconstructive and cosmetic operations that were selected based on interest, need, and frequency. The contributors for each chapter were selected based on talent, ability, reputation, and a commitment to the educational process. The final product represents a compendium of breast operations that the plastic surgeon should be able to perform and master.

There are several individuals that I would like to thank for, without them, completion of the text would not have been possible. The first is Gregory R. D. Evans, MD who invited me to be the principal editor of the section on breast surgery. Greg and I were residents together at Johns Hopkins and have maintained a friendship since. Greg has always been a source of inspiration because he works as hard as anyone I know. I would also like to thank the staff at Elsevier for their hard work and commitment towards publishing a truly outstanding series on Procedures in Reconstructive Surgery. Finally, I would like to thank my family, Anissa, Danielle, and Sophia, for their support, patience, and understanding during the many hours spent in the preparation of this work.

M.Y.N.

Contributors

Siamak Agha-Mohammadi, MD, PhD
Clincial Assistant Professor of Surgery
(Plastic)
University of Pittsburgh Medical School
Hurwitz Center for Plastic Surgery
Pittsburgh, PA
USA

Diane Z. Alexander, MD, FACS
Artisan Plastic Surgery
Atlanta, GA
USA

Bernadette Wang Ashraf, MD, FACS
Artisan Plastic Surgery
Atlanta, GA
USA

Kristin A. Boehm, MD, FACS
Clinical Professor, Emory University
Paces Plastic Surgery
Atlanta, GA
USA

Bernard W. Chang, MD
Chief of Plastic Surgery
Mercy Medical Center;
Associate Professor of Surgery
Johns Hopkins School of Medicine
Plastic and Reconstructive Surgery at
Mercy
Baltimore, MD
USA

David W. Chang, MD, FACS
Professor of Surgery
Department of Plastic Surgery
The University of Texas M.D. Anderson
Cancer Center
Houston, TX
USA

Mark W. Clemens, MD
Resident
Department of Plastic Surgery
Georgetown University Medical Center
Washington, DC
USA

Steven P. Davison, MD, DDS, FACS
Associate Professor of Surgery
Department of Plastic Surgery
Georgetown University Medical Center
Washington, DC
USA

Joseph H. Dayan, MD
Chief Resident
Georgetown University Hospital
Washington, DC
USA

Joseph J. Disa, MD, FACS
Associate Attending Surgeon
Memorial Sloan-Kettering Cancer Center
Plastic and Reconstructive Surgery Service
New York, NY
USA

Matthew D. Goodwin, MD
Plastic and Reconstructive Surgeon
Boca Raton, FL
USA

Elizabeth J. Hall-Findlay, MD, FRCSC
Private Practice
Mineral Springs Hospital
Banff, AB
Canada

Moustapha Hamdi, MD
Associate Professor of Plastic Surgery
Department of Plastic and Reconstructive
Surgery
Gent University Hospital
Gent
Belgium

Dennis C. Hammond, MD
Center for Breast and Body Contouring
Grand Rapids, MI
USA

John Hijjawi, MD
Stephen Kroll Clinical Fellow, 2006
Department of Plastic and Reconstructive
Surgery
Gent University Hospital
Gent
Belgium;

Assistant Professor of Plastic Surgery
Department of Plastic Surgery
Medical College of Wisconsin and
Froedtert Hospital
Milwaukee, WI
USA

Dennis J. Hurwitz, MD, FACS
Clinical Professor of Surgery (Plastic)
University of Pittsburgh Medical School
Hurwitz Center for Plastic Surgery
Pittsburgh, PA
USA

Steven J. Kronowitz, MD, FACS
Associate Professor of Plastic Surgery
Department of Plastic Surgery
The University of Texas M.D. Anderson
Cancer Center
Houston, TX
USA

Colleen M. McCarthy, MD, MSc, FRCSC
Fellow
Memorial Sloan-Kettering Cancer Center
Plastic and Reconstructive Surgery Service
New York, NY
USA

Ali N. Mesbahi, MD
Resident in Plastic Surgery
Department of Plastic Surgery
Georgetown University Hospital
Washington, DC
USA

Maurice Y. Nahabedian, MD, FACS
Associate Professor of Plastic Surgery
Georgetown University
Washington, DC
USA

Foad Nahai, MD, FACS
Clinical Professor
Emory University;
Paces Plastic Surgery & Recovery Center
Atlanta, GA
USA

Kenneth C. Shestak, MD
Plastic Surgery Service
Magee Women's Hospital
Pittsburgh, PA
USA

Scott L. Spear, MD
Chairman
Department of Plastic Surgery
Georgetown University Hospital
Washington, DC
USA

Michael R. Zenn, MD, FACS
Associate Professor
Division of Plastic and Reconstructive
Surgery
Duke University Medical Center
Durham, NC
USA

Breast Reconstruction with Tissue Expanders and Implants

Maurice Y. Nahabedian and Ali N. Mesbahi

INTRODUCTION

Prosthetic devices for breast reconstruction following mastectomy have been available since the 1980s, and the use of expanders and implants is arguably the most commonly used technique. Over the past decade there have been significant advancements regarding the devices themselves and the methods of insertion that have promoted the safety and efficacy of this technique. This chapter focuses on many of the salient aspects of breast reconstruction using tissue expanders and/or implants. Emphasis will be placed on patient selection, device selection, one- versus two-stage reconstruction, immediate versus delayed reconstruction, delayed-immediate reconstruction, expander–implant reconstruction in the setting of radiation therapy, expander–implant reconstruction using bioprosthetic materials, and the management of complications.

INDICATIONS AND CONTRAINDICATIONS

Patient selection

Patient selection is becoming increasingly recognized as an important consideration when deciding on reconstructive options. As the techniques and methods to reconstruct a breast have improved, so have patient expectations been enhanced. It is no longer acceptable to merely create a mound on the chest wall: most women are interested in both volume and contour symmetry following either unilateral or bilateral reconstruction. With the variety of devices currently available, the ability to create a breast with symmetry of volume, position, and contour has increased.

Perhaps one of the most important aspects of patient selection is to understand their expectations. It is critical for women interested in breast reconstruction to understand that the reconstructed breast will not look exactly like the natural breast. The appearance may improve or it may not: the point is that it will be different. Women should understand that breast reconstruction is a staged procedure and that sometimes, several procedures will be necessary before a final desirable outcome can be achieved. Complications can occur regardless of the method of reconstruction selected. These may be minor or major and can include bleeding, infection, and reconstructive failure, which in the case of prosthetic devices includes premature removal, rupture, and capsular contracture.

Current options for women interested in breast reconstruction include autologous tissue or prosthetic devices. Although there is significant overlap in the criteria that would allow these procedures to be performed in a given woman, various factors should be considered that may result in the selection of one method rather than another. It is important to recognize that just about any size breast can be reconstructed with a prosthetic device. The most commonly used method of assessing breast size is via bra size. Although there are more quantifiable methods to make this assessment, such as three-dimensional imaging techniques, most women have a reasonable understanding of breast volume using bra sizing mechanics.

Relative contraindications for breast reconstruction with tissue expanders and implants are recognized. Body habitus will usually correlate with breast size. Morbid obesity is a relative contraindication for prosthetic reconstruction because the outcomes are often less satisfactory than in women with a moderate body habitus. In these situations, the expander or implant will have a significant volume that is below the projecting surface of the chest wall and will result in a breast with poor projection and contour. The delivery of radiotherapy before breast reconstruction with prosthetic devices is also a relative contraindication because the fibrosis that occurs following radiotherapy will often make breast expansion difficult. When making these decisions, it is important to assess patient expectations and recognize the inherent strengths and limitations of a given technique.

During the initial consultation with a woman regarding options for breast reconstruction following mastectomy, it may become very evident that she is interested in a procedure that is relatively quick, results in little downtime, and is associated with minimal morbidity. For many women considering prosthetic reconstruction, it is important to resume activities of daily living quickly, or to be able to continue with their physical activity with little disruption. Prosthetic devices are excellent in this regard because there are no additional operative sites, which facilitates postoperative recovery. In addition, women who choose to proceed with prosthetic reconstruction will continue to remain candidates for autologous reconstruction in the event of prosthetic failure or patient desire.

Prosthesis selection

The traditional patient for breast reconstruction with prosthetic devices is one who is generally thin, with small breasts, and with none or only mild breast ptosis. Fortunately, with the variety of implantable devices now available, these characteristics have expanded and can include women with a variety of body and breast shapes. It is now possible to create a breast with natural contours using prosthetic devices with volumes based on bra cup sizes ranging from A to D. Plastic surgeons have the luxury of a large number of devices at their disposal that will allow the creation of a breast with good to excellent aesthetic outcomes. The implants that are currently available vary in shape, surface texture, size, and filler material (Figs 1.1–1.3) Selection of the optimal device can at times be perplexing; however, there are several principles and concepts to facilitate the process. In general, decisions regarding the shape of the device are based on the physical appearance of the natural breast and patient expectations. Contoured and high-profile devices will usually enhance breast projection, whereas round and mild to moderate-profile devices will result in less projection and have the potential for increased ptosis. A textured surface is used for contoured devices to prevent malrotation. A smooth surface is usually used for round implants and will permit increased mobility of the breast. Silicone gel devices will more closely mimic the natural 'feel' of the breast compared to saline-filled devices. They also improve appearance because there is usually less wrinkling and rippling associated with silicone gel than with saline. Breast implant size is guided by patient expectations but optimized based on the volume, base diameter, and surface characteristics of the natural breast as well as the body habitus.

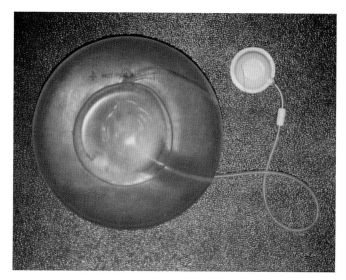

FIGURE 1.2 Postoperatively adjustable expander/implant. This device can be used for one-stage reconstruction or as the permanent implant during the second stage of a two-stage reconstruction. The remote valve is secured to the chest wall and removed as a separate procedure when postoperative volume symmetry is achieved.

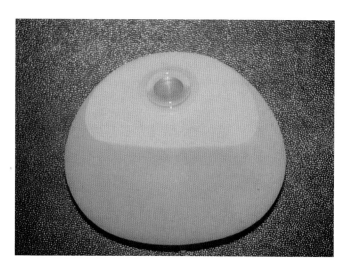

FIGURE 1.1 Contour profile tissue expander. This is the most common type of tissue expander used for the first stage of a two-stage breast reconstruction. It has a textured surface, an integrated fill valve, and is filled with saline.

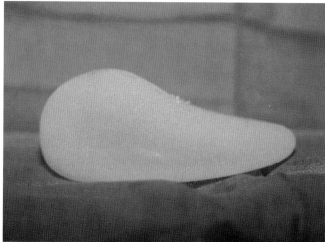

FIGURE 1.3 Contour profile implant. These devices are ideal for the second stage of a two-stage reconstruction. The highly cohesive silicone gel implants are form-stable and can promote ideal breast contours.

The use of silicone gel implants for breast reconstruction has been receiving increasing attention. These devices have been available since 1963, but since 1990 have been subject to significant controversy and debate, especially in the United States. Since that time, there have been hundreds of scientific studies and publications supporting the safety and efficacy of these devices. Currently, silicone gel implants are available to all women for breast reconstruction, and in this author's practice are preferred by the majority because of their superior qualities. Improvements in gel cohesiveness and shell integrity, as well as scientific and epidemiologic studies demonstrating no adverse health consequences, have resulted in widespread acceptance of these devices.

The consultation

There are many important issues that must be discussed before proceeding with prosthetic breast reconstruction. These points are the opinion of the primary author and may not apply to everyone. One of the first is that prosthetic devices can result in a beautiful reconstruction. However, the devices will not last forever. They all have a finite lifespan and will more likely than not have to be removed or replaced at some future date. Reasons for failure include capsular contracture, rupture, infection, and poor aesthetic outcome. In general, implant-based breast reconstruction tends to deteriorate over time because of the body's response to foreign substances.

The issue of patient expectations is important to reiterate. It must be understood that more than one operation may be necessary before the final result is achieved. Secondary operations are usually spaced apart by at least 3 months to allow for the previous procedure to mature. The reconstructed breast can look good, but it will be different from the non-operated breast.

Pre- and postoperative photographs should be reviewed in order to review possible outcomes, which may be excellent, average, or poor. Some women are under the impression that breast reconstruction with implants is similar to breast augmentation with implants. It must be explained that the reconstructed breast will usually project more and feel different from the natural breast, because the implant is essentially responsible for 90–95% of the projecting volume, whereas with augmentation a much larger percentage of the projecting volume is natural breast tissue. Following a mastectomy there is very little subcutaneous fat remaining. The photographs will also help women to understand the nature and location of the scars, as well as the fact that they may be pink to red for 1 or 2 years after the operation.

OPERATIVE APPROACH

Immediate breast reconstruction using prosthetic devices

Immediate reconstruction using prosthetic devices is currently the most commonly performed breast reconstruction

---

BOX 1.1 Two-stage immediate breast reconstruction with expanders and implants

- The amount of skin preserved at the time of mastectomy correlates inversely with the need for expansion: the more skin envelope present, the less need for volume or expansion.
- Options for expander placement include total muscular coverage, 'dual-plane' technique, and pectoralis extender method with bioprosthetic material.
- Potential pitfalls associated with total muscular coverage include patient discomfort during the expansion process and the potential for superior displacement of the device due to muscle spasm.
- Consider potential for adjuvant radiation and chemotherapy.

---

technique for women following mastectomy. The reasons for this are multifactorial and include a relatively simple operation, facilitated recovery, and little downtime. Many women are averse to removing tissues from remote parts of their body resulting in additional scars, potential donor site morbidity, and prolonged recovery. The technology and practice of breast reconstruction with prosthetic devices have significantly changed and improved over the recent past, but controversies have always existed and still continue. There has always been debate over whether to proceed with one- or two-stage reconstruction using prosthetic devices. The reality is that both methods are appropriate and acceptable in certain situations, and will be reviewed here.

Two-stage breast reconstruction with expanders and implants

Two-stage prosthetic reconstruction is arguably more commonly performed than its one-stage counterpart. The principle behind two-stage reconstruction is that the mastectomy skin is first expanded with a temporary device or tissue expander in order to attain the desired volume. During the second stage the tissue expander is removed and a permanent implant inserted. This creates a breast that is optimally shaped, contoured, and positioned (Fig. 1.4). One-stage immediate breast reconstruction can be performed when there is little need to expand the skin following the mastectomy, for example after mastectomy with nipple/areolar preservation, or following skin-sparing mastectomy in a woman with a small or non-ptotic breast. Both techniques are capable of delivering an acceptable outcome. Outcome is ultimately linked to proper patient selection, device selection, and surgeon experience.

Planning: Stage 1

In formulating a plan for breast reconstruction using a tissue expander, various factors should be considered. These include the type of mastectomy (nipple/areolar sparing, skin sparing, or non-skin sparing), type of implant (profile height, length and volume of implant), quality of the mastectomy

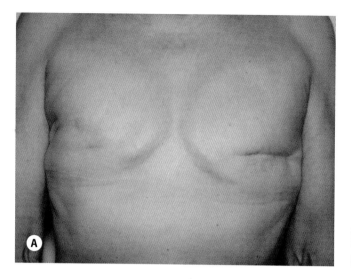

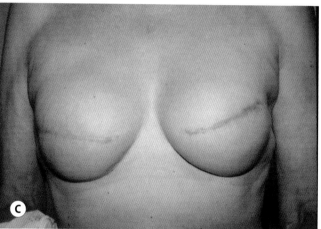

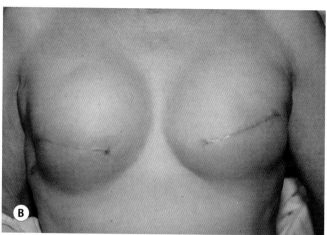

FIGURE 1.4 A Preoperative photograph following bilateral mastectomy. **B** The first stage of a two-stage reconstruction using a 450 mL tissue expander. A breast mound is created, but the inframammary fold is poorly defined. **C** The second stage of a two-stage reconstruction is completed. A 400 mL smooth, round permanent implant has been inserted. The inframammary fold has been recreated using a thoracoepigastric advancement.

skin flaps, history of prior or upcoming radiation therapy, and whether or not to use biosynthetic materials such as acellular dermal matrix. Most mastectomies today are performed using a skin-sparing pattern in which only the nipple–areolar complex and glandular tissue are excised. The advantage of this is that the majority of the skin envelope is preserved and will minimize the amount of expansion required, facilitating the obtaining of contour and volume symmetry.

Selection of the tissue expander is based upon preoperative measurements of the breast, including the base diameter, tissue compliance, and volume. Current methods of expander selection are primarily based on the base diameter of the breast. This dimension should correlate with the base diameter of the implant. This will permit the device to be optimally positioned along the anterior chest wall and inframammary fold, and to more closely mimic the size of the natural breast. It is important to assess patient expectations and determine whether the reconstructed breast should be larger, smaller, or equal to the natural breast in terms of size. Volume assessment is important because a given base diameter can correlate with a variety of implant shapes and heights. Volumes can be estimated in the office or deter-

mined in the operating room based on the weight of the mastectomy specimen.

Stage 1 using a tissue expander only

The preoperative markings include the sternal midline, the inframammary and lateral mammary folds, and delineation of a proposed mastectomy incision. Rather than performing a circular incision around the nipple–areolar complex, a small elliptical incision incorporating the complex is preferred in order to facilitate closure. Skin-sparing mastectomies are beneficial because as the quantity of the natural breast skin envelope is increased, the amount of relative expansion is reduced. In addition, a greater amount of saline can be instilled into the expander during this initial operation.

Following the mastectomy, the plastic surgeon has two options for expander placement. The first is total muscular coverage under the pectoralis major muscle, and the second is partial muscular coverage under the pectoralis major. This second method is currently referred to as the 'dual-plane' technique, in which the upper two-thirds of the expander is covered by the pectoralis major and the lower one-third is covered by the lower mastectomy skin flap. A third option is possible involving the use of bioprosthetic materials to serve as a pectoralis extender. This will be described later.

It is important to review the fundamental concepts regarding the handling of tissue expanders and implants. Many of the specifics are the preferred methods of the primary author, whereas others are recommended by the manufacturers (Mentor Corporation, Santa Barbara, CA and Allergan Corporation (formerly Inamed), Irvine, CA). Sterility must be maintained during the insertion. Gloves should be changed or washed with an antibiotic solution. Sharp objects and cautery devices should not come in contact with the implants. Following the removal of the expander from its container it is soaked in an antibiotic–saline solution. All air is evacuated from the expander using a large syringe with an appropriate needle. It is the authors' practice to partially fill the expander with 50 mL of saline prior to insertion into the subpectoral space.

Total muscular coverage of the tissue expander has been commonly performed by many plastic surgeons. This achieves stable coverage of the expander but often results in an uncomfortably high-riding device that frequently encroaches on the clavicle. This has been thought to be secondary to muscle spasm and contraction, which has the effect of pushing the expander superiorly. The dual-plane technique has obviated many of the shortcomings of total muscular coverage by positioning the base of the expander at the inframammary fold. With this technique, the pectoralis major muscle is draped over the expander and secured via marionette sutures or via direct sutures to the dermis or to the subcutaneous tissues of the lower mastectomy skin flap. When properly performed, the dual-plane technique essentially eliminates the risk of a high-riding expander. The technique is illustrated in Figure 1.5. In the event of a narrow chest wall and a tissue expander with a larger base diameter than that of the subpectoral pocket, it may be necessary to undermine along the lateral border of the serratus anterior muscle in order to create a cul-de-sac to prevent lateral displacement of the expander. One to two drains are used and usually remain in place for 1 week.

Following completion of the operation, patients are usually discharged home on postoperative day 1 with a prescription for oral antibiotics. Serial inflation of the tissue expander is performed in the office and begun 2 weeks after the operation. Generally 50–100 mL are instilled weekly until the desired volume is obtained. In the event of adjuvant therapy such as chemotherapy or radiation, it is the authors' practice to discontinue the expansion process. However, studies have demonstrated that expansion can be safely continued during chemotherapy if so desired. In the event of radiation therapy, ongoing expansion is contraindicated during treatment to avoid disturbance of dosimetry and the target site. Some radiation oncologists recommend that the partially inflated tissue expander be deflated during radiation treatment. Once all adjuvant treatments are completed and the tissue expander is optimally filled, the expander may be exchanged for a permanent implant. When no radiation therapy was administered, this usually occurs 1 month after the final expansion. When radiation therapy has been administered, this usually occurs 3–6 months following the final expansion, or when the skin has sufficiently healed and softened.

Stage 1 with a tissue expander and bioprosthetic material

Perhaps one of the most significant advancements in breast reconstruction using tissue expanders has resulted from the application of bioprosthetic materials. These are composed of decellularized cadaveric dermis in the form of a tissue matrix. The advantage of this material is that, when properly used, it will revascularize and integrate into the surrounding tissues and assume the tissue characteristics of the host. The most recognized and used bioprosthetic material today is AlloDerm (LifeCell Corporation, Branchburg, NJ). AlloDerm has been used in a variety of clinical scenarios and most recently in breast reconstruction. Its role as a 'pectoralis extender' is becoming widely accepted as a means of improving outcomes.

The technique of tissue expander placement using AlloDerm is straightforward but does require additional steps. The AlloDerm comes in variously sized sheets, but the two sizes currently in use for this purpose measure 4 × 16 cm and 6 × 16 cm. AlloDerm requires hydration in a saline solution until it is soft and pliable, usually for approximately 10–20 minutes, according to the thickness of the material. Therefore, the hydration process should be begun at the start of the reconstruction procedure.

The technique of AlloDerm insertion to be described is that used by the primary author (Fig. 1.6). There may be differences in technique based on surgeons' preference. Following the mastectomy, the inferior border of the pectoralis major muscle is detached using electrocautery and extended laterally towards its humeral insertion. The AlloDerm is inserted adjacent to the inferior border of the pectoralis major and should be orientated with its basement membrane (shiny) side up. This is the side that will tend to revascularize with the greatest efficiency and therefore should be in contact with the lower mastectomy skin flap. The medial border of the AlloDerm is sutured to the inferomedial corner of the pectoralis major using a 2/0 monofilament absorbable suture. The inferior border of the AlloDerm is then sutured to the inframammary fold using the same technique. The tissue expander filled with 50 mL of saline is inserted in the dual-plane position at this time. The suture points of the AlloDerm along the lateral chest wall are also adjusted at this time. The location along the lateral chest wall where the AlloDerm is attached to recreate the lateral mammary fold is based on both the diameter of the tissue expander and the delineated natural position of the lateral mammary fold. Sometimes the length of AlloDerm is excessive and shortening is required. It is important to compartmentalize the expander and not allow for lateral or medial displacement. Once set, two closed suction drainage tubes are inserted. The first is placed between the AlloDerm and the tissue expander, and the second between the AlloDerm and the lower mastectomy skin flap. The upper border of the AlloDerm is sutured to the lower border of the pectoralis major. Additional saline is instilled into

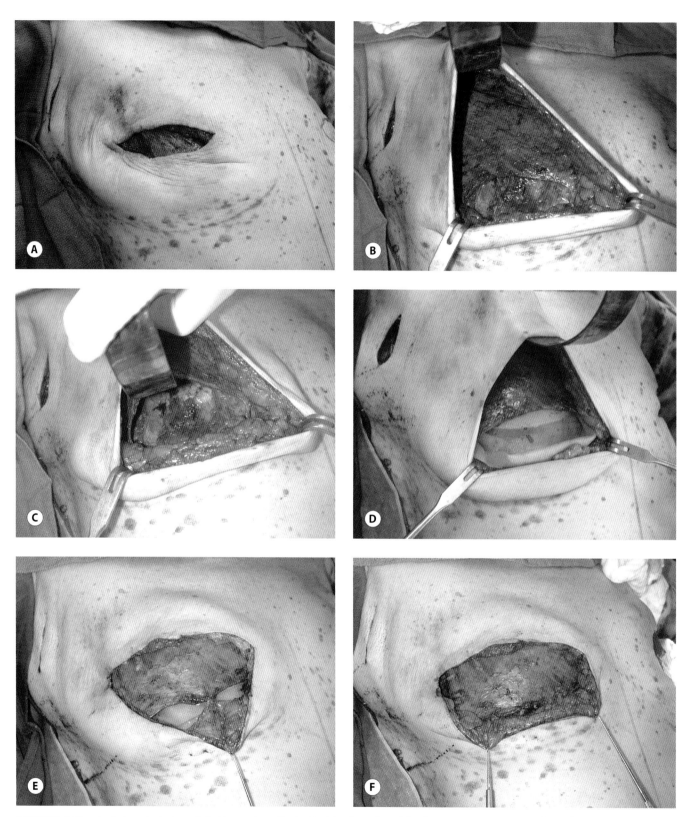

FIGURE 1.5 The dual-plane technique **A** A skin-sparing elliptical incision is preferred for the mastectomy pattern. This will permit linear closure with minimal 'dog-ear' formation. **B** The inferior border of the pectoralis major muscle is incised extending from its medial origin and extending to its inferolateral origin. **C** The subpectoral pocket is created with sufficient space to accommodate the tissue expander. The lateral border of the serratus anterior muscle is sometimes elevated to create a lateral cul-de-sac for the expander. **D** The tissue expander is inserted into the subpectoral space. The base of the expander is positioned at the inframammary fold. When the fold has been undermined during the mastectomy, it must be reapproximated. **E** The inferior border of the pectoralis major muscle is sutured to the subcutaneous tissue of the lower mastectomy skin flap using absorbable sutures. **F** The entire inferior border of the pectoralis major muscle is sutured to the lower mastectomy skin flap. The upper portion of the expander is covered by muscle and the lower portion by subcutaneous tissue.

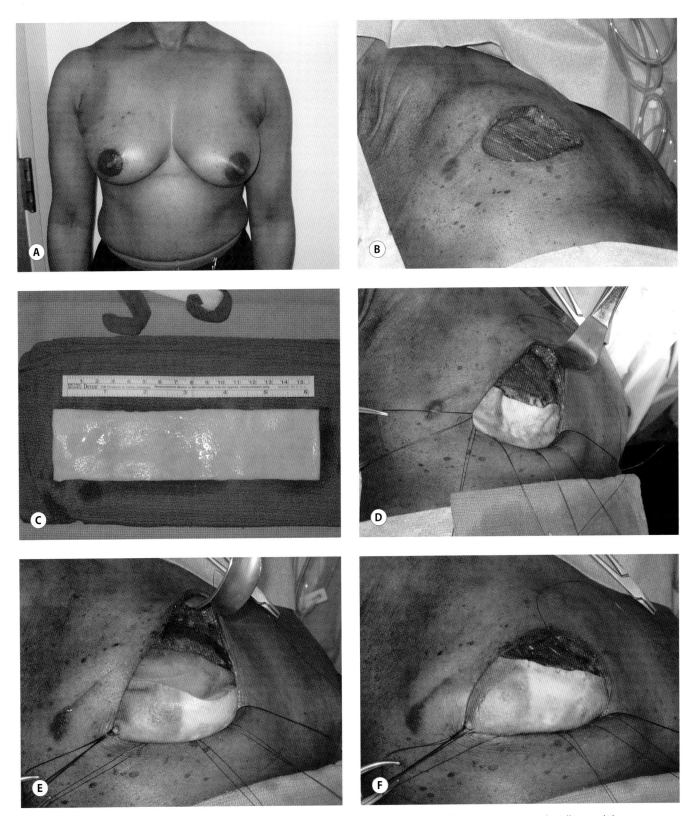

FIGURE 1.6 Technique of AlloDerm insertion. **A** Preoperative photograph. The important landmarks are the sternal midline and the inframammary folds. The inframammary fold is measured to assist with AlloDerm sizing. **B** Following the mastectomy, the inferior and lateral borders of the pectoralis major muscle are elevated. The serratus anterior muscle is undisturbed. **C** The AlloDerm is hydrated in a warm saline solution. **D** The AlloDerm is inserted and oriented horizontally with the basement membrane side up. The medial border of the AlloDerm is sutured to the inferomedial corner of the pectoralis muscle. The inferior border of the AlloDerm is sutured to the inframammary fold. The lateral border of the AlloDerm is trimmed and adjusted to accommodate the base dimension of the expander. **E** The tissue expander is aspirated of all air, filled with 50 mL saline, and inserted into the subpectoral pocket in the dual plane. **F** The inferior border of the pectoralis major muscle is temporarily stapled to the superior border of the AlloDerm. Additional saline is instilled until mild to moderate tension is achieved.

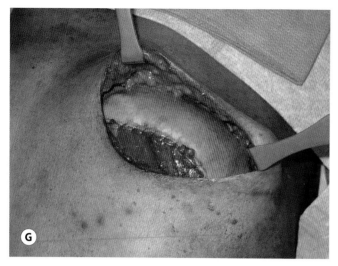

FIGURE 1.6, cont'd G The pectoral muscle and AlloDerm are sutured and the staples removed. Two drains are inserted, one above and one below the AlloDerm.

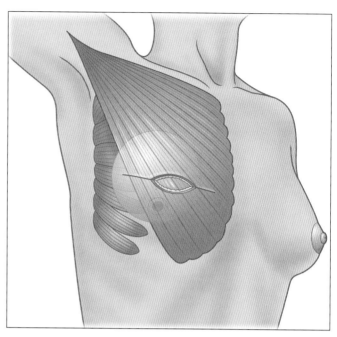

FIGURE 1.7 Second-stage implant exchange. The mastectomy scar is incised. The inferior border of the pectoralis major muscle is incised and the expander removed. A permanent implant is inserted with or without a remote port.

the expander at this time, the amount varying depending on the implant size, degree of internal tension, and amount of mastectomy skin present.

Stage 2 – the permanent implant

The advantage of breast reconstruction in two stages is that during stage 1, the tissue expander will effectively stretch the skin and underlying structures, and during stage 2 is replaced by a permanent implant to optimize the aesthetic outcome. The decision as to which permanent device to select can be perplexing, especially when one considers that the shape can be round or contoured, the surface can be textured or smooth, and the filler can be saline or silicone gel. The benefit of using silicone gel devices is most appreciated following the second stage of a breast reconstruction in which a silicone gel device has been selected as the permanent implant. It is important to appreciate that the permanent implant following a mastectomy is responsible for 95% of the contour, appearance, and feel of the reconstructed breast. For these reasons, it is the authors' opinion that silicone gel-filled implants have an advantage over saline-filled devices. Silicone gel mimics the natural feel of the breast more closely than saline. In addition, there is less rippling and wrinkling associated with silicone gel implants. Currently, silicone gel implants are available as smooth round devices and as textured contoured devices. Both can achieve excellent aesthetic results and can be selected based on surgeon recommendation, patient acceptance, and patient expectations.

The second stage of the two-stage reconstruction is technically simpler than stage 1 but requires attention to detail. It is explained that during this procedure the location and position of the implant will be optimized, the feel of the device will be improved as the scar tissue is released and a new implant inserted, and the aesthetic appearance of the breast will be enhanced. The technical aspects of an implant exchange are relatively straightforward. The previous incision scar is usually excised. The dissection proceeds toward the inferior edge of the pectoralis major muscle (Fig. 1.7). The capsule of the implant is incised and the expander removed. The remaining capsule is incised or excised as necessary. All breast specimens are sent to pathology to rule out carcinoma. The permanent implant is inserted and a drain is usually used.

Postoperative recovery is characterized by drain care instructions, oral antibiotic therapy for 5–7 days, and restriction of physical exercise for 4–6 weeks. This is necessary in order for the newly inserted device to settle into its new position with minimal risk of displacement. Patients are permitted to shower on postoperative day 2 or 3. Drains are usually removed between postoperative days 5 and 7, although extra time may be necessary depending on the drains' output.

Clinical outcomes following immediate breast reconstruction in two stages can be excellent. Because the natural breast landmarks are preserved, the re-establishment of the inframammary and lateral mammary folds is facilitated. In the case of unilateral reconstruction, contralateral procedures may be necessary. However, following bilateral reconstruction, symmetry is the rule rather than the exception. Figures 1.8 and 1.9 illustrate the outcome following unilateral and bilateral reconstructions.

One-stage reconstruction with implants

An alternative method to two-stage reconstruction using prosthetic devices is the one-stage technique. This method does not require the use of the classic tissue expander

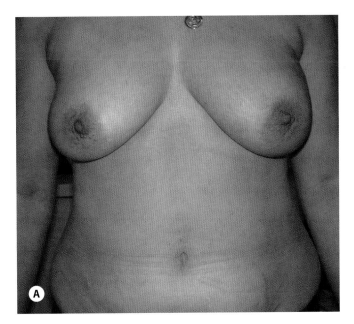

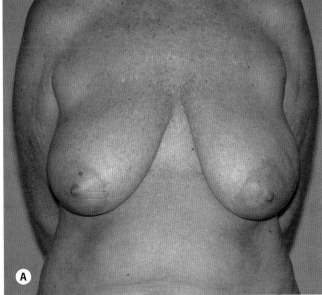

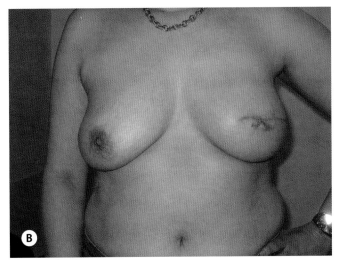

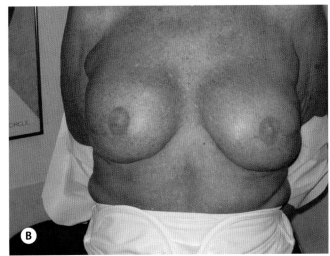

FIGURE 1.8 Immediate unilateral two-stage breast reconstruction. **A** Preoperative photograph demonstrating grade 2 ptosis and symmetry. **B** Following the second stage, grade 2 ptosis is re-established and breast symmetry is achieved without a contralateral procedure.

FIGURE 1.9 Immediate bilateral two-stage breast reconstruction. **A** Preoperative photograph demonstrating grade 2/3 ptosis. **B** Following two-stage reconstruction, there is a slight contour asymmetry with an overall outcome rated as excellent by the patient.

> **BOX 1.2 One-stage immediate breast reconstruction with implants**
>
> - Typically employs the use of devices that are postoperatively adjustable through a remote port.
> - Candidates are women with small breasts and minimal ptosis, or other cases in which the need for expansion is minimal, such as nipple- or skin-sparing mastectomy.
> - One-stage reconstruction is usually limited to women who will have immediate reconstruction.

but rather uses a permanent implant that is adjustable postoperatively.

The adjustable implant with a remote port is ideally designed for women who desire or are candidates for one-stage reconstruction. In general, these include women with small breasts and minimal ptosis as well as women following nipple- or skin-sparing mastectomy, in which the need to expand the mastectomy skin flaps is minimal. The adjustable implants that are available for this purpose include both saline and silicone gel devices, such as the Spectrum and the Becker implants (Mentor Corporation, Santa Barbara, CA) (Fig. 1.10). Spectrum implants are saline devices that are available in a smooth or textured surface and in a round or contoured shape. The Becker implant is a dual-compartment device in which the outer

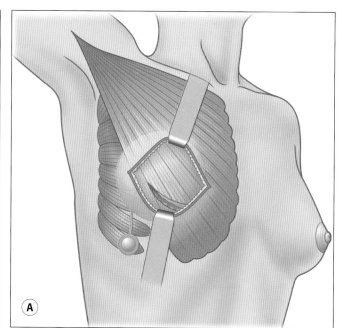

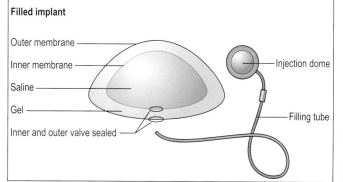

Filled implant

Outer membrane
Inner membrane
Saline
Gel
Inner and outer valve sealed

Injection dome
Filling tube

FIGURE 1.10 Postoperatively adjustable implants. The Spectrum and Becker implants are characterized by the remote port. The Becker implant is compartmentalized. The outer non-adjustable compartment is silicone gel and the inner adjustable compartment is saline.

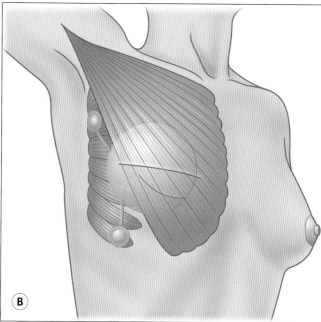

FIGURE 1.11 Remote valve position. Through the mastectomy opening, the lower border of the pectoralis major is incised, the subpectoral plane is created, and the postoperatively adjustable implant is inserted. The remote valve can be positioned along the inframammary fold (**A**) or along the lateral mammary fold (**B**).

lumen is composed of silicone gel and the inner lumen of saline. The advantage of the Becker implant is that the device will feel like a silicone gel implant and have the adjustability of a saline implant. Use of these implants for one-stage reconstruction is usually limited to women who will have immediate reconstruction. For women interested in delayed reconstruction using prosthetic devices the two-stage technique is usually recommended.

The technique for one-stage reconstruction using adjustable implants is similar to the first phase of the two-stage reconstruction. Following the mastectomy, the subpectoral plane is created. The implant, with the attached remote port, is positioned such that its inferior base is at the level of the inframammary fold. The dual-plane technique is the authors' preferred method of implant placement. In cases where the mastectomy results in substantial undermining of the inframammary fold, absorbable sutures are used to

reposition and secure this important anatomic landmark. The remote port is then sutured to a stable base. In these cases, this is usually to the lateral chest wall or to the anterior chest wall just below the inframammary fold (Figs 1.11, 1.12). The inferior edge of the pectoralis major muscle is then secured as previously described using either Allo-Derm or suture ligation to the inferior mastectomy skin flap. The implant is then filled with saline. Devices prefilled with silicone gel can also be used for one-stage breast recon-

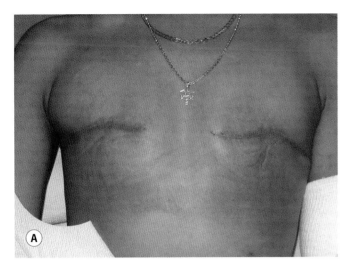

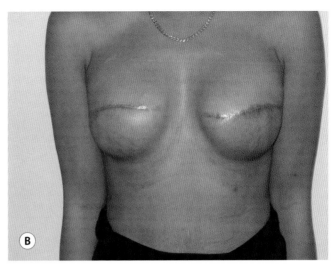

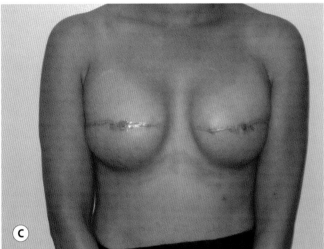

FIGURE 1.12 Delayed bilateral two-stage breast reconstruction. **A** Preoperative photograph following bilateral mastectomy without radiation therapy. **B** Stage 1 of the reconstruction using 350 mL tissue expanders. **C** The tissue expander has been removed and replaced with a 350 mL contour profile silicone gel implant.

struction; however, subpectoral insertion can be compromised by considerations of volume.

DELAYED BREAST RECONSTRUCTION USING TISSUE EXPANDERS AND IMPLANTS

When immediate breast reconstruction is not recommended for women with breast cancer following mastectomy, delayed reconstruction is often a possibility. Many women are not considered good candidates for immediate reconstruction because of advanced tumor stage, cutaneous involvement, or the need for aggressive tumor surveillance. In these women, the oncologic considerations take precedence over the aesthetic and psychological advantages of immediate reconstruction.

The approach to prosthetic reconstruction in the delayed setting is different from the immediate setting. In the immediate setting the normal breast landmarks, such as the inframammary fold, the lateral mammary fold, and the cutaneous envelope, are well defined and present. In the delayed setting, the inframammary and the lateral mammary folds are obliterated. The soft, supple breast is replaced by a layer of scar. There is also a skin deficit following excision

of the cutaneous envelope of the breast. Thus two-stage reconstruction is the rule rather than the exception for delayed reconstruction with prosthetic devices. The role of the tissue expander in the woman having delayed reconstruction is amplified because of the need to stretch the limited amount of remaining skin.

Delayed breast reconstruction: preoperative considerations

Delayed reconstruction can pose different challenges to the surgeon because the primary landmarks of the breast are usually no longer present and the cutaneous envelope has been removed. The goal is therefore to create a three-dimensional breast from a two-dimensional surface. This is best achieved following a two-stage breast reconstruction using a combination of tissue expanders and implants.

During the preoperative evaluation it is important to assess the quality of the chest wall skin following the mastectomy. Ideally it should be soft and supple, but in the event of pre- or post-mastectomy radiation this may not be the case. Delayed breast reconstruction using tissue expanders and implants is not usually recommended in the setting of previous radiation therapy because of the difficulties encountered with skin expansion. The skin has compromised vascularity and a relative inelasticity due to the radiation fibrosis that has ensued. Contrary to the irradiated chest wall, the non-irradiated chest will expand easily and is very amenable to tissue expansion. The size of the implant required is best determined by measuring the base width of the opposite breast or by estimating the base width of the chest wall based on the distance between the anterior axillary line and the medial border of the sternum.

Operative approach

Delayed breast reconstruction – stage 1

Before entering the operating room, the landmarks of the breast are delineated, including the lateral and inframammary folds as well as the sternal midline. In the operating room, the mastectomy scar is excised and submitted to pathology. Dissection proceeds posteriorly to the level of the pectoralis major, and then inferiorly along the adipopectoral plane to the inferior border of the pectoralis major. Usually this is a very short distance, ranging from 1 to 2 cm. Dissection proceeds in the subpectoral plane and a space is created to accommodate the expander that conforms to the delineated breast landmarks. The expander is prepared as previously described. The use of bioprosthetic material can be considered for delayed breast reconstruction, but in the primary author's practice is not normally used. Use of a single drain is recommended to prevent the accumulation of a seroma and to prevent rotation of the contoured expander. Once the expander is inserted, the pectoral muscle is either reapproximated or sutured to the lower mastectomy skin flap using absorbable sutures. Skin closure is the final step. Additional sterile saline can be instilled as tolerated, based on skin elasticity. The usual amount ranges from 50 to 100 mL in this setting.

Postoperative recovery is much as for immediate reconstruction with an expander. The drains are usually removed after 5–7 days, or when the output is less than 30 mL/day. Expansion is commenced after 2 weeks and continues up to the maximum permitted, based on expander volume or when the patient is happy with the volume. It is advised to expand 50–100 mL beyond the final desired volume because there will be some skin contraction when the expander is removed. The additional skin can be used to create a better inframammary fold during the second stage.

Delayed breast reconstruction – stage 2

The technical aspects of the second stage of delayed breast reconstruction are similar to those of the second stage of an immediate reconstruction. The main difference is that the cutaneous envelope has been more stretched than in the latter. This will result in some degree of elastic recoil when the expander is removed. Overexpansion will be beneficial in these situations for the reasons given above. The primary objective of the second stage is to ensure adequate breast volume and projection; however, a secondary objective is to recreate the inframammary fold adequately.

Breast volume and projection are best achieved in this setting using contoured implants or high-profile round implants. These can be saline or silicone gel-filled. In the primary author's practice the silicone gel devices have provided the best outcomes based on appearance and texture. There is less rippling and wrinkling, and the breast reconstructed with silicone gel devices mimics the natural breast more closely. Before inserting these devices, the soft tissue capsule created by the tissue expander is scored or excised depending on its thickness and the degree of contracture. The authors' preferred technique is to score the capsule circumferentially at the base and then to score the lower and/or upper poles of the expanded skin envelope radially. This will effectively increase the elasticity of the cutaneous envelope and allow for enhanced breast shaping and positioning.

The inframammary fold is best recreated by undermining the thoracoepigastric soft tissue plane slightly below the level of the proposed fold. The tissue is advanced in a cephalad direction and then sutured to the inframammary fold. This effectively provides additional skin that can be used to create breast ptosis at the level of the fold.

Outcomes following delayed reconstruction can be excellent for both unilateral and bilateral reconstructions. The creation of an inframammary fold can be difficult but is best achieved with a thoracoepigastric advancement flap. In the event of a unilateral reconstruction, a contralateral procedure is sometimes necessary and may include breast augmentation or reduction. Clinical examples are illustrated in Figs 1.12–1.14.

DELAYED-IMMEDIATE BREAST RECONSTRUCTION

The technique of delayed-immediate breast reconstruction was introduced in 2004 and has proved very useful because of the increasing trend for post-mastectomy radiation therapy following immediate breast reconstruction with autologous tissue. The untoward effects of radiation on an autologous reconstruction are well known and include flap shrinkage, fat necrosis, generalized fibrosis, progressive distortion, and contour abnormalities. The effects of radiation on the quality of prosthetic reconstruction can be equally deleterious, and include capsular contracture, delayed

---

BOX 1.3 Delayed-immediate breast reconstruction

- Placement of a tissue expander when immediate autologous tissue reconstruction is desired but the need for post-mastectomy radiation is uncertain.
- If radiation is necessary, expander is inflated beforehand, allowing expansion of the cutaneous envelope and preservation of normal breast landmarks. Autologous reconstruction can be completed after the radiation is complete.
- Final outcome will resemble that of an immediate reconstruction despite being performed on a delayed basis.

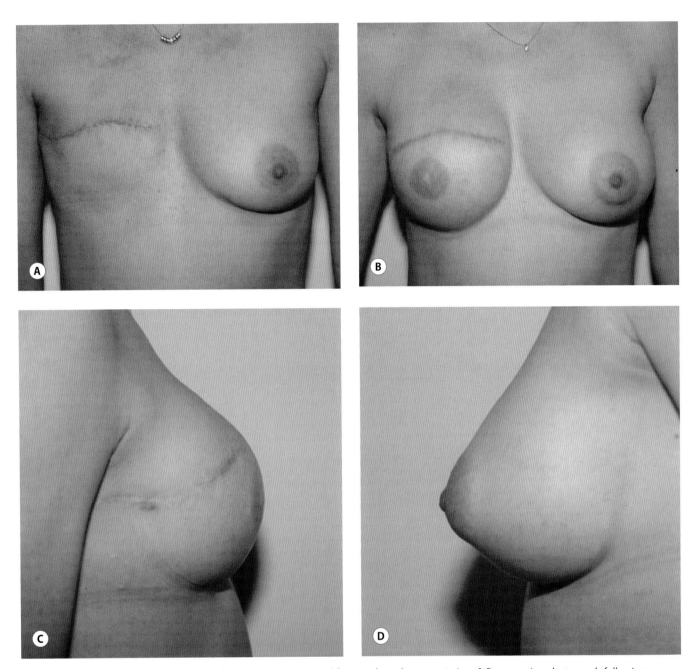

FIGURE 1.13 Delayed unilateral two-stage breast reconstruction with contralateral augmentation. **A** Preoperative photograph following unilateral mastectomy without radiation therapy. **B** Postoperative photograph following right breast reconstruction and left breast augmentation. **C** Lateral view of the right breast following reconstruction. **D** Lateral view of the left breast following augmentation.

healing, infection, progressive distortion, and premature removal. The difference between autologous reconstruction and prosthetic reconstruction is that the first is permanent and the second can be temporary. The radiated tissue expander can easily be removed, whereas the flap cannot.

The premise of delayed-immediate reconstruction is that when immediate breast reconstruction with autologous tissue is being considered or desired and the need for post-mastectomy radiation therapy is uncertain, a tempo-rary tissue expander can be inserted immediately after the mastectomy. Once the final pathology and tumor staging are completed, usually 1 week after the operation, the decision to proceed or not with radiation therapy is clear. If radiation is not necessary, the patient can be scheduled for autologous reconstruction as soon as possible. If radiation is necessary, the expander can be inflated beforehand. Following the radiation, the tissue expander is removed and replaced with autologous tissue. The reason to proceed in

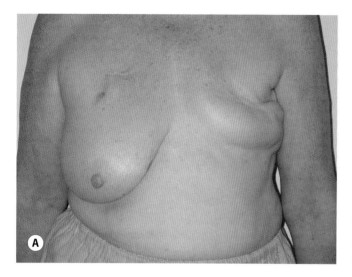

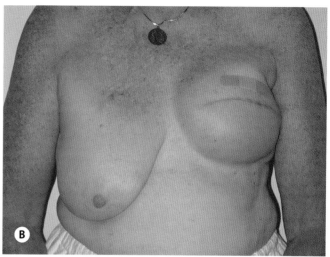

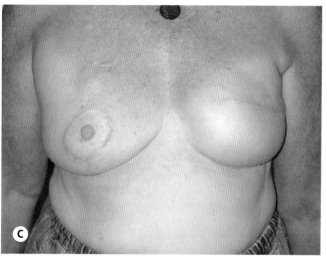

FIGURE 1.14 Delayed unilateral two-stage breast reconstruction with contralateral reduction mammoplasty. **A** Preoperative photograph following left mastectomy without radiation therapy. **B** Following the tissue expansion of the left breast, there is significant asymmetry. **C** Following stage 2, the left expander is removed and replaced with a permanent implant and the right breast is reduced to achieve volume and contour symmetry.

BOX 1.4 Two-stage delayed breast reconstruction with expanders and implants

- Often more challenging owing to loss of normal breast landmarks, such as the inframammary fold, and scarring of the cutaneous envelope.
- Goal is to create a three-dimensional breast from a two-dimensional surface.
- Potential pitfall: expansion of an irradiated chest wall has the potential for higher complication rates and difficult expansion due to the lack of skin elasticity. Autologous tissue reconstruction is preferred in such cases.
- Second stage generally involves more breast shaping with capsule manipulation and recreation of the inframammary fold.

this fashion is because the final outcome resembles that of an immediate reconstruction despite the fact that it is delayed. This is because the inframammary fold is preserved and the cutaneous skin envelope stretched prior to radiation.

Operative approach

The patient is marked as previously described. A skin-sparing mastectomy is preferred when possible. Following the mastectomy, the technique is identical to that of immediate tissue expansion without the use of bioprosthetic materials. Despite the temporary nature of this procedure, subcutaneous placement of the expander is not recommended. Delayed healing can occur and has resulted in premature removal of the temporary expander, hence the subpectoral position is preferred. After radiation the patient will have a choice between continuing with prosthetic reconstruction or changing to autologous reconstruction. Should implant reconstruction be selected, the expander is removed and replaced with a permanent implant. The specifics of this are described in the section on technique of second-stage implant reconstruction. If flap reconstruction is desired, the salient features are described. The expander is removed, and the pectoralis major muscle separated from the superior mastectomy skin flap. The muscle is reinserted inferiorly using absorbable sutures to reapproximate its natural position. Autologous reconstruction then proceeds as desired by the patient and directed by the surgeon.

COMPLICATIONS

As with all surgical procedures, complications are possible and must be explained and reviewed with the patient preoperatively. They include bleeding, infection, scars, delayed healing, premature removal of the device, rippling and wrinkling, capsular contracture, fill port failure, implant rupture, pain, seroma, distortion, asymmetry, and secondary procedures.

BOX 1.5 Potential advantages of prosthetic reconstruction

- A simpler surgical procedure.
- Use of adjacent tissue of similar color, texture and sensation.
- Less donor site morbidity.
- Less incisional scarring.
- Shorter operative time and postoperative recovery.
- Leaving autologous tissue for a later date.
- The psychological benefit of a more rapidly reconstructed breast.

BOX 1.6 Indications and contraindications

- Patient preference
- Patients who do not have sufficient autologous donor site tissue
- Women interested in a quicker recovery for return to activities of daily living and physical activity
- Bilateral mastectomies in which symmetry can be more readily achieved

Contraindications
- Radiation therapy a relative contraindication to implant reconstruction alone
- Failed previous prosthetic reconstructions: relative contraindication
- Morbid obesity: relative contraindication

Patient selection
- Patient preference
- Patient expectations

BOX 1.7 Optimizing outcomes

- Consider likelihood of postoperative radiation or chemotherapy
- Evaluate opposite breast in unilateral reconstructions for symmetry procedures such as augmentation, mastopexy, or breast reduction
- Reserve immediate reconstruction for those cases in which the likelihood of skin healing is not in question
- Proper device and patient selection are important components affecting final outcome

---

Implant rupture

The main limitation of all implants is that they are mechanical devices and as such will not last forever. The long-term failure rate is directly proportional to the length of time the device has been in place. Failure can be the result of technical factors related to the surgical procedure, shell characteristics of the implant, and the body's response to a foreign substance. Implants that are filled with less than the recommended volume are at increased risk for rupture due to fold fatigue of the shell. The shells are relatively thin to allow for a soft implant, but are subject to the pressure, shear, and stress forces exerted from capsules, surrounding tissues, and activities of daily living.

Ruling out a rupture can sometimes be difficult, especially with the newer cohesive gel implants. Silent rupture is a known entity and is best diagnosed with magnetic resonance imaging (MRI). The classic 'linguini sign' (Fig. 1.15) is characteristic of rupture in an early-generation silicone gel implant, whereas the 'teardrop sign' is characteristic of rupture in current devices. Rupture of saline implants, on the other hand, is relatively easy to diagnose because the breast will flatten or shrink as the implant deflates and the saline is absorbed. In either case, the implant should be removed and replaced as desired. With silicone gel ruptures, all implant material, including the capsule, should be removed.

Capsular contracture

Capsular contracture is a well-described occurrence with a poorly understood etiology. Etiologic factors include subclinical infection, blood products around the implant, and a normal body reaction to a foreign material. Capsular contracture is known to increase over time and often causes distortion and hardening of the breast mound (Fig. 1.16). Techniques to prevent or minimize its occurrence are related to meticulous handling of the implant, ensuring

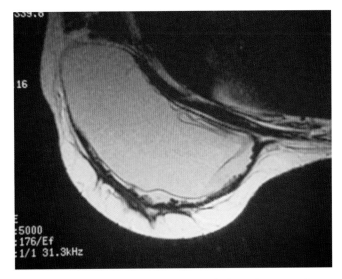

FIGURE 1.15 Linguini sign. The classic MRI finding of a ruptured silicone gel implant is the linguini sign representing folds in the implant shell.

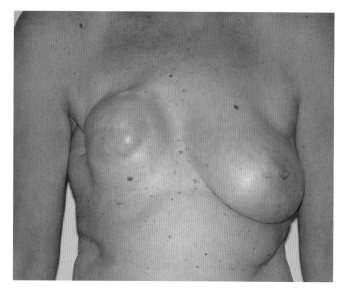

FIGURE 1.16 Capsular contracture. The right breast is severely distorted and painful, which is characteristic of a grade IV capsular contracture.

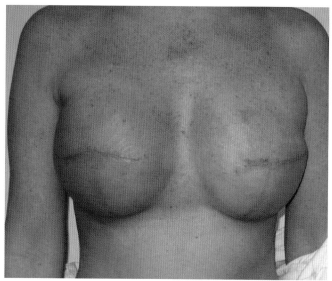

FIGURE 1.17 Cellulitis around breast implant. In this patient following bilateral mastectomy and implant reconstruction, the right breast is characterized by redness and swelling, which is consistent with cellulitis.

a bloodless operative field, and antibiotics. The debate between textured surface devices resulting in less capsular contracture than smooth shell devices has been ongoing for many years but has yielded no significant differences from the current devices in use today.

The management of capsular contracture is surgical and may include capsulotomy, partial capsulectomy, and total capsulectomy. Patients who are predisposed to severe capsular contracture or who have recurrences may be better candidates for autologous reconstruction.

Implant infection

Infection following breast reconstruction with prosthetic devices can be a devastating complication. Fortunately this is not a common event, occurring in probably less than 5% of patients. Common presenting signs and symptoms include cellulitis, pain, and swelling (Fig. 1.17); fever and elevated leukocytosis may also occur. The most common bacteria associated with infection is *Staphylococcus epidermidis*, but other bacteria may also be implicated. The difficulty with this diagnosis is differentiating the superficial skin infection from deep space infections. The management of implant-related infection is immediate hospitalization and broad-spectrum intravenous antibiotics. Superficial infections will usually subside by 24–48 hours, but deep infections will not. For these patients, operative exploration is necessary. It is the authors' opinion that the infected breast implant must be removed, especially when purulence is encountered (Fig. 1.18). Secondary prosthetic reconstruction should be deferred for at least 6–12 months.

Fill port failure

Problems and complications specific to the adjustable implant are primarily related to the fill port. In some women

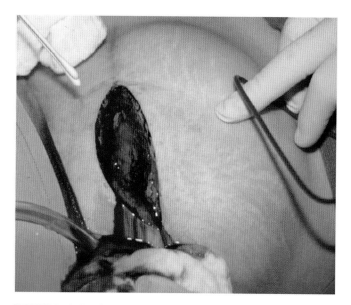

FIGURE 1.18 Purulence around breast implant. Following incision and drainage, purulent fluid is demonstrated. The implant was removed.

the port can become dislodged from the subcutaneous pocket in which it was placed, resulting in an inability to access it. This has been observed despite suturing the port to the chest wall and closing the opening to the pocket with sutures. Kinking of the fill port tubing is possible when it is too long and tortuous. Twisting of the tube that connects the remote port to the implant can result in a tear and deflation of the implant (Fig. 1.19). This has been observed following dislodgement and repeated twisting of the remote port. The management of fill port dysfunction usually

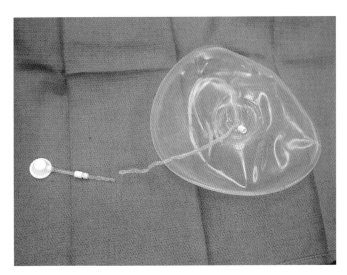

FIGURE 1.19 Fill tube failure. Dislodgment with repeated twisting of the remote port and tubing eventually resulted in failure of the device.

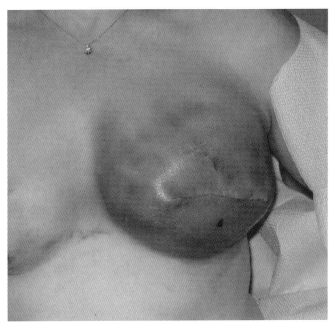

FIGURE 1.20 Hematoma complicating tissue expansion. A postoperative hematoma occurred after breast reconstruction with a tissue expander. The hematoma was surgically evacuated.

requires a surgical procedure. The implant is usually replaced with a permanent device.

Hematoma

Postoperative hematoma following breast reconstruction with prosthetic devices is uncommon and may complicate the reconstruction in 1–2% of cases (Fig. 1.20). The use of closed suction drainage tubes is very helpful in preventing and diagnosing this problem. Left untreated, a hematoma will organize and promote the formation of a thick, disfiguring, and uncomfortable capsule. Therefore, it is recommended that all patients with a hematoma be prepared for surgical evacuation following diagnosis. On exploration some patients will have a bleeding vessel along the surface of the pectoralis muscle or subcutaneous tissue. Other patients may have a previously undiagnosed bleeding disorder and will benefit from an appropriate workup. Most of the time the bleeding has subsided on its own and all that is necessary is clot evacuation, thorough irrigation, and placement of new closed suction drains.

Seroma

The seroma that follows breast reconstruction with a prosthetic device can be troubling. This is usually caused either by lymphatic fluid that accumulates following lymph node removal, or by excess production of serous fluid following the operation. The drainage tubes are usually very effective in controlling excess fluid production and are normally removed after 1–2 weeks. In some cases the fluid production persists, necessitating use of the drainage tubes for 2–4 weeks. In the event that the drainage tubes are removed and a fluid collection accumulates, it is the authors' practice to allow the seroma to resorb spontaneously. This may require 1–2 months and may be associated with rotation of the expander. The other option is to return to the operating

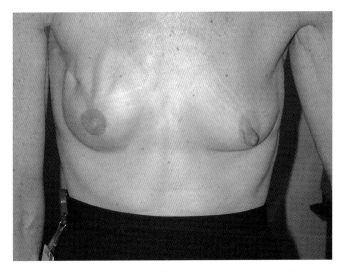

FIGURE 1.21 Rippling and wrinkling are sometimes seen with implants and are due to thin skin and the nature of the prosthetic device.

room and place a new drain. If persistent, lymphoscintigraphy may be needed to identify and clip the source.

Rippling and wrinkling

Rippling and wrinkling are sometimes observed following breast reconstruction with prosthetic devices (Fig. 1.21), more commonly with permanent implants rather than tissue expanders. It becomes evident once the soft tissue edema and swelling has subsided and is usually visible in the upper mastectomy flap, and sometimes palpable in the lower mastectomy flap. It has been observed that textured

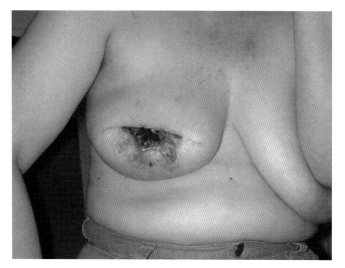

FIGURE 1.22 Soft tissue necrosis. Delayed healing due to poor vascularity of the mastectomy skin flaps.

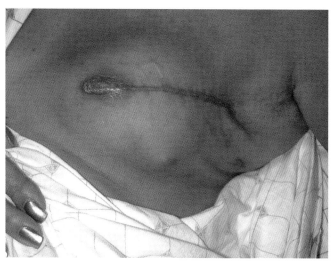

FIGURE 1.23 Impending implant exposure. Delayed healing due to increased internal pressure, poor skin quality, and localized infection.

and saline devices are more prone to this phenomenon, although it can occur with any type of implant. Treatment can be difficult, especially in women with thin skin.

The simplest solution is to remove a textured-surface or saline-filled device and exchange it for a silicone-filled or smooth-surfaced one. It is often tempting to insert a larger device, thinking that the added compartment pressure will fill out the wrinkles and ripples. Unfortunately, these will become evident as the skin stretches, and so upsizing is not recommended. Another option is to use non-vascularized autologous fat transfer in the form of a graft to add to the thickness of the cutaneous envelope. This technique is currently being studied and the reader is referred to the appropriate sources. In the event that all attempts to correct this are unsuccessful, autologous tissue can be considered.

Delayed healing

Delayed healing can complicate any prosthetic-based breast reconstruction but is most prevalent following immediate reconstruction using tissue expanders or permanent implants (Figs 1.22, 1.23). Delayed healing is most often attributed to the poor vascularity of the remaining skin flaps following the mastectomy. Most surgeons will perform a skin-sparing mastectomy, and some will routinely undermine below the level of the inframammary fold, across the sternal midline, and up to the clavicle. This will compromise the vascularity of the remaining mastectomy skin flaps. Determining the perfusion of these skin flaps can be difficult. Techniques include assessment of dermal edge bleeding that includes both arterial and venous flow; assessment of skin color for signs of congestion, ecchymosis, or pallor; and fluorescein lamps. In all cases non- or poorly perfused skin should be excised to minimize skin necrosis and delayed healing.

If healing is delayed, it must be ascertained whether the process is superficial or deep. Superficial wounds, such as

a minor cutaneous dehiscence of skin ulceration, can be managed conservatively with local care and oral antibiotics. More advanced wounds involving the deep structures should be managed aggressively with surgical debridement. The decision as to whether or not to retain the implant is based on the judgment of the operating surgeon.

CONCLUSIONS

Breast reconstruction using prosthetic devices has improved dramatically over the past several years. With the acknowledgment and acceptance that these devices are safe and effective, further refinements will be made to enhance outcomes. It is hopefully recognized that proper patient and device selection, as well as adherence to the basic principles, concepts, and techniques, will allow surgeons to deliver predictable and reproducible results.

FURTHER READING

1. Salzberg CA. Nonexpansive immediate breast reconstruction using human acellular tissue matrix graft (AlloDerm). Ann Plast Surg 2006; 57: 1–5.
2. Breuing KH, Warren SM. Immediate bilateral breast reconstruction with implants and inferolateral AlloDerm slings. Ann Plast Surg 2005; 55: 232–239.
3. Spear SL, Mesbahi AN. Implant based reconstruction. Clin Plast Surg 2007; 34: 63–73.
4. Cordeiro PG, McCarthy CM. A single surgeon's 12 year experience with tissue expander/implant breast reconstruction: part 1. A prospective analysis of early complications. Plast Reconstruct Surg 2006; 118: 825–831.
5. Cordeiro PG, McCarthy CM. A single surgeon's 12 year experience with tissue expander/implant breast reconstruction: part 2. An analysis of long-term complications, aesthetic outcomes, and patient satisfaction. Plast Reconstruct Surg 2006; 118: 832–839.
6. McCarthy CM, Pusic AL, Disa JJ, et al. Unilateral chest wall radiotherapy in bilateral tissue expander/implant reconstruction patients: A prospective outcomes analysis. Plast Reconstruct Surg 2005; 116: 1642–1647.

7. Nahabedian MY, Tsangaris T, Momen B, Manson PN. Infectious complications following breast reconstruction with expanders and implants. Plast Reconstruct Surg 2003; 112: 467–476.

8. Nahabedian MY. Symmetrical breast reconstruction: analysis of secondary procedures following reconstruction with implants and with autologous tissue. Plast Reconstruct Surg 2005; 115: 257–260.

9. Disa JJ, Ad-El DD, Cohen SM, et al. The premature removal of tissue expanders in breast reconstruction. Plast Reconstruct Surg 1999; 104: 1662.

10. Krueger EA, Wilkins EG, Strawderman M, et al. Complications and patient satisfaction following expander/implant breast reconstruction with and without radiotherapy. Int J Radiation Oncol Biol Phys 2001; 49: 713.

11. Forman DL, Chiu J, Restifo RJ, et al. Breast reconstruction in previously irradiated patients using tissue expanders and implants: A potentially unfavorable result. Ann Plast Surg 1998; 40: 360.

12. Spear SL, Majidian A. Immediate breast reconstruction in two stages using textured, integrated-valve tissue expanders and breast implants: A retrospective review of 171 consecutive breast reconstructions from 1989 to 1996. Plast Reconstruct Surg 1998; 101: 53.

13. Tallet AV, Salem N, Moutardier V, et al. Radiotherapy and immediate two-stage breast reconstruction with a tissue expander and implant: complications and esthetic results. Int J Radiation Oncol Biol Phys 2003; 57: 136.

14. Ascherman JA, Hanasono MM, Newman MI, Hughes DB. Implant reconstruction in breast cancer patients treated with radiation therapy. Plast Reconstruct Surg 2006; 117: 359.

15. Spear SL, Pelletiere CV. Immediate breast reconstruction in two stages using textured integrated valve tissue expanders and implants. Plast Reconstruct Surg 2004; 113: 2098–2103.

16. Kronowitz SJ, Hunt KK, Kuerer HM, et al. Delayed-immediate breast reconstruction. Plast Reconstruct Surg 2004; 113: 1617–1628.

17. Nahabedian MY. The adjustable breast implant. In: Jackson IT, Noone RB, eds. Innovation in breast surgery. Vol. 1. St Louis: Quality Medical Publishing, 2005; 109–121.

18. Becker H. Breast reconstruction using an inflatable breast implant with a detachable reservoir. Plast Reconstruct Surg 1984; 73: 678–683.

Pedicled TRAM Flap
Breast Reconstruction

Dennis C. Hammond

INTRODUCTION

Breast reconstruction after mastectomy has become an important part of the overall recovery process for women undergoing treatment for breast cancer. To that end, the results of breast reconstruction have improved steadily over the past 20 years as experience with the various techniques has grown. Perhaps the most important development to dramatically influence these improved results was the description of the transverse rectus abdominis musculocutaneous or TRAM flap.[1,2] By using the patient's own tissues to fashion the reconstructed breast mound without the need for a prosthetic device, outstanding results can be obtained with few long-term complications.

The original description of the TRAM flap based the blood supply to the skin and fat of the lower abdomen on an arteriovenous pedicle which passed along the length of the rectus abdominis muscle, running from under the costal margin to the perforators located in the lower abdomen. This technique involved elevating the rectus abdominis muscle in continuity with the skin and fat of the lower abdomen to preserve the vascular supply. This direct communication between the flap and the muscle led to the term 'pedicled' TRAM flap breast reconstruction.[2] Over the years, alternative microsurgical methods of manipulating the vascular inflow to the flap have been developed, including the free TRAM flap as well as the deep inferior epigastric artery perforator or DIEP flap. Although these procedures are associated with several advantages, including improvement in blood supply to the flap and fewer donor site complications, many surgeons are reluctant to incorporate these more complicated and technically intensive procedures into their breast reconstruction armamentarium. As a result, the pedicled TRAM flap remains a very important method of autogenous breast reconstruction.[3]

INDICATIONS AND CONTRAINDICATIONS

Because the technique is autogenous in nature, TRAM flap breast reconstruction is the single best method for obtaining high-quality, long-lasting results.[1] Because no prosthetic device is required, all of the complications associated with breast implants are obviated. However, the potential complications associated with TRAM flap reconstruction are significant and every effort must be made to perform the procedure safely on appropriately selected patients using sound surgical technique. To understand which patients might be the best candidates for pedicled TRAM flap breast reconstruction, it is helpful to review the most common complications associated with the procedure, so that the variables that lead to complications can be identified and controlled.

Perhaps the most damaging of complications regarding pedicled TRAM flap breast reconstruction relates to insufficient blood supply to the flap. When a significant portion of the flap necroses, the short-term wound healing issues and the long-term breast shape issues that result can severely detract from the overall success of the procedure. For this reason, any condition associated with diminished cutaneous blood supply must be considered a relative contraindication to the use of a pedicled TRAM flap. Examples include a history of hypertension, diabetes mellitus, connective tissue disease, or any general debilitating condition that could be considered a stressor to the patient's overall vitality. It is the author's practice to reserve the use of a pedicled TRAM flap for those patients who are in excellent health. All other patients are considered for other methods of reconstruction, including free tissue transfer techniques, combined latissimus dorsi with expander/implant techniques, or expander/implant techniques alone. Thus the best chance of success can be ensured with a minimum of complications.

Special mention must be made of the issue of smoking. It has been demonstrated in many studies that a history of smoking generally doubles the complication rate of many types of procedure.[4] This is particularly true for flap procedures, and a smoking history, no matter how brief or intense, must be considered a relative contraindication for a pedicled TRAM flap. At the very least, full informed consent must be given before patient and surgeon embark upon a pedicled TRAM flap procedure in the face of a smoking history.

Obesity is also a variable that must be carefully considered when choosing the pedicled TRAM flap technique. Certainly there must be a relative excess of lower abdominal skin and fat to permit a breast of sufficient volume to be reconstructed. However, in patients with significant obesity the risk for insufficient vascular inflow to the excess amount of fat present in the TRAM flap, as well as in the abdominal donor site, is high. Therefore, although successful pedicled TRAM flap breast reconstruction can be performed in the obese, it must be realized that the potential for vascular inflow-related complications with tissue necrosis and wound healing problems can be significant.[5]

PREOPERATIVE HISTORY AND CONSIDERATIONS

Apart from questions concerning the general health of the patient and documentation of any smoking history, several anatomic factors can affect the use of a pedicled TRAM flap for reconstruction. Specifically, it must be ascertained whether or not any previous abdominal surgery has been performed. Perhaps the most obvious potential problem relates to the patient who has had an open cholecystectomy: clearly, a scar across the right upper quadrant should alert the surgeon that the rectus muscle has probably been divided, thereby cutting the peripheral extension of the superior epigastric artery through the muscle down to the lower abdominal skin and fat. In such cases the use of a left pedicled TRAM flap is still possible, as is the use of a free TRAM flap or a DIEP flap. Also, any scar that runs from the umbilicus down to the pubis in the midline will probably adversely affect the ability of cutaneous blood flow to pass across the midline when a unipedicled TRAM flap technique is used. In patients who have undergone cardiac bypass, the left – and less commonly both – internal mammary artery can be divided as they are rerouted into the coronary vessels. In these patients, although the intercostal vessels can provide some inflow to the superior epigastric system, the pressure head must be considered to be severely diminished, making a pedicled TRAM flap a much less attractive option. Also, any midline scar raises the suggestion that the continuity of one or both rectus muscles could potentially be divided, thereby cutting the blood supply to a pedicled TRAM flap. In these circumstances, a clear understanding of the previous surgical procedures must be elicited to ensure that the superior epigastric system is intact.

Special mention must be made regarding scars from a cesarian section. This is an exceedingly common clinical scenario, and in the vast majority of patients such scars have no bearing on the successful use of a TRAM flap. In fact, in some circumstances it can prove helpful, as some obstetricians/gynecologists will tie off the inferior epigastric vessels in the course of exposing the abdominal cavity. This essentially constitutes a delay procedure, which can greatly enhance the likelihood that the superior epigastric circulation will be dominant and will provide vigorous vascular support to the pedicled TRAM flap. Obtaining previous surgical notes may help clarify these issues to allow appropriate preoperative surgical planning.

OPERATIVE APPROACH

Anatomy

The TRAM flap is a musculocutaneous flap that takes advantage of the lower abdominal vascular territory served by perforators of the superior and inferior epigastric arteries and veins as they course through the rectus abdominis muscle.[6,7] The paired muscle originates from the ventral aspect of the conjoined medial lower rib cartilages on each side, and inserts via a narrow tendon into the superior border of the pubis. At variable intervals along the length of the muscle, two to four fibrous confluences or inscriptions separate it into distinct compartments that are usually paired. These inscriptions create the widely recognized contour breaks in the surface of the muscle that can be seen through the thin abdominal fatty layer in fit individuals, creating the so-called 'six pack.'

The superior epigastric artery is the terminal branch of the very robust internal mammary artery. It exits from under the rib margin approximately one to two fingerbreadths lateral to the xiphoid process and curves laterally to run along the underside and down the length of the rectus muscle. The artery will arborize variably within the muscle as it passes inferiorly. In selected cases the artery can be large and distinct enough to be visualized as an identifiable vessel passing along the junction of the lateral third and the medial two-thirds of the muscle. In other cases the vascular pedicle arborizes quickly within the substance of the muscle. The inferior epigastric artery enters the lower lateral margin of the rectus four to five fingerbreadths below the umbilicus and runs along the underside of the muscle. Again, the main substance of the pedicle runs along the junction of the lateral third and the medial two-thirds of the muscle, where it then variably arborizes with the superior epigastric pedicle. Along the way, laterally based intercostal branches course to the pedicle axis, where they join up with the vascular arcade. These intercostal branches consist of an artery, vein, and nerve that contain sympathetic, parasympathetic, and autonomic fibers.[8] Soon after the inferior epigastric pedicle enters the underside of the muscle, a separate umbilical branch courses superomedially toward the umbilicus, where it then courses through the fascia to the underside of the abdominal wall. With this as a basic vascular framework, several distinct perforators arise from this combination vascular arcade to serve the overlying skin and fat. Laterally, very typically a 'key perforator' arises from the vascular axis at the inscription of the rectus muscle located at the level of the umbilicus. Below this, separated by 2–3 cm, arise two or three additional perforators that tend to be slightly smaller than the key perforator. These two to four perforators form the vascular basis of a pedicled TRAM flap. There are also very typically additional perforators that arise from the umbilical branch, again with a prominent perforator being noted at the level of the umbilical inscription of the rectus abdominis muscle. These perforators can add additional vascular support to a pedicled TRAM flap. Above the level of the umbilical muscle inscription, scattered perforators arise from the muscle. However, these tend to be so small as to be of little value compared to the main perforators running directly from the epigastric vascular axis (Fig. 2.1).

The clinical significance of this vascular arrangement directly affects the vascularity of a pedicled TRAM flap. The main vascular supply to the soft tissues of the lower abdomen is the inferior epigastric vascular arcade. Once the muscle is dissected free and the inferior epigastric pedicle is divided, the continued viability of the flap will depend on the superior epigastric arcade effectively communicating with the inferior system through the choke region located just above the umbilical inscription. If this communication is robust, a pedicled TRAM flap will survive reliably. If the communication is tenuous, the skin and fat of the flap might be at risk for ischemia. Fortunately, in the majority of cases the communication between the superior and inferior vascular arcades is sufficient to maintain flap viability. However, in at-risk patients such as smokers or diabetics, the ability of the superior circulation to supply the flap adequately can be limited, and many surgeons will use free tissue transfer techniques instead.

The vascular supply to the skin occurs predominantly through the lateral perforators. Once in the soft tissue, fairly distinct zones of perfusion can be identified that can variably overlap. Typically, the perforators coming through the rectus abdominis muscle on one side will serve mainly the skin and fat on that side of the abdomen, and there will be variable and often diminished collateral flow across the midline to the other side of the flap.[9] This has clinical implications for operative planning when the entire flap will be needed to reconstruct the breast. Because of the uncertainty over the vascular supply to the flap across the midline, many surgeons will use a double pedicle flap to accomplish the reconstruction. In my experience, a double pedicle TRAM flap provides the same level of reliability as a free TRAM flap as far as vascular perfusion is concerned. The disadvantage is centered on the need to harvest both rectus muscles and the subsequent donor site complications that can ensue.

The fascial anatomy of the rectus muscle plays a key role in successfully elevating a TRAM flap without creating donor site morbidity. The muscle itself is surrounded by an anterior and a posterior rectus sheath. At each inscription, the anterior rectus sheath attachments are densely adherent to the inscription, creating a prominent crease running horizontally along the width of the muscle. Laterally the confluence of the internal and external oblique muscles merges with the lateral margin of the rectus sheath to provide a firm support layer for the abdominal wall. Several centimeters below the level of the umbilicus, the orientation of the rectus sheath changes and the posterior sheath switches location and merges with the anterior sheath. As a result, a prominent crease is formed at the inferiormost portion of the posterior rectus sheath, called the 'line of Douglas.' Recognizing and reconstituting these relationships is important in achieving closure of the abdominal wall donor site after TRAM flap elevation.[10,11]

Marks

The main aim of the marking procedure is to identify the landmarks that define the location of the muscle, and to outline the cutaneous vascular territory of the perforators. It is best to mark the patient in the standing position to ensure symmetric application of the skin pattern. Also, it is in this position that the vertical width of the flap can be best estimated. The major focus of the marking procedure is to correctly identify the margins of the skin paddle. Typi-

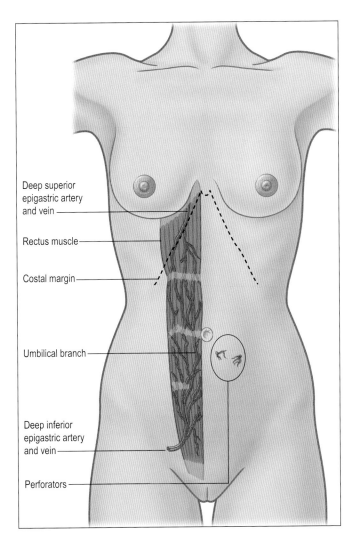

Deep superior epigastric artery and vein

Rectus muscle

Costal margin

Umbilical branch

Deep inferior epigastric artery and vein

Perforators

FIGURE 2.1 The vascular anatomy of the epigastric vessels in relation to the rectus abdominis muscle.

cally, a mark is made just above the umbilicus and extended laterally in a curvilinear fashion to the lateral aspect of the abdominal wall. Near the midline, the mark jogs slightly superiorly to ensure that the tissues surrounding the 'key' perforator are included in the flap. The exact location of the lateral flap extension varies according to the soft tissue relationships of the skin and fat of the lower abdominal wall. The goal is to draw the flap in such a way as to minimize the creation of a lateral dog-ear after closure of the skin donor site. Once the lateral limits of the flap are determined, the lower border is estimated based on the elasticity of the skin and the tissue requirements of the reconstructed breast. Typically this line will course just above the hair-bearing portion of the pubic area.

Once the limits of the flap location have been determined, the muscle location as well as the estimated location of the perforators is diagrammed. Ultimately, the origin of the muscle along the costal margin will be released, and the location of the costal cartilages is palpated and marked for future reference. The location of the tunnel that will be used to pass the flap is drawn, and orientation marks are made on the flap that will subsequently assist in planning its shape. The skin pattern for the mastectomy is also drawn. In immediate cases a skin-sparing mastectomy pattern is used and applied according to the dictates of breast volume as well as the size of the skin envelope. In delayed cases, the dimensions of the planned breast are outlined using the old mastectomy scar as an access incision (Fig. 2.2).

If the opposite breast requires alteration, either to provide symmetry or to improve the overall esthetic result, this procedure is performed along with the first-stage TRAM flap reconstruction and the breast is marked accordingly. In this fashion, any postoperative settling that may occur in the normal breast after mastopexy, reduction, or augmentation can stabilize during the postoperative recovery period. Then, at the second-stage procedure, the normal breast will function as a stable construct against which the reconstructed breast can be matched.

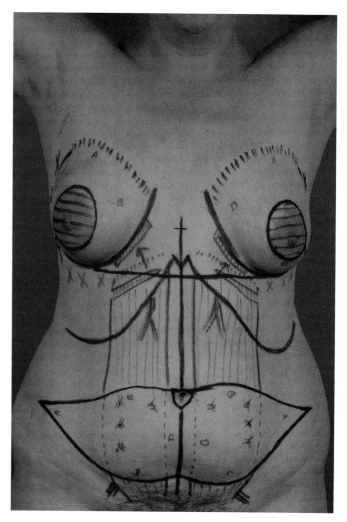

FIGURE 2.2 Marks in preparation for bilateral TRAM flap breast reconstruction.

Operative technique

Single-pedicle TRAM flap

In cases of immediate reconstruction, the dimensions of the mastectomy defect and the condition of the mastectomy flaps and the inframammary fold are assessed after the mastectomy has been completed. If the fold has been lowered, it is best to resuspend it back into the proper position using permanent sutures placed along the midline of the fold and extending laterally. This will avoid the medial inframammary corner where the communicating tunnel will ultimately be located. If necessary, fluorescein can be used to assess the viability of the mastectomy flap, and debridement can be performed as indicated. The goal of this assessment is to stabilize the mastectomy defect so that appropriate decisions can be made during subsequent elevation and insetting of the TRAM flap. In some cases it is possible to begin working on TRAM flap elevation even as the oncologic surgeons are removing the breast, in an effort

to save time and shorten the duration of the procedure. This is an excellent strategy; however, once the mastectomy has been completed, it is recommended to assess the mastectomy flap as described to optimize further operative planning.

In cases of delayed reconstruction, the mastectomy scar is excised and the flaps elevated to the proper dimension to set the proposed borders of the reconstructed breast. Any scar tethering in the mastectomy flaps is released by scoring the underside as needed to create a soft, pliable flap. Once the defect has been re-created, the TRAM flap can be elevated.

Flap elevation begins by incising the skin at the upper border and dissecting down to the abdominal wall at a slight angle, directed superiorly to increase the eventual volume of the flap. The upper abdominal panniculus is elevated away from the abdominal wall up to a level up and over the costal margin on each side. Communication is then made with the mastectomy defect through the inferomedial corner of the inframammary fold, creating a tunnel of sufficient width to allow the hand to easily be inserted. The upper panniculus is then pulled down to the lower proposed TRAM flap mark to be certain that the donor site abdominal wound will be closed without difficulty. The patient can be elevated to about 20° at the waist to assist in this determination. Once the location of the lower incision has been confirmed, the skin is incised and the dissection carried straight down to the abdominal wall, through the two fatty layers of the abdomen separated by Scarpa's fascia. As well, the umbilicus is released from the flap to allow eventual umbilical relocation.

It is my preference to use an ipsilateral pedicle for reconstruction of a single breast.[12–14] With this in mind, the attachments of the flap to the overlying muscle on the side of the reconstructed breast are identified and preserved as the lateral wings of the flap are elevated away from the abdominal wall. On the opposite side of the abdomen, away from the muscle perforator zone, the flap is elevated from the underlying rectus muscle and dissection proceeds across the midline until the medial perforators on the target muscle are identified. On the muscle side, the flap is elevated laterally from the abdominal fascia until the lateral row of perforators is identified coming up from the underlying rectus muscle. This dissection identifies the segment of fascia that must be taken with the muscle to preserve the perforators passing up into the flap (Fig. 2.3). Above and below this perforator zone the zone of fascial harvest is tapered off to allow a contoured closure of the fascia once the muscle is released. The proposed fascial incisions are then made, and superiorly the remaining segment of anterior rectus sheath is divided in the midline to allow access to the muscle. The medial and lateral anterior rectus sheath flaps are then elevated from the underlying rectus muscle, and the muscle itself is carefully released from any deeper

attachments, particularly along the area of the inscriptions. Laterally the intercostal branches are divided up to the level of the costal margin. Inferiorly, the inferior epigastric vascular pedicle is divided and the muscle is released from the pubis through the smaller but well-delineated tendinous area just above the pubic attachment. The muscle is sutured to the underside of the TRAM to prevent inadvertent traction injury to the perforators, and any remaining attachments of the muscle are released as the muscle is lifted away from the fascial bed. Superiorly the lateral portion of the rectus muscle is divided above the costal margin, with release extending superomedially until only 2–3 cm of muscle remain attached just lateral to the xiphoid. This release is completely safe, as the superior epigastric pedicle lies deeper under the costal margin and is not in danger of injury as long as muscle release is performed on top of the cartilaginous border. This maneuver offers significant advantage in easing the arc of rotation of the flap without creating excessive bunching or kinking at the rotation point. The flap is then passed through the subcutaneous tunnel created previously by turning the muscle 180°, such that the deep portion of the muscle stays deep as the adipocutaneous portion is passed to the mastectomy defect. This is as opposed to a double flip of the muscle, which can potentially create a kink resulting in flap ischemia. Once the flap is positioned in the mastectomy defect, it is temporarily inset with staples and allowed to recover from the shock of elevation that is associated with the newly oriented vascular patterns.

Abdominal closure begins by reapproximating the anterior rectus sheath incision directly with a 0 or #1 sized permanent monofilament suture. By beginning above at the level of the xiphoid process and below at the level of the pubis, and running toward the center of the incision, a direct approximation of the fascial edges can be obtained. It is important to be sure that the fascial edge of the internal oblique is included in the closure, particularly inferiorly, as it tends to separate away from the combined fascial edge of the anterior rectus sheath. It is also usually necessary to 'overdo' the closure above and below the area of fascial harvest to prevent the creation of a fascial dog-ear. The opposite anterior rectus sheath is then plicated as needed to further reinforce the abdomen and create a contoured abdominal profile. This maneuver also serves to pull the umbilicus back to the midline and prevent umbilical malposition. Using this fascial sparing strategy it will always be possible to accomplish primary fascial repair using a unipedicled TRAM flap. No mesh is needed, and adding an onlay mesh to reinforce the closure is unnecessary. Two drains are placed in the abdominal dissection space, and the lower skin incision is closed in layers. The umbilicus is inset into the abdominal flap to complete the abdominal closure.

Double-pedicle TRAM flap–bilateral TRAM flap

In cases of bipedicled TRAM flap breast reconstruction or bilateral breast reconstruction, both rectus abdominis muscles will be harvested to supply one or both flaps. Because of this, the perforator zone over each muscle must

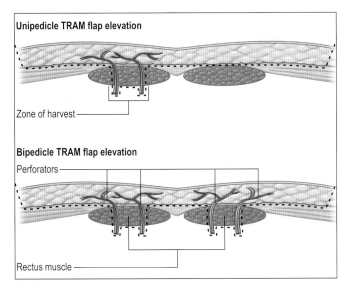

FIGURE 2.3 Schematic diagram comparing the perforator and fascial dissections required for a unipedicled and bipedicled TRAM flap elevation. The zone of fascial harvest is dictated by the location of the medial and lateral perforators.

be preserved during the dissection. In bilateral cases this is easily accomplished, as the flap is divided in the midline and the medial perforators from each muscle are directly exposed. In a bipedicled procedure, a dissection tunnel is created under the midline of the flap as the medial perforators are identified and the fascial incisions are made. Flap elevation then proceeds exactly as for a single-pedicle TRAM flap. In bilateral procedures the two hemiflaps are simply passed to the mastectomy defects as before, and in bipedicled procedures the entire flap is passed to one side. In either circumstance, the flaps are rotated and not flipped as described previously. In bipedicled procedures, the two muscles can create more bulk at the costal margin rotation point. This effect can be minimized by appropriate muscle release at the costal margin, as described previously.

The major difference between unipedicled and bipedicled TRAM flap procedures is in the abdominal closure. Even when the fascial sparing technique is used as described, in some patients it will be difficult to close the fascial edges directly. If both anterior rectus sheaths cannot be closed primarily, it is my practice to close one and then use a Marlex mesh interposition fascial replacement in the other. Typically, the mesh is placed exactly in the area where the

fascia was harvested to preserve the integrity of the perforators. Using this strategy, reliable fascial closure of the abdomen can be accomplished with a very low incidence of TRAM flap hernia formation or bulging. In all other respects flap elevation, transfer, and skin closure are the same.

TRAM flap shaping

If flap elevation represents the technical side of TRAM flap breast reconstruction, shaping represents the artistic side. Basically, the goals of TRAM flap shaping include completely filling the mastectomy defect and adequately restoring the integrity of the skin envelope. Skin envelope issues mainly become a concern in cases of delayed reconstruction. All of this must be done with an eye to creating an esthetic shape.

Once the TRAM flap has been transferred to the mastectomy defect, there are three orientations that can be used to position the volume of the flap anatomically in such a way as to create an esthetic breast shape: transverse, oblique, and vertical (Fig. 2.4A–C).

- **Transverse** This orientation is best used when a wide-base diameter is required and the vertical height of the breast is not excessive. Typically with this type of breast,

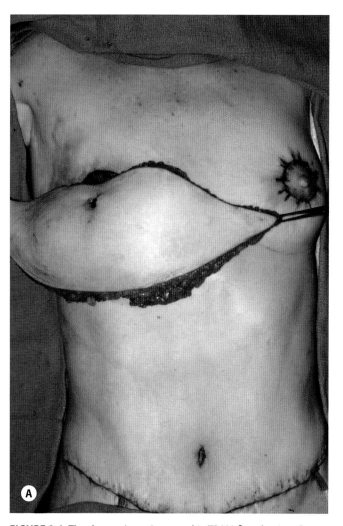
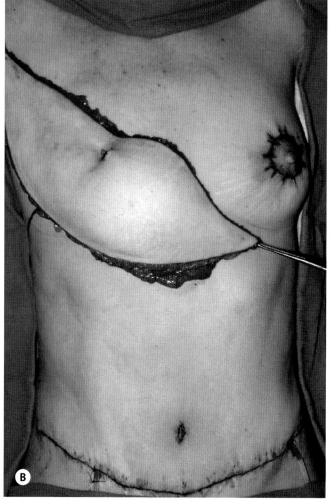

FIGURE 2.4 The three orientations used in TRAM flap shaping. **A** transverse; **B** oblique; **C** vertical.

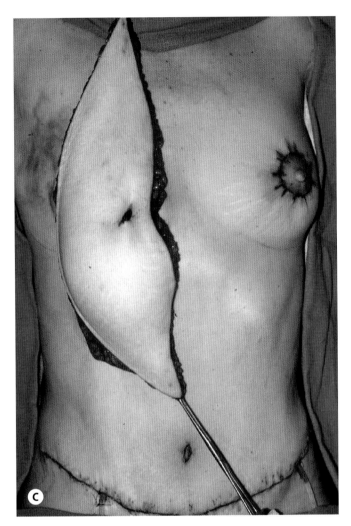

FIGURE 2.4, cont'd

a significant volume requirement exists and it is most commonly used with a bipedicled TRAM flap.

- **Oblique** This orientation can be used in either single- or double-pedicle procedures and is a very versatile way to shape a flap. By slightly orienting the flap such that the tip is in the upper outer quadrant of the breast, appropriate vertical height can be created in the reconstructed breast in a way that preserves an appropriate base width. The oblique orientation is a reasonable 'compromise' position that allows both parameters to be controlled in many patients.

- **Vertical** The vertical orientation is perhaps the easiest and most versatile for TRAM flap shaping. The basic anatomy of the flap sets up well for the task, as the thin lateral tip of the flap is inset into the superior portion of the reconstructed breast. As a result, a smooth and contoured upper pole can be created very easily. The triangularly shaped flap can then be trimmed at the corners to create rounded contours and a very esthetic breast shape. Also, the muscle bulk sutured to the inferior portion of the flap further accentuates the projection of the flap. Finally, vertical orientation does not require any excess twisting of the flap that might result in positional ischemia.

The borders of the TRAM flap must be inset into the mastectomy defect in a way that creates smooth contours. One very effective technique for this is to use the de-epithelialized edges of the cutaneous portion of the flap as a scaffold to suspend it from the chest wall. By suturing these flap edges into the margin of the mastectomy defect, the entire defect can be filled without creating any stepoffs. This is as opposed to suturing the fatty layers of the TRAM into the margins, as this can create a ridge along the peripheral borders of the reconstructed breast. Once the periphery of the mastectomy defect has been esthetically controlled, the remainder of the flap is inset as needed to hold the flap in the correct position. Once the position of the flap has been set, the requirements for the skin island can be finalized and the appropriate areas of the flap de-epithelialized. Insetting of the skin island over a drain completes the procedure.

Postoperative recovery generally proceeds uneventfully. A hospital stay of usually 3–5 days is required to allow sufficient recovery for discharge. Typically an abdominal binder is worn for several weeks to provide comfort and a sense of support to the abdominal wall. By 6 weeks the patient has generally returned to full normal function.

Second-stage procedure

Whereas first-stage TRAM flap surgery requires both a technical and an artistic eye, it is as a result of the second-stage revision that truly outstanding results are created. The second-stage procedure is performed after the edema associated with the first procedure has resolved. This occurs anywhere from 4 to 6 months after the initial operation. At this procedure, any alteration in the reconstructed breast that will improve the overall result is performed. Very commonly this will include liposuction to the reconstructed breast, excision of redundant skin, resetting of the contours of the breast including the inframammary fold, and finally reconstructing the nipple–areolar complex (NAC). Alterations in the abdominal donor site can also be made, including scar revision, dog-ear correction, and liposuction recontouring.[15] Occasionally reinforcement of the abdominal wall is necessary in cases where abdominal laxity, bulging, or more uncommonly hernia formation has occurred. This is typically performed under general anesthesia as an outpatient procedure and in most instances requires no more than 1 week of recovery time.

RESULTS

Because the breast is reconstructed with autologous tissue, once the initial healing has occurred the size and shape of the reconstructed breast remain stable as long as the body habitus of the patient does not change dramatically. It is for this reason that the TRAM flap is widely recognized as the most attractive option for breast reconstruction. All the potential complications associated with implant-based techniques are avoided; the technique can applied in cases of unilateral or bilateral reconstruction,[16,17] either immediate or delayed, and is generally very compatible with the delivery of postoperative chemotherapy. Special circumstances, including reconstruction after subcutaneous or partial mastectomy, can be easily managed with the technique, and skin-sparing mastectomy strategies complement the procedure and combine to give outstanding results for many patients (Figs 2.5–2.7).

COMPLICATIONS

Although most patients tolerate TRAM flap breast reconstruction without difficulty, several well-recognized complications can occur and may require operative attention. These can be either related to the flap itself or to the donor site.

Flap-related complications

These relate almost exclusively to the vascularity of the flap. If any portion of the skin or fat of a TRAM flap necroses, the result will suffer. Small areas of fat or skin necrosis can simply be managed conservatively and allowed to heal by secondary intention during the recovery from the initial procedure. Larger areas may require intervention to debride necrotic skin or fat and achieve a healed wound. In either circumstance, revision can be performed at the second stage to remove necrotic fat, revise scars and reshape the breast. Should the tissue loss be extensive, restoration of a pleasing breast contour can be accomplished with the addition of a latissimus dorsi flap.[18] In this fashion, the autologous nature of the procedure is preserved.

Abdominal complications

Necrosis of skin and fat can also occur in the abdomen. Typically, such areas are allowed to heal by secondary intention and are then revised later at the second stage. Occasionally laxity or bulging of the abdominal wall is noted, and second-stage reinforcement of these areas via suture placation, with or without the addition of mesh, can be performed to restore abdominal competence. Rarely, a patient can present with persistent abdominal pain after a TRAM flap procedure. In these cases, point injections with local anesthetic mixed with steroid can confirm and potentially treat the condition. Operative exploration can be

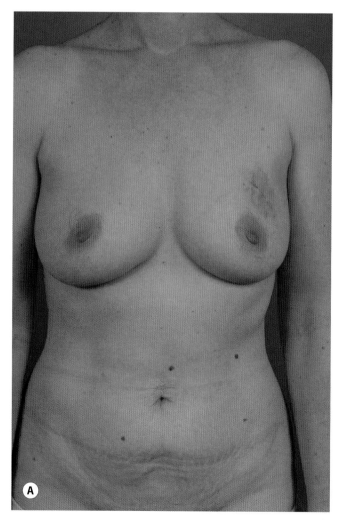

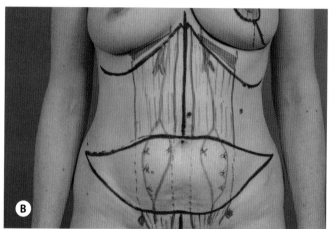

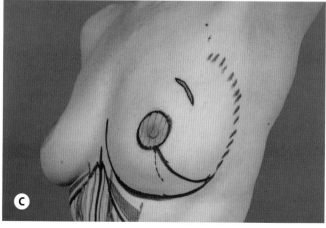

FIGURE 2.5 A Preoperative appearance of a patient who presents with a left-sided intraductal breast carcinoma. **B, C** Preoperative marks in preparation for skin-sparing modified radical mastectomy followed by immediate bipedicled TRAM flap breast reconstruction.

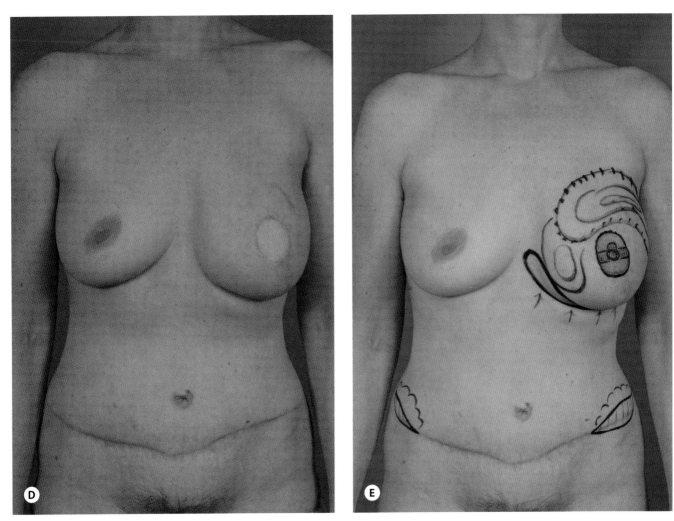

FIGURE 2.5, cont'd D Appearance after first-stage reconstruction. **E** Marks in preparation for second-stage reconstruction, which will include liposuction contouring of the reconstructed breast, reconstruction of the NAC, and revision of the TRAM scar.

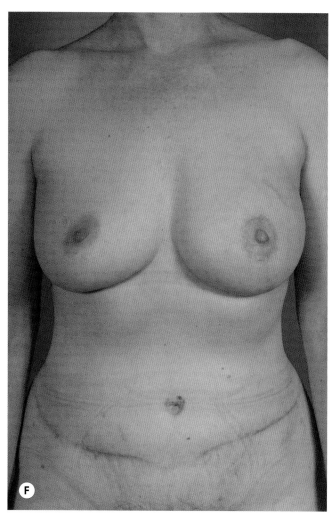

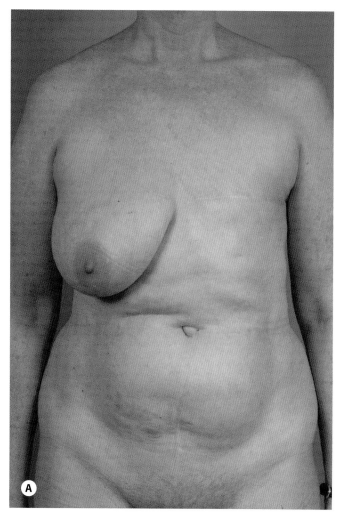

FIGURE 2.5, cont'd F One-year postoperative appearance demonstrating an esthetic and symmetric result.

FIGURE 2.6 A Preoperative appearance of a patient after previous modified radical mastectomy.

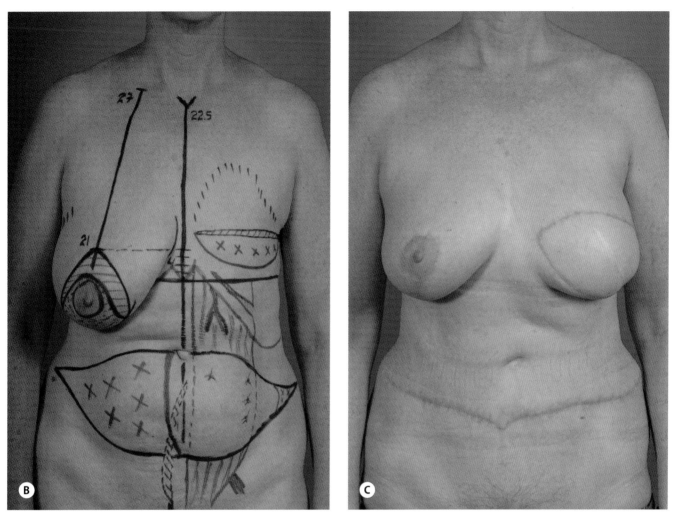

FIGURE 2.6, cont'd B Preoperative marks in preparation for left unipedicled TRAM flap breast reconstruction along with right-sided breast reduction. **C** Appearance after first-stage reconstruction.

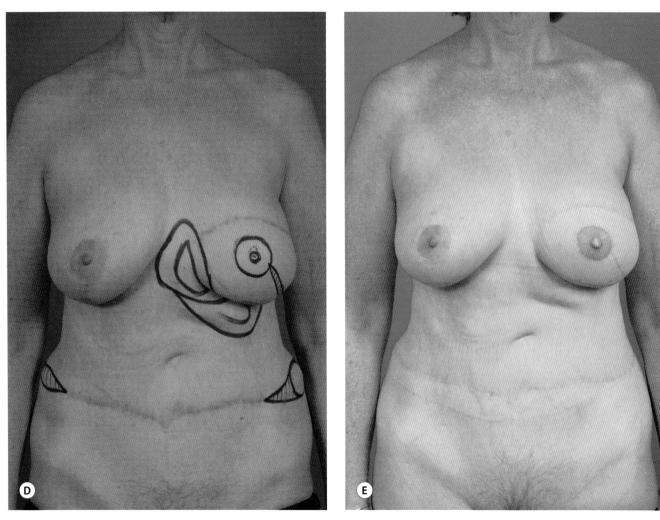

FIGURE 2.6, cont'd D Second-stage marks. **E** One-year postoperative appearance.

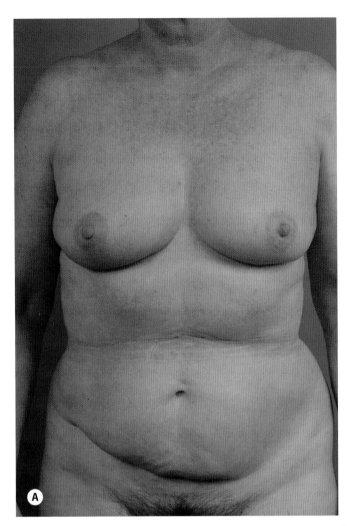
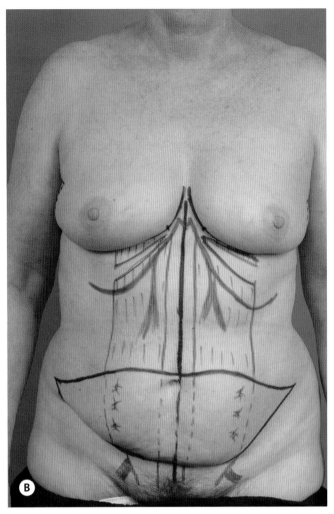

FIGURE 2.7 A Preoperative appearance of a patient with a strong family history of breast cancer who desired prophylactic mastectomy with immediate TRAM flap breast reconstruction. **B** Preoperative marks in preparation for bilateral subcutaneous mastectomy followed by pedicled TRAM flap breast reconstruction.

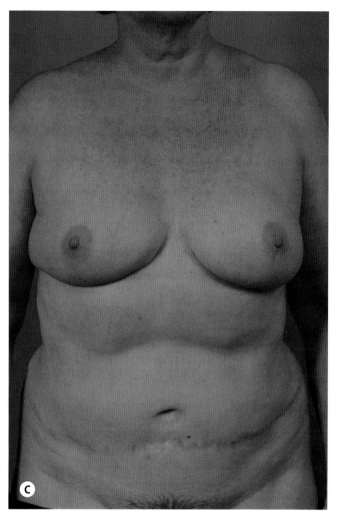

FIGURE 2.7, cont'd C Three-year postoperative appearance.

performed in the event of failure of conservative measures to potentially release a cut nerve trapped in scar, repair any scar tethering that may be present, or even reinforce a weak area in the abdominal wall.

CONCLUSIONS

The pedicled TRAM flap remains one of the procedures of choice for many patients seeking breast reconstruction after mastectomy. The procedure is technically straightforward, reliable, and can provide outstanding results in appropri-

ately selected patients. It remains a mainstay of treatment in the armamentarium of breast reconstruction techniques for many surgeons.

REFERENCES

1. Kroll SS. Why autologous tissue? Clin Plast Surg 1998; 25: 135–143.
2. Scheflan M, Hartrampf CR, Black PW. Breast reconstruction with a transverse abdominal island flap. Plast Reconstruct Surg 1982; 69: 908–909.
3. Jones G. The pedicled TRAM flap in breast reconstruction. Clin Plast Surg 2007; 34: 83–104.
4. Padubidri AN, Yetman R, Browne E, et al. Complications of postmastectomy breast reconstruction in smokers, ex-smokers, and nonsmokers. Plast Reconstruct Surg 2001; 107: 350–351.
5. Kroll SS, Netscher DT. Complications of TRAM flap breast reconstruction in obese patients. Plast Reconstruct Surg 1989; 84: 886–892.
6. Moon HK, Taylor GI. The vascular anatomy of rectus abdominis musculocutaneous flaps based on the deep superior epigastric system. Plast Reconstruct Surg 1988; 82: 815–832.
7. Taylor GI, Corlett RJ, Boyd JB. The versatile deep inferior epigastric (inferior rectus abdominis) flap. Br J Plast Surg 1984; 37: 330–350.
8. Hammond DC, Larson DL, Severinac RN, Marcias M. Rectus abdominis muscle innervation: implications for TRAM flap elevation. Plast Reconstruct Surg 1995; 96: 105–110.
9. Yamaguchi S, De Lorenzi F, Petit JY, et al. The 'perfusion map' of the unipedicled TRAM flap to reduce postoperative partial necrosis. Ann Plast Surg 2004; 53: 205–209.
10. Kroll SS, Schusterman MA, Mistry D. The internal oblique repair of abdominal bulges secondary to TRAM flap breast reconstruction. Plast Reconstruct Surg 1995; 96: 100–104.
11. Reece GP, Kroll SS. Abdominal wall complications: Prevention and treatment. Clin Plast Surg 1998, 25: 225–227.
12. Olding M, Emory RE, Barrett WL. Preferential use of the ipsilateral pedicle in TRAM flap breast reconstruction. Ann Plast Surg 1998; 40: 349–353.
13. Clugston PA, Gingrass MK, Azurin D, et al. Ipsilateral pedicled TRAM flaps: the safer alternative? Plast Reconstruct Surg 2000; 105: 77–82.
14. Marin-Gutzke M, Sanchez-Olaso A, Fernandez-Camacho FJ, Mirelis-Otero E. Anatomic and clinical study of rectus abdominis musculocutaneous flaps based on the superior epigastric system: ipsilateral pedicled TRAM flap as a safe alternative. Ann Plast Surg 2005; 54: 356–360.
15. Maxwell GP, Andochick SE. Secondary shaping of the TRAM flap. Clin Plast Surg 1994; 21: 247–253.
16. Simon AM, Bouwense CL, McMillan S, et al. Comparison of unipedicled and bipedicled TRAM flap breast reconstructions: assessment of physical function and patient satisfaction. Plast Reconstruct Surg 2004; 113: 136–140.
17. Wagner DS, Michelow BJ, Hartrampf CR Jr. Double-pedicle TRAM flap for unilateral breast reconstruction. Plast Reconstruct Surg 1991; 88: 987–997.
18. Hammond DC, Simon AM, Khuthaila DK, et al. Latissimus dorsi flap salvage of the partially failed TRAM flap breast reconstruction. Plast Reconstruct Surg 2007; 120: 383–389.

Breast Reconstruction with Free TRAM Flaps

David W. Chang

INTRODUCTION

Since it was first described in 1979, the free transverse rectus abdominis myocutaneous (TRAM) flap has become one of the most popular and reliable methods of microsurgical breast reconstruction.[1] The free TRAM flap has many features that make it well suited for breast reconstruction.[2-5] Most patients have adequate lower abdominal skin and subcutaneous tissue available for incorporation into the flap to reconstruct a breast. Its vascular pedicle is large, long, constant, and reliable. The robust blood supply of the free TRAM flap reduces the risk of fat necrosis and also enables aggressive folding, trimming, and shaping of the flap to optimize the aesthetic outcome of breast reconstruction. In addition, in most cases the free TRAM flap requires minimal donor site sacrifice. And finally, the flap can be harvested with the patient in a supine position, while mastectomy is being performed.

Over the years, variations on the free TRAM flap, including the free muscle-sparing (MS) TRAM flap, the deep inferior epigastric perforator (DIEP) flap, and the free superficial inferior epigastric artery (SIEA) flap, have been developed to further minimize donor site morbidity by harvesting less muscle and less anterior rectus fascia.[6,7] Each flap transfers the same lower abdominal skin and subcutaneous tissue and is able to provide an aesthetically pleasing breast reconstruction.

INDICATIONS AND CONTRAINDICATIONS
(Box 3.1)

Indications

A free TRAM flap can be used for breast reconstruction in the overwhelming majority of mastectomy patients.[8] A possible candidate for reconstruction with a free TRAM flap is a healthy patient with moderate amounts of abdominal skin laxity and fat, and a minimal to moderate volume requirement for breast reconstruction. The patient must be willing to undergo a long, complex procedure with possible prolonged postoperative recovery. She must understand and accept additional scars in the abdomen and potential donor site morbidities.

Contraindications

Contraindications to the use of a free TRAM flap are:
- A patient who is unwilling to accept additional donor site scars and potential donor site morbidities.
- A patient who is unwilling to undergo a long, complex procedure with prolonged postoperative recovery.
- An abdominal donor site that cannot be closed primarily because the patient is too thin or has a pot-belly habitus.
- A previous TRAM flap or an abdominoplasty.
- A previous abdominal operation in which the deep inferior epigastric vessels were divided or damaged.
- Significant medical comorbidities that make the patient a poor surgical candidate.

High-risk patients
Smokers
Because of the free TRAM flap's excellent blood supply, a history of smoking is not by itself an absolute contraindication. In our experience, the use of a free TRAM flap reconstruction in tobacco smokers is not associated with a significant increase in the rates of vessel thrombosis, flap loss, or fat necrosis compared to rates in non-smokers.[9] However, smokers are at significantly higher risk for mastectomy skin flap necrosis, abdominal flap necrosis, and hernia than non-smokers. These smoking-related

---

BOX 3.1 Indications and contraindications

- A healthy patient with an adequate abdominal donor site

Contraindications
- Inadequate abdominal donor site
- A poor surgical candidate because of medical co-morbidities

---

complications can be significantly reduced when the patient stops smoking at least 4 weeks before surgery.

Obese patients

The decision about whether to use a free TRAM flap for breast reconstruction in an obese patient should be individualized. In our experience, obese patients have significantly higher flap and donor site complications than normal-weight patients.[10] Specifically, compared to normal-weight patients, obese patients have significantly higher rates of total flap loss, flap seroma, mastectomy skin flap necrosis, abdominal hernia, donor site infection, and seroma. In fact, there appears to be an almost linear relationship between complications of all kinds and body weight. Thus, for markedly and morbidly obese patients (body mass index = 40), TRAM flap breast reconstruction should probably be avoided if possible. For patients who are obese but not markedly or morbidly so (body mass index = 30 but <40), free TRAM flap reconstruction may be considered if they are otherwise in good health and well informed of the increased risk of flap failure and complications. Obese patients undergoing delayed breast reconstruction should be encouraged to reduce the risk by losing weight prior to the surgery.

Previous abdominal suction-assisted lipectomy

There is debate about whether a free TRAM flap can be reliably used following abdominal liposuction. The obvious concern is that the perforating vessels to the flap and the microvasculature to the flap may have been damaged by the prior suction-assisted lipectomy (SAL) procedure, which could compromise the viability of the flap. However, a few cases of free TRAM flap breast reconstruction following SAL of the abdomen have been reported.[11] When this is being considered, preoperative Doppler ultrasonography can be used to confirm the presence and the patency of the perforating vessels of the abdominal wall. Additionally, the surgeon should consider incorporating the maximum number of perforators into the flap to render it more robust for transfer.

PREOPERATIVE CONSIDERATIONS

Free flap procedures impose major surgical stress on the patient. Fluid loss is considerable with two operative sites, and patients tend to become hypothermic because of the lengthy nature of these procedures. Thus candidates for free flap reconstruction must have their cardiac, pulmonary, and renal status carefully evaluated preoperatively.

Patients must be advised to abstain from smoking preoperatively to reduce the risks of anesthetic complications and wound-healing problems. Avoiding aspirin-containing products for 2 weeks before surgery is also important so that the baseline coagulation status is normal.

Preoperatively, the patient's abdomen should be evaluated to make sure that she is a good candidate for a TRAM flap. In particular, the abdomen should be examined for any scars. If there are scars, their location, length, duration, and cause must be considered to determine whether a free TRAM flap can be performed safely. The abdomen should be examined with the patient in a supine position with the knees flexed to ensure that the abdomen can be closed primarily after harvesting of the flap. In addition, the integrity of the abdominal wall must be examined for the presence of hernias and for pot-belly habitus.

Once it is determined that the patient is a good candidate for a free TRAM flap, the design of the flap is marked with the patient standing. The inframammary folds are marked bilaterally. The TRAM flap is designed in the lower abdomen with a transverse skin flap. The upper marking is usually just at or above the umbilicus, and the lower marking is just above the pubis, generally following the natural skin fold there. The design of the flap is then tapered to the anterior superior iliac spine so that closure of the donor site will not result in a dog ear (Fig. 3.1).

ANATOMY

Rectus abdominis muscle

The rectus abdominis muscles are a pair of long, straight muscles that flex the spine and tighten the intra-abdominal wall. They arise from the symphysis pubis and the pubic crest and insert on the linea alba and at the fifth, sixth, and seventh costal cartilages. Each rectus abdominis muscle is subdivided by two to five tendinous inscriptions, with the most caudal one at the level of the umbilicus.[12] The tendinous inscriptions are adherent to the overlying anterior rectus sheath but not to the posterior sheath. The inscriptions do not usually extend completely through the muscle and may pass only halfway across it.[13]

Rectus sheath

The rectus abdominis muscles are enclosed by a thick sheath, except for the posterior part below the arcuate line. The rectus sheath is attached to the anterior aspect of the muscles by fusion to the tendinous inscriptions. The aponeurotic extensions of the muscles of the intra-abdominal wall merge to form the anterior portion of the rectus sheath fascia.

An important transition is in the posterior sheath at the arcuate line (semicircular line, or arc of Douglas). The arcuate line is generally located halfway between the umbilicus and symphysis pubis, though this is variable. The arcuate line marks the transition point where the internal oblique aponeurosis ceases to split and the aponeuroses of all three muscles pass ventral to the rectus abdominis. The

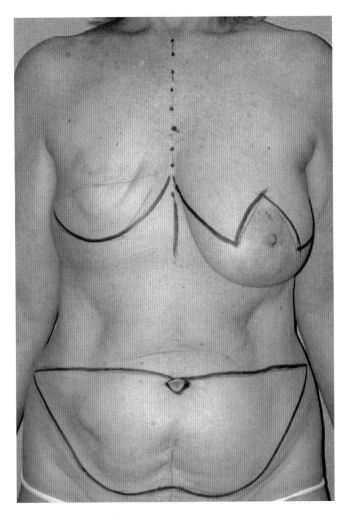

FIGURE 3.1 A TRAM flap design.

transversalis fascia is the only layer present below the arcuate line, and is thus a region of weakness and potential herniation after flap dissection.

The linea alba represents the decussation of the fused aponeuroses in the midline. The linea alba is wider in the region of the xiphoid process and narrows to a fine line below the umbilicus. The lateral border of the rectus sheath is often discernable externally and is referred to as the linea semilunaris.

Blood supply

The rectus abdominis muscle has two vascular pedicles, one composed of the deep superior epigastric artery (DSEA) and the other of the deep inferior epigastric artery (DIEA).[12] The DSEA and DIEA pedicles arborize as they approach each other under the surface of the rectus abdominis. These two systems connect above the umbilicus through a system of small-caliber vessels that Taylor and Palmer[14] refer to as 'choke' vessels.

The DSEA arises from the internal mammary artery at the level of the sixth intercostal space. It generally has two venae comitantes. There is a small branch of the DSEA that courses along the costal margin to join the intercostal artery lateral to the rectus sheath.[15]

The DIEA usually originates 1 cm above the inguinal ligament from the medial aspect of the external iliac artery, directly opposite the deep circumflex iliac artery. The main DIEA pierces the transversalis fascia and enters the rectus sheath just below the arcuate line. It then ascends obliquely and medially between the rectus abdominis muscle and the posterior wall of the sheath. Generally, the DIEA divides into two or three large branches below the level of the umbilicus. Through cadaveric studies, the degree of arborization of the DIEA has been classified into three different types. In type 1, the DIEA does not divide and remains as a single vessel as it courses under the surface of the rectus abdominis (29%). Type 2 refers to a DIEA that divides into two dominant branches (57%). The type 3 pattern is a trifurcation of the DIEA (14%).[15]

The DIEA has two venae comitantes, which usually join to form a single vein prior to their junction with the external iliac vein. In the study by Boyd et al., the deep inferior epigastric veins (DIEV) entered the external iliac vein as a single trunk in 68% of cases and as a double trunk in 32%.[15]

Perforators

The deep arteries supply the TRAM flap's overlying abdominal skin by a system of perforators. These vessels are terminal branches of the DIEA and DIEV. Cadaveric studies by Taylor and Palmer[14] demonstrated a rich connection between the DIEA system and the abdominal wall skin. Many perforating arteries emerge through the anterior rectus sheath, but the highest concentration is in the periumbilical area. The fewest number of perforators is found in the suprapubic area. The branches of the periumbilical perforators have the appearance of the radiating spokes of a wheel whose hub is located at the umbilicus. Thus, incorporation of the periumbilical perforators permits the harvesting of a skin flap with virtually any orientation from the midline.[16]

The perforators communicate with the other regional superficial vessels through a system of choke vessels that link these territories and allow the design of large skin islands based on the DIEA. The dominant connections between these systems occur within the subdermal plexus.

TRAM flap

The blood supply to the TRAM flap is a two-tiered arrangement of muscular and subcutaneous networks (Fig. 3.2). The superior and inferior epigastric artery systems form a deep longitudinal blood supply that is linked to the lower six intercostal vessels and the ascending branch of the deep circumflex iliac artery within the muscles of the abdominal wall. The DIEA is the dominant vessel of the rectus abdominis muscle and the TRAM flap. Injection of this vessel with dye will stain the abdominal wall as high as midway between the umbilicus and xiphoid process, whereas injection of the DSEA with dye rarely results in staining below the umbilicus. The subcutaneous network consists

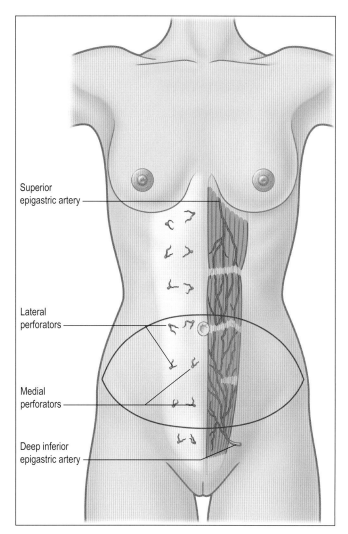

FIGURE 3.2 The blood supply to the TRAM flap (Redrawn from Schusterman MA (ed) Microsurgical reconstruction of the cancer patient. Lippincott-Raven, 1997).

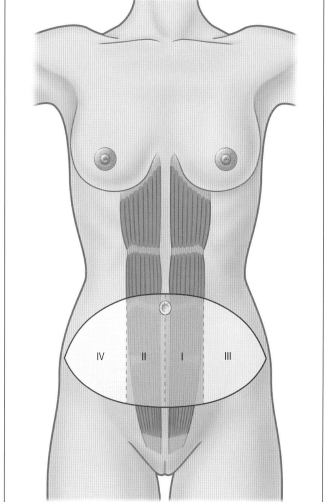

FIGURE 3.3 Four zones of a TRAM flap based on vascularity (Redrawn from Schusterman MA (ed) Microsurgical reconstruction of the cancer patient. Lippincott-Raven, 1997).

of branches of the superficial epigastric artery, superficial circumflex iliac artery, external iliac artery, superficial superior epigastric artery, and the intercostal arteries. The subcutaneous and deep systems are connected by perforators that traverse the rectus abdominis muscles.

Extensive studies of the venous circulation of the TRAM flap have revealed both superficial and deep systems.[17] The veins of the superficial system are above Scarpa's fascia and communicate extensively across the midline. The superficial veins drain into the deep venous system by way of the veins accompanying the musculocutaneous arterial perforators. Valves located in the connecting veins regulate the direction of blood flow from the superficial towards the deep system.

A TRAM flap incorporates skin from the entire lower abdomen. Four different skin zones can be included in a TRAM flap (Fig. 3.3).[18] Zone 1 refers to the skin overlying each lateral rectus abdominis muscle. Zone 2 denotes skin of the contralateral lower abdomen overlying the opposite rectus abdominis muscle. The skin territory on each side

of the abdomen lateral to the linea semilunaris is referred to as zone 3, and the skin lateral to the opposite linea semilunaris is zone 4. The blood supply to zone 4 is the most tenuous.

Innervations

The rectus abdominis muscles are innervated in a segmental fashion from the lower six intercostal nerves, derived from T7–T12, which traverse the plane between the transversus abdominis and the internal oblique muscles. These mixed motor and sensory nerves provide innervation to the rectus abdominis muscles and sensory supply to the overlying skin. The intercostal nerves enter the mid-portion of the rectus muscles at the posterior surface.[16]

OPERATIVE APPROACH (see also Box 3.2)

All flap and recipient site dissection is done under loupe magnification, and the author finds it useful to wear a headlight for optimal visualization of the operative field.

BOX 3.2 Optimizing outcomes

- Careful patient selection
- Understand patient's goals and expectations of breast reconstruction
  - Evaluate and address patient's risk factors
- A precise and meticulous surgical technique
  - Atraumatic dissection of recipient and donor vessels, including perforators
  - Minimal sacrifice of rectus fascia
  - Minimal dissection of rectus muscle
  - Maximize preservation of innervations to the remaining rectus muscle
- Use only well-vascularized portion of the flap for breast reconstruction
  - Discard zone 4
- Ensure optimal and error-free microvascular anastomoses
  - Focus on proper set-up so that microvascular anastomoses can be performed in a comfortable position
  - Ensure that the vascular pedicle is not twisted or kinked
  - Use atraumatic and precise microsurgical technique
- Optimal donor site closure
  - The fascia repair should be tension-free
  - Do not leave dog ears
  - Pay attention to details such as the size, the location and the type of an umbilical repair
- Attempt to create a breast that is aesthetically optimal and natural, yet easy to revise if needed
  - Focus on creating an adequate cleavage volume
  - Better to create a breast that is slightly larger than too small

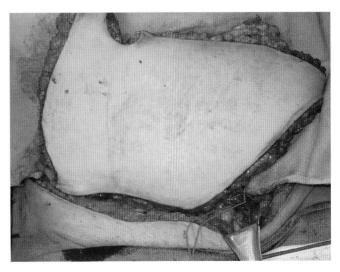

FIGURE 3.4 The superficial inferior epigastric vein (SIEV) and artery (SIEA) are identified and preserved.

Patient positioning

The patient should be placed supine, lying symmetrically and straight on the table. Her waist should be at the proper bend of the table so that she can be placed in a sitting position during flap insetting and shaping. With most operating tables, in order to place the patient in a sitting position the table needs to be reversed so that her head is at the table's foot. The patient's arms are extended out and placed on arm boards, with ample foam padding at the elbows and wrists. Both arms are then secured to the boards with gauze rolls. This allows the surgeons access to the axilla for lymph node dissection if necessary.

For immediate reconstruction, the flap harvest and the breast resection are accomplished simultaneously to reduce operating time. For delayed reconstruction, the recipient site preparation and the flap harvest can be performed simultaneously by two teams of surgeons.

The first step of flap harvest is to dissect out the umbilicus. It helps to make four small stab incisions with a #11 blade at the 12, 3, 6, and 9 o'clock positions. Skin hooks are then placed into the incisions to provide retraction while incisions are made to connect the stab incisions. Using a tenotomy scissors, the umbilical stalk is dissected down to its base. There is no need to make the umbilical stalk overly thin or thick. A marking stitch is placed at the 12 o'clock position of the umbilicus for use as a guide

during the insetting of the umbilicus and to prevent twisting of the stalk.

The border of the skin island is incised down to the abdominal wall. The superficial inferior epigastric vein (SIEV) and SIEA are identified and preserved (Fig. 3.4). If the SIEA is significant in size, and if the patient is a good candidate, an SIEA flap can be used for breast reconstruction. Even if an SIEA flap is not planned, it is important to preserve and dissect out the SIEV for about 4–5 cm. With the increasing use of DIEP and free MS-TRAM flaps with fewer and smaller perforators being included with the flap, occasionally the SIEV needs to be used as a second means of venous drainage if the deep venous drainage alone is not adequate.

Full-muscle TRAM flap

For patients with high-risk factors such as smoking and obesity, a priority is to optimize perfusion to the flap by including as many major perforators as possible. In these instances, a full-muscle TRAM flap may be the best choice.

The TRAM flap is carefully dissected off the rectus sheath, preserving all major perforators on the preferred side (Fig. 3.5). A fascia-sparing technique is used to open the rectus sheath fascia, incorporating only a small cuff of fascia around the perforators and then connecting these islands of fascia to each other (Fig. 3.6). When the fascia is opened in this manner only a minimal amount is sacrificed, facilitating primary closure of the fascia without tension or the use of synthetic mesh. The rectus sheath incision is extended inferiorly and laterally to expose the underlying rectus abdominis muscle.

The anterior rectus sheath fascia is dissected off the underlying rectus abdominis and its tendinous inscriptions. The rectus sheath attachments are divided to the medial and lateral borders of the muscle. Care must be taken when separating the inscriptions to the anterior rectus sheath,

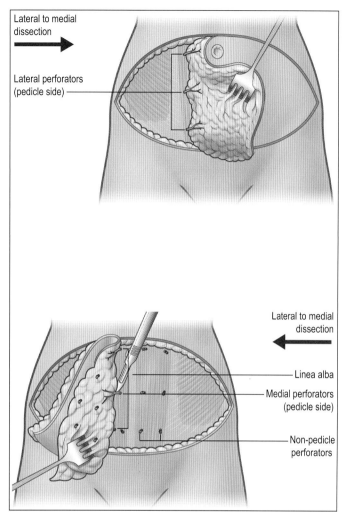

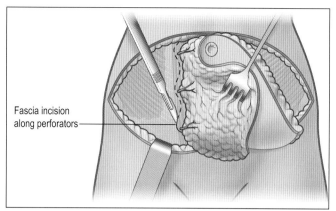

FIGURE 3.6 A fascia-sparing technique is used to open the rectus sheath fascia (Redrawn from Schusterman MA (ed) Microsurgical reconstruction of the cancer patient. Lippincott-Raven, 1997).

FIGURE 3.5 The TRAM flap is carefully dissected off the rectus sheath, preserving all major perforators (Redrawn from Schusterman MA (ed) Microsurgical reconstruction of the cancer patient. Lippincott-Raven, 1997).

where they are densely adherent. Several intercostal nerves and vessels will be seen on the surface of the posterior rectus sheath. The intercostal branches are isolated and ligated. The lateral border of the muscle is identified and dissected inferiorly, where the DIEA pedicle is found at the lateral border of the lower part of the muscle above the pubic tubercle. The rectus abdominis muscle is separated from the posterior sheath.

The rectus abdominis muscle is then gently retracted to expose the deep inferior epigastric vessels that course beneath it. Once the vascular pedicle has been identified and isolated, the inferior muscle attachment at the symphysis pubis and pubic crest is detached to facilitate exposure and dissection of the deep inferior epigastric pedicle. This is then traced toward its origin at the external iliac vessels to obtain optimal vascular pedicle length. The upper muscle attachment is divided, and the superior epigastric artery and vein are ligated. Superiorly, the muscle can be divided at any level above the perforators to the flap, even at its insertion at the costal margin if necessary. The deep

inferior epigastric pedicle is left intact until the recipient site is prepared.

Once the recipient vessels are dissected and the mastectomy pocket is prepared, the TRAM flap harvesting is completed by individually ligating the DIE artery and veins using either hemoclips or suture ligatures. After the flap is harvested, the muscle is secured to the overlying flap with several sutures so as to minimize any undue tension or twisting of perforators.

MS-TRAM flap

The skin and subcutaneous tissues are elevated off the anterior rectus sheath from lateral to medial until the lateral perforators are seen. At this time, the lateral perforators from both the right and the left side are evaluated, and the decision is made as to which will be kept. The size, number, and orientation of the perforators should be considered when making this evaluation. The lateral row of perforators on the side that will not be used are hemoclipped and divided, and then the flap is elevated to expose the medial row of perforators. Once again, perforators on both sides are evaluated and the preferred ones are kept; the others are hemoclipped and divided. This maneuver is continued until two or more of the best perforators remain, having been selected for inclusion in the flap. All things being equal, the author prefers medially located perforators on the contralateral side of the abdomen to the breast defect. Medial perforators provide longer pedicles and their harvest results in less functional damage to the remaining rectus muscle, as the muscle is innervated from lateral to medial. Also, compared to the laterally located perforators, more medially located perforators may provide better perfusion to the tissues across the midline of the flap. Generally, two or three moderate to large perforators will provide sufficient circulation to the TRAM flap.

The anterior rectus sheath fascia is dissected off the underlying rectus abdominis muscle and its inscriptions, and the orientation and course of the perforators within the rectus muscle are evaluated. The decision to perform an

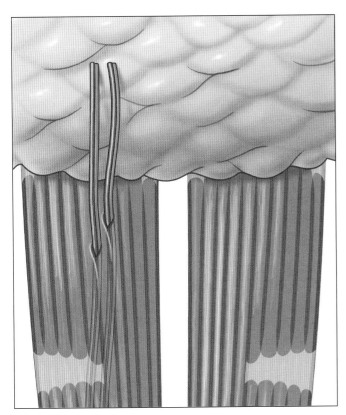

FIGURE 3.7 A DIEP flap is selected when there is a single large perforator, or when two or more perforators are located within the same intramuscular septum (Redrawn from Bajaj AK, Chevray PM, Chang DW. Comparison of donor-site complications and functional outcomes in free muscle-sparing TRAM flap and free DIEP flap breast reconstruction. Plast Reconstruct Surg 2006; 117: 737–746).

MS-TRAM or a DIEP flap is based on the number, caliber, and location of perforators as well as their orientation and course within the rectus muscle. A DIEP flap is selected when there is a single large perforator, or when two or more perforators are located within the same intramuscular septum (Fig. 3.7). If the perforators are located in different intramuscular layers, the muscle fibers between them would need to be divided for a DIEP flap; under these circumstances, a small cuff of muscle fibers between and around the perforators is incorporated, and a free MS-TRAM flap is performed (Fig. 3.8A,B). The author prefers to perform a DIEP flap only if it can be harvested without significant damage to the rectus abdominis muscle.

Three types of free MS-TRAM flap can be performed (Fig. 3.9). The medial portion of the rectus abdominis muscle can be preserved and a lateral portion of the rectus muscle harvested with the flap (MS-1M).[6,7] A lateral portion of the muscle can be preserved and the medial portion of the rectus muscle harvested with the flap (MS-1L). Finally, a small cuff of muscle around the perforators can be harvested with the flap, leaving the majority of the muscles intact (MS-2).

The type of free MS-TRAM flap harvested depends for the most part on the location and orientation of the

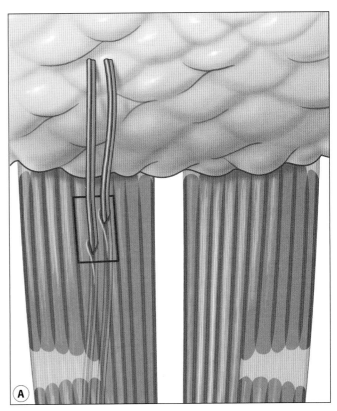

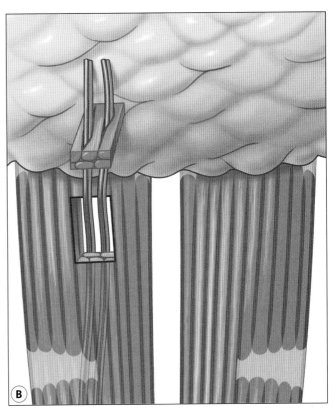

FIGURE 3.8 A, B If the perforators are located in different intramuscular layers, a small cuff of muscle fibers between and around the perforators is incorporated, and a free MS-TRAM flap is performed (Redrawn from Bajaj AK, Chevray PM, Chang DW. Comparison of donor-site complications and functional outcomes in free muscle-sparing TRAM flap and free DIEP flap breast reconstruction. Plast Reconstruct Surg 2006; 117: 737–746.)

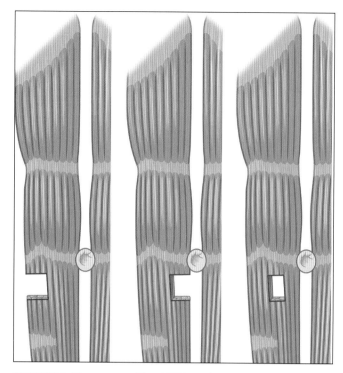

FIGURE 3.9 Three types of free MS-TRAM flap can be performed (Redrawn from Bajaj AK, Chevray PM, Chang DW. Comparison of donor-site complications and functional outcomes in free muscle-sparing TRAM flap and free DIEP flap breast reconstruction. Plast Reconstruct Surg 2006; 117: 737–746.)

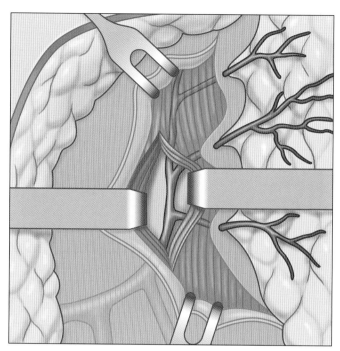

FIGURE 3.10 The muscle is split in the direction of its fibers within the intramuscular septum medially and laterally down to the posterior rectus sheath (Redrawn from Schusterman MA (ed) Microsurgical reconstruction of the cancer patient. Lippincott-Raven, 1997.)

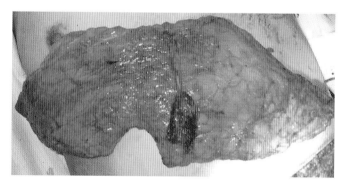

FIGURE 3.11 A free MS-TRAM flap.

perforators. If the perforators are located very medially, then the MS-1L is usually used. If the perforators are located in the middle of the muscle, usually the MS-2 is used. If the perforators are located laterally, then the MS-1M can be harvested. Also, the orientation of the perforators within the rectus muscle is a determining factor in how much of the rectus abdominis will be taken with the perforators. If the perforators are coming directly up through the muscle, then only a small amount of muscle needs to be sacrificed. However, if the perforators are coursing obliquely through the muscle, then more muscle will need to be sacrificed.

Once the extent of the muscle that needs to be taken with the flap is decided, the muscle is split in the direction of its fibers within the intramuscular septum medially and laterally down to the posterior rectus sheath (Fig. 3.10). Under the rectus abdominis muscle, the main branch to the perforators can usually be visualized at this time. Inferior to the most inferior perforator, the muscle fibers between the lateral and medial dissected plane are then divided. The author prefers to use a bipolar device for dividing the muscles to minimize bleeding. All vascular branches should be either hemoclipped or cauterized with the bipolar device. It is important to maintain a hemostatic, clean operative field to optimize visualization and exposure. Once the inferior portion of the muscle is divided, the main pedicle should be exposed. The rectus muscle fibers are then split inferiorly to further expose and dissect out the main pedicle. With a free MS-TRAM or a DIEP flap, the pedicle does not usually need to be dissected all the way down to the origin, as it is already fairly long. Finally, the muscle fibers at the superior aspect of the perforators are divided between the medially and laterally dissected planes of the rectus muscle. At this time, the superior blood supply to the rectus muscle is seen and ligated (Fig. 3.11).

Once the recipient vessels are dissected and the mastectomy pocket is prepared, the flap harvesting is completed by individually ligating the DIE artery and veins using either hemoclips or suture ligatures. After the flap is harvested, the muscle is secured to the overlying flap with several sutures so as to minimize any undue tension or twisting of perforators.

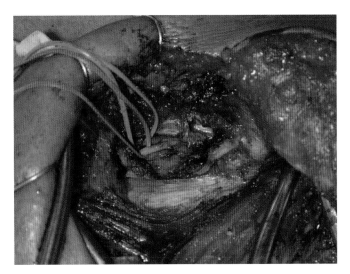

FIGURE 3.12 The internal mammary vessels as the primary recipients of choice.

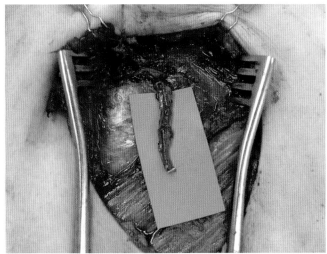

FIGURE 3.13 The internal mammary perforator vessels.

Preparation of the recipient site

For immediate reconstruction, after the mastectomy is completed the mastectomy skin flap and defect are carefully evaluated before the recipient vessels are dissected. For delayed reconstruction, the previous mastectomy scar is excised and sent for pathologic evaluation. The skin flap is then elevated off the pectoralis major muscle superiorly and inferiorly to recreate the mastectomy defect. Inferiorly, careful attention is paid to avoid excessive dissection, which would create a low inframammary fold.

Currently, the author uses the internal mammary vessels as the primary recipients of choice (Fig. 3.12). The intercostal spaces are palpated to find an optimal space that is wide and readily accessible for comfortable microvascular anastomoses. This is usually at the second or third intercostal space. Then, the region above the pectoralis muscle is scanned to identify any perforator vessels that may be usable as recipients. Occasionally, fairly large perforator vessels can be seen medially coming out of the pectoralis muscle fibers (Fig. 3.13). Usually, perforating veins are large with a very thin wall, and perforating arteries are small. Furthermore, most perforators will pose a size mismatch with the main DIEA and DIEV, making anastomoses challenging. Only experienced microsurgeons who are comfortable with these types of anastomosis should use perforators as recipient vessels.

If no suitable perforators are noted above the pectoralis major muscle, then the pectoralis muscle at the desired intercostal space is split in the direction of its fibers to expose the intercostal space. There is no need to detach the pectoralis muscle from the sternum. Usually, more perforators can be seen underneath the pectoralis coming out of the intercostal muscles. Again, the perforators are evaluated for their suitability, and if the surgeon feels they are large enough they can be used as recipient vessels.

To expose the internal mammary vessels, the overlying intercostal muscle fibers are carefully divided layer by layer with a bipolar device. Usually, within 1–3 cm from the edge of the sternum the internal mammary vein and artery are identified. If there is a single vein, it is medial to the artery. If there are two veins, then the artery is between the veins. It is critical to keep the operative field bloodless for optimal exposure. Extreme care must be taken to control bleeding from small branches. Adjacent cartilage does not need to be removed routinely; however, if the intercostal space is narrow or deep, making anastomoses difficult, then the overlying cartilage should be removed to better expose the vessels. Either the cartilage above or that below can be resected. To accomplish this, the perichondrium is incised and dissected off the cartilage, 2–3 cm of cartilage is removed directly over the internal mammary vessels using a rib dissector or rongeur, and then the perichondrium is carefully dissected off the internal mammary vessels. Once again, extreme care must be taken to control bleeding from all small branches. Final preparation of the recipient vessels is best performed under a microscope.

Flap insetting and shaping

The overall goal of autologous tissue breast reconstruction is to transfer well-vascularized tissue to the mastectomy site and create a breast mound that appears as anatomically and aesthetically normal as possible.

The author prefers to place the TRAM flap vertically for breast reconstruction. This is best done using a flap from the contralateral side of the abdomen (Fig. 3.14). That way, the flap lies vertically on the chest with the vascular pedicle oriented medially, in an anatomically natural position, toward the internal mammary recipient vessels. The SIEV will also be oriented medially, so that if a second source of venous drainage is needed the SIEV can be anastomosed to an internal mammary perforator vein or to a second internal mammary vein. The thin zone 3 tissue is inset in the superior region, and the tissue of zones 1 and 2, the thickest portion of the flap, is at the mound of the reconstructed breast. The corner of the flap from zone 3 is usually

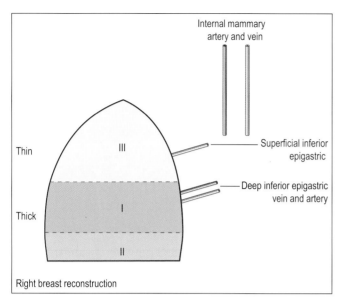

Internal mammary
artery and vein

Thin

III

Superficial inferior
epigastric

Deep inferior epigastric
vein and artery

Thick

I

II

Right breast reconstruction

FIGURE 3.14 The author prefers to place the TRAM flap vertically for breast reconstruction.

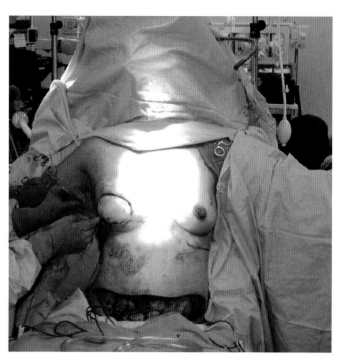

FIGURE 3.15 The patient is placed in a sitting position for insetting and the shaping of the TRAM flap.

discarded, and zone 4 is always discarded. In certain situations, zone 2, i.e., the flap across the midline, can be folded to increase the flap's projection or to create a ptotic-appearing breast.

During the insetting and the shaping of the flap the surgeon must always be aware of the tension, the rotation, and the status of the vascular pedicle. Some surgeons like to secure the flap to the chest wall, but I find this is unnecessary in most cases and that the sutures create an unnatural contour of the reconstructed breast. Usually, the mastectomy skin flap alone will provide good support for the TRAM flap. However, when the flap is significantly smaller than the mastectomy defect, it needs to be secured medially and superiorly so that it does not fall down within the pocket, which can also cause excessive tension on the vascular pedicle.

The TRAM flap is temporarily placed into the mastectomy defect, and the mastectomy flap is draped over the TRAM flap. The mastectomy flap is then temporarily secured over the TRAM flap with skin staples. The patient is placed in a sitting position, and the TRAM flap is shaped into a breast (Fig. 3.15).

When shaping a TRAM flap for breast reconstruction, it is important to focus on the superior and medial areas of the breast to ensure adequate cleavage volume (Fig. 3.16A,B). A slightly overcorrected cleavage region can be easily revised with SAL. However, undercorrected cleavage, resulting from deficient tissue volume in the superior and medial portions of the breast, can be difficult to correct; usually, the flap needs to be re-elevated and advanced to fill the hollow area, which can be a major procedure.

It is better to make the initial breast mound volume slightly larger than the contralateral breast. In most instances, mild shrinkage of the reconstructed breast will occur. Furthermore, a slightly too-large breast can usually be readily revised with SAL or direct excision. However, an overzealous attempt at achieving a 'perfect' volume match at the time of initial reconstruction can sometimes result in a breast that is smaller than desired. If the initial reconstructed breast is significantly smaller than the opposite breast, this can be corrected only by augmentation of the reconstructed breast or reduction of the opposite native breast. Attention also needs to be paid to make sure the inframammary fold is placed in the correct location, as it is very difficult to adjust this later on.

Once the optimal size and shape have been achieved compared to the contralateral breast, the skin paddle is marked. The patient is then placed back in a supine position, and the buried portion of the skin is de-epithelialized. One drain is placed underneath the flap.

In unilateral breast reconstruction, the contralateral native breast is used as a guide to achieve volume and shape symmetry for the reconstructed breast. When immediate reconstruction is performed following skin-sparing mastectomy, the remaining mastectomy skin envelope can facilitate the shaping of the flap for breast reconstruction.

In delayed breast reconstruction, the surgeon must decide how to manage the inferior portion of the mastectomy skin flap. If the skin flap is abundant and soft, the author prefers to preserve it and use it for the breast reconstruction, as this allows for more 'natural'-appearing shape. If the skin flap is fibrotic due to irradiation, it may be better to discard it and replace that area with TRAM flap skin.

One of the most difficult parts of delayed breast reconstruction is achieving an optimal inframammary fold. A careful and accurate preoperative marking with the patient in a standing position is essential to create an inframammary fold in the proper location. A fold that is created too

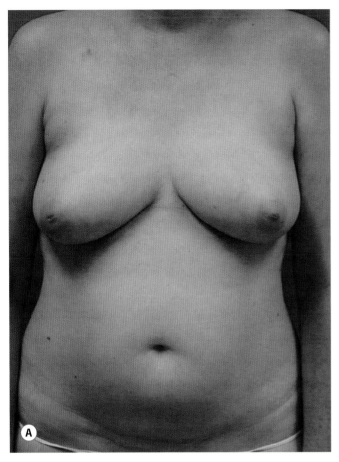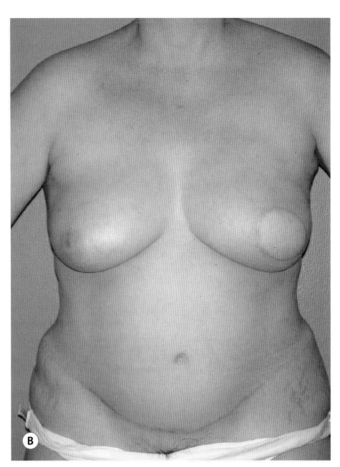

FIGURE 3.16 A, B When shaping a TRAM flap for breast reconstruction, it is important to focus on the superior and medial areas of the breast to ensure adequate cleavage volume.

high or too low during the initial reconstructive procedure is often difficult to correct. However, it is probably better to err on the side of making the fold slightly too high than too low. I personally find it easier to lower an inframammary fold that is too high than to move up an inframammary fold that is too low.

Management of the donor site

Meticulous closure of the donor site defect is necessary to prevent weakening or herniation of the anterior abdominal wall. If the fascia was harvested using a fascia-sparing technique, the medial and lateral cuffs of the anterior rectus sheath can be closed primarily where it was split longitudinally without creating any tension, even in cases of bilateral flap harvest. The rectus fascia sheath is closed primarily with non-absorbable sutures using an interrupted and running technique (Fig. 3.17A,B). However, if the integrity of the overlying fascia is poor, or if a significant amount of fascia was harvested and tension-free primary closure is difficult, synthetic mesh is used to reinforce the closure. Synthetic mesh can be placed using an inlay or onlay technique, depending on the surgeon's preference. The anterior rectus sheath should be carefully repaired below the level of the arcuate line where herniation is more likely to occur,

as the posterior rectus sheath is deficient in this area. Closed-suction drains are placed above the fascia closure in the subcutaneous tissue.

After the abdomen is closed, the umbilicus is brought out through an incision made in the midline of the abdominal flap and secured with sutures. Care should be taken to ensure that the umbilicus is in the correct anatomic location in the midline and that it is not twisted at its stalk. There are many different ways to inset the umbilicus. The author prefers to make a 'frown' incision and to resect a small wedge from the inferior portion of the umbilicus for a more youthful appearance (Fig. 3.18).

COMPLICATIONS

Flap loss

The success of even the most elegantly designed free TRAM flap breast reconstruction is ultimately dependent on the success of the arterial and venous anastomoses. The most common cause of vessel thrombosis leading to flap loss is probably technical error during the microvascular anastomoses. Thus, it is critical that the surgeon have a thorough understanding of the physiologic factors that

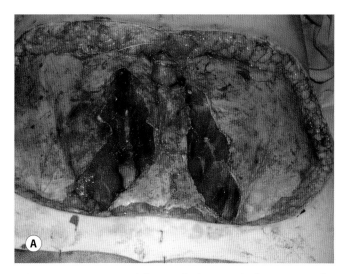
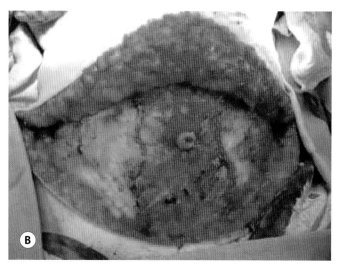

FIGURE 3.17 Donor sites following the harvest of a free MS TRAM flap (**A**) and a DIEP flap (**B**). The rectus fascia sheath is closed primarily with non-absorbable sutures using an interrupted and running technique.

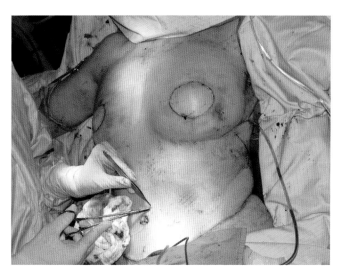

FIGURE 3.18 For the umbilicus, the author prefers to make a 'frown' incision and to resect a small wedge from the inferior portion of the umbilicus.

affect anastomotic patency, technical competence, and sound clinical judgment gained from experience.

Fat necrosis/partial flap loss

Fat necrosis and partial flap loss result from inadequate perfusion to a portion of the flap. The best ways to minimize this are to ensure that the perfusion to the flap is optimal and that any poorly perfused area is discarded. This includes any areas of the flap that do not have bright red bleeding. In almost all cases zone 4 tissue should be discarded. Usually, a small portion from the corner of zone 3 is also discarded.

As many perforators as necessary should be included to provide optimal perfusion to the flap. In many cases only two or three perforators, and occasionally even a single large perforator, will provide sufficient perfusion. However, in higher-risk patients, such as smokers or the obese, the surgeon should consider including more perforators to reduce the risk of significant fat necrosis or partial flap loss.

Proper selection of recipient vessels is also important to ensure optimal blood inflow and outflow. It is elegant to use perforators as recipient vessels, but the surgeon must be careful to consider the vessel size match and the size of the flap being used for breast reconstruction to minimize complications.

Abdominal bulge/hernia

The driving force behind the development of free TRAM flap variants, such as the MS-TRAM and DIEP flaps, has been the desire to reduce abdominal donor site morbidity, particularly hernia or bulge. One way to do this is to ensure optimal tension-free fascial closure. The author prefers to use a fascia-sparing technique for harvesting most free TRAM flaps, regardless of how much rectus abdominis muscle is sacrificed. Thus, even in bilateral cases the rectus fascia sheath can be closed primarily with minimal tension. However, if the overlying fascial integrity is poor, or if tension-free primary closure is difficult, synthetic mesh can be used to reinforce the closure.

POSTOPERATIVE CARE

In most cases no special vasodilators or anticoagulation agents are needed after surgery. A support bra is used to help support and maintain the position of the reconstructed breast medially. The patient is placed in a flexed position to minimize tension at the abdominal donor site. The flap is checked every hour by the nursing and/or surgical staff. The patient refrains from oral intake on the day of surgery. The next morning, if the flap is doing well, the diet is advanced as tolerated. Early postoperative ambulation is encouraged. Exercise that involves the abdomen may be resumed approximately 6 weeks after surgery.

Revisions

After creation of the breast mound, a second-stage operation may be needed to revise the reconstructed breast to achieve the final desired size and shape. Occasionally, surgical intervention on the opposite breast will be needed as well. Other procedures that may be done during this second stage include excision of fat necrosis, correction of inframammary fold asymmetry, scar revisions, minor touch-ups to the abdominal donor area, and nipple–areolar reconstruction.

During the initial reconstruction it is often not possible to make a breast that exactly matches the size and shape of the opposite breast. One reason is the position of the patient. Even if the breast is shaped with the patient in a sitting position as much as possible, the full effect of gravity when the patient is standing cannot be duplicated on the operating table. Also, there are limitations as to how much shaping can be performed without jeopardizing the blood supply and the viability of the flap. Finally, the initially reconstructed breast rarely, if ever, completely retains its original shape or size. Thus, it is reasonable to expect that the final product will need some touch-ups in many or even most cases. As the flap and the surgical site heal together, the reconstructed breast's size and shape continue to evolve. For these reasons, some revision of the reconstructed breast is often necessary.

The extent of revision surgery needed can vary from minor outpatient surgery with local anesthesia to major intervention requiring general anesthesia. Often the type and extent of the revision can be planned during the initial reconstruction. That is, during the initial reconstructive surgery, insetting and shaping of the flap can be performed in such a way that the second-stage revision surgery, if needed, will be minor.

CONCLUSIONS

The free TRAM flap is one of the most popular and reliable methods of microsurgical autologous tissue breast reconstruction and has spawned several variations, including the free MS-TRAM flap, free DIEP flap, and free SIEA flap. With proper patient selection and safe surgical technique, each of these flaps can transfer the lower abdominal skin and subcutaneous tissue to provide an aesthetically pleasing breast reconstruction with minimal donor site morbidity.

REFERENCES

1. Holmstrom H. The free abdominoplasty flap and its use in breast reconstruction. Scand J Plast Reconstruct Surg 1979; 13: 423.
2. Schusterman MA, Kroll SS, Weldon ME. Immediate breast reconstruction: Why the free TRAM over the conventional TRAM flap? Plast Reconstruct Surg 1992; 90: 255.
3. Elliott LF, Eskenazi L, Beegle PH. Immediate TRAM flap breast reconstruction: 128 consecutive cases. Plast Reconstruct Surg 1993; 92: 217.
4. Grotting JC. Immediate breast reconstruction using the free TRAM flap. Clin Plast Surg 1994; 21: 207.
5. Pennington DG, Pelly AD. The rectus abdominis myocutaneous free flap. Br J Plast Surg 1980; 33: 277.
6. Bajaj AK, Chevray P, Chang DW. Comparison of donor site complications and functional outcomes in free muscle-sparing TRAM flap and free DIEP flap breast reconstruction. Plast Reconstruct Surg 2006; 117: 737–746.
7. Nahabedian MY, Momen B, Galdino G, Manson PN. Breast reconstruction with the free TRAM or DIEP flap: Patient selection, choice of flap, and outcome. Plast Reconstruct Surg 2002; 110: 466–475.
8. Lipa JE, Youssef AA, Kuerer HM, et al. Breast reconstruction in older women: Advantages of autogenous tissue. Plast Reconstruct Surg 2003; 111: 1110–1121.
9. Chang DW, Reece G, Wang B, et al. Effect of smoking on complications in patients undergoing free TRAM flap breast reconstruction. Plast Reconstruct Surg 2000; 105: 2374–2380.
10. Chang DW, Wang B, Robb G, et al. The effect of obesity on flap and donor site complications in free TRAM flap breast reconstruction. Plast Reconstruct Surg 2000; 105: 1640–1648.
11. Kim JYS, Chang DW, Temple C, et al. Free TRAM flap breast reconstruction in patients with prior abdominal suction-assisted lipectomy. Plast Reconstruct Surg 2004; 113: 28e.
12. Moon H, Taylor GI. The vascular anatomy of the rectus abdominis musculocutaneous flaps based on the deep superior epigastric system. Plast Reconstruct Surg 1988; 82: 815.
13. Mathes S, Nahai F. Clinical applications for muscle and musculocutaneous flaps. St Louis: CV Mosby, 1982; 44.
14. Taylor G, Palmer J. The vascular territories (angiosomes) of the body: experimental and clinical applications. Br J Plast Surg 1987; 40: 113.
15. Boyd JB, Taylor GI, Corlett R. The vascular territories of the superior and deep inferior epigastric systems. Plast Reconstruct Surg 1984; 73: 1.
16. Duchateau J, Declety A, Lejour M. Innervation of the rectus abdominis muscle: implications for rectus flaps. Plast Reconstruct Surg 1988; 82: 223.
17. Carramenha E, Costa M, Carriquiry C, et al. An anatomic study of the venous drainage of the transverse rectus abdominis musculocutaneous flap. Plast Reconstruct Surg 1987; 79: 208.
18. Scheflan M, Hartrampf CR, Black PW. Breast reconstruction with a transverse abdominal island flap. Plast Reconstruct Surg 1982; 69: 908–909.

CHAPTER

Breast Reconstruction-Perforator Flaps (DIEP, SIEA)

4

Moustapha Hamdi and John Hijjawi

INTRODUCTION

Hartrampf et al introduced the transverse rectus abdominis myocutaneous (TRAM) flap in the early 1980s and with it the use of the lower abdomen for autologous breast reconstruction. The TRAM flap quickly gained the reputation as the gold standard in breast reconstruction for many plastic surgeons and their patients. Technical advances since then have been directed towards improving aesthetic outcomes and minimizing donor site morbidity for patients undergoing reconstruction with lower abdominal tissue. These goals also include improving the reliability of all lower abdominal flaps transferred to the chest for breast reconstruction, and maintaining the excellent aesthetic results achieved with the pedicled TRAM flap.[2-4]

A major advance toward these goals has been the development of 'perforator' flaps, most notably the deep inferior epigastric artery perforator (DIEaP) flap[5-10] and the superficial inferior epigastric artery (SIEA) perforator flap.[11-13] The use of these flaps in autologous breast reconstruction is the subject of this chapter. The introduction and popularity of the perforator flap concept has its roots in the field of microvascular breast reconstruction. The reduction in donor site morbidity of the DIEP and SIEA flaps over the TRAM flap has been well established.[14-16]

INDICATIONS AND CONTRAINDICATIONS

The DIEaP and SIEA flaps are excellent choices for breast reconstruction in any woman with an immediate or delayed mastectomy defect who has an adequate volume of lower abdominal donor tissue supplied by appropriate vessels (Figs 4.1–4.5).

The DIEaP flap is contraindicated in patients who have already had cosmetic abdominoplasty. Relative contraindications for DIEaP reconstruction include smoking, previous abdominal liposuction, lack of adequate tissue volume, and

poor overall medical condition.[31-33] However, a DIEaP free flap can still be harvested if intact and appropriately sized perforators are confirmed by preoperative imaging techniques such as Duplex ultrasound or computed tomographic (CT) scan.[34] In such cases two pedicles, such as bilateral DIEA or DIEA/SIEA, may be required to ensure the viability of required zones of the abdominal flap to reconstruct even a unilateral breast defect. Obviously, a bipedicled DIEaP/DIEaP gives the greatest latitude in flap shaping because of the length of the pedicle (Fig. 4.6).

Use of the SIEA free flap may be limited by the anatomical considerations previously outlined. This flap is more suited to clinical situations where only a moderate amount of tissue (located in zones I and II) is required for unilateral or bilateral breast reconstruction. Indeed, bilateral reconstruction is an ideal indication for the SIEA flap because it allows a shorter operative procedure without intramuscular dissection relative to the DIEaP or TRAM flap options. Another good indication is in partial breast reconstruction, where a limited volume of tissue is required to correct a secondary breast deformity following breast-conserving surgery (tumorectomy and radiotherapy).[35]

The absence or interruption of the SIEA vessels due to previous abdominal surgery (e.g. Pfannenstiel incision or inguinal hernia repair) is an absolute contraindication to the SIEA flap. The vein should also be explored carefully in cases of previous saphenous vein surgery in case it is interrupted at this level.

PREOPERATIVE CONSIDERATIONS

Surgical anatomy

The skin and fat of the lower abdominal wall are lax, with zones of adherence at the linea alba and the umbilicus. The soft consistency of the fat is ideal for breast reconstruction, **49**

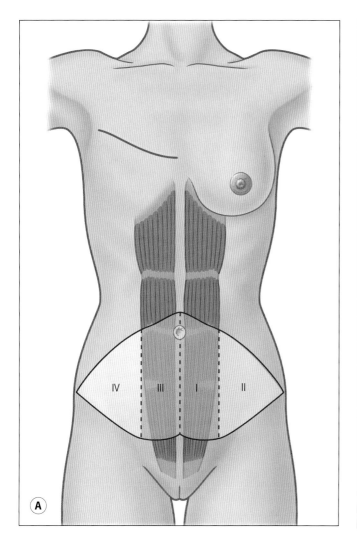
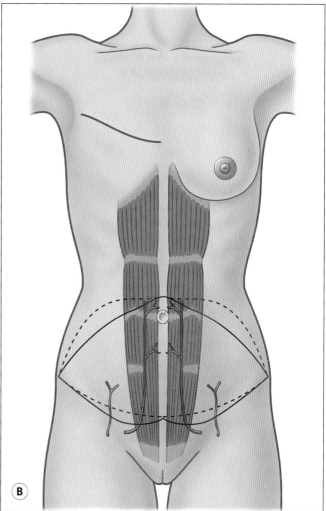

FIGURE 4.1 Flap territory and design. **A** The vascular territory of the lower abdomen is divided into four zones (I–IV). **B** The DIEaP design (dotted line) compared to the SIEA flap design (dark line). **C** The SIEA vascular territory (dotted zone) is limited to the ipsilateral lower abdomen (zones I and II) with some extension to half of the contralateral zone III.

as it allows the creation of a soft, pliable breast mound. The blood supply to the lower abdominal wall which is of interest in free abdominal flap breast reconstruction arises primarily from the external iliac artery. A variety of elliptical flaps can be harvested from the tissue between the umbilicus and the pubis. However, this abdominal region is traditionally divided into four zones (I, II, III, and IV) depending on an ipsilateral blood supply.[17] Zone IV is most remote from the pedicle and is not usually included in the flap (Fig. 4.7A).

Primary blood supply

The deep inferior epigastric artery, which is the major blood supply to the lower abdominal wall, is a branch of the external iliac artery arising 1 cm cranial to the inguinal ligament. The pedicle traverses deep to the transversalis fascia in a superomedial direction and comes into close contact with the posterior surface of the rectus abdominis muscle as it passes superficial to the arcuate line. In most patients, and at a variable distance cranial to the arcuate line, the main pedicle bifurcates into a lateral and a medial

branch prior to penetrating the rectus muscle. In about 28% of patients there is no bifurcation, and in these cases the vessel takes a central course. As the pedicle courses through its intramuscular course it gives off muscular branches.[18] An average of two to eight 'major' perforators, defined as being more than 0.5 mm in diameter, penetrate the anterior rectus sheath per side in an area extending between 2 cm cranial to the umbilicus and 6 cm caudal to it, and 1–6 cm lateral to the umbilicus.[19,20] The lateral branch, or lateral row, perforators may be larger and easier to dissect, but the midline perforators supply better blood flow to zone IV, which is farthest from the vascular pedicle.[21,22] As such, the medial row perforators perfuse larger areas than lateral row perforators, but the dissection must be carried out over a longer intramuscular course with more extensive longitudinal muscle splitting. Perforators that pass through the rectus muscle at the level of the tendinous insertions are generally large, with few side branches. At this location, the distance from the anterior rectus sheath to the main pedicle is also shorter, which reduces the complexity of the dissection. The perforators branch either immediately above the

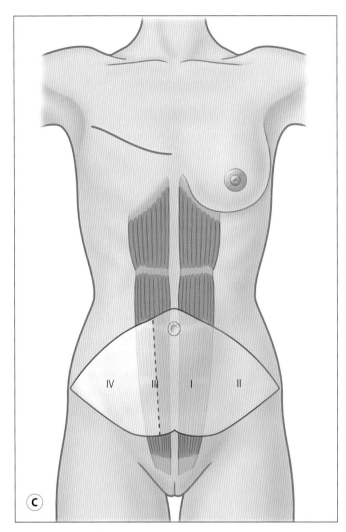

FIGURE 4.1, cont'd

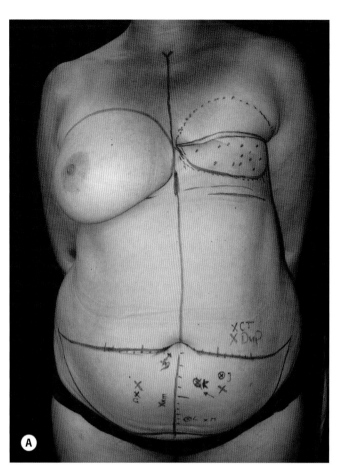

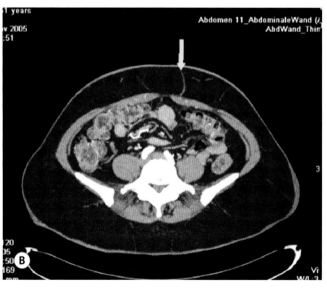

FIGURE 4.2 A 51-year-old patient who planned for a secondary breast reconstruction on the left side. **A** The DIEaP flap markings and the perforators are marked on the lower abdomen. **B** The MDCT findings in a different section and then transferred at the abdomen skin in a 3D image. The best perforator is (K) at the left side (ipsilateral) side.

anterior rectus sheath, just below Scarpa's fascia, or above Scarpa's fascia. When branching occurs just above the anterior rectus sheath, one needs to be cautious when performing the suprafascial dissection around the circumference of the perforator (see below) to avoid injuring any important draining veins that may not be visible from a lateral perspective. Once dissected, the pedicle is approximately 10.3 cm long, with an average diameter of 3.6 mm at the origin of the vessel. Whereas perforators arising from the medial branch of the DIEA have a longer intramuscular course, they also tend to be more dominant and so allow one to carry a greater bulk of tissue from the contralateral abdomen without concern over fat necrosis.

Secondary blood supply

The SIEA, which is one of the secondary blood supplies to the lower abdomen, has several anatomical variations, as reported by Taylor and Daniel.[23] The SIEA arises from the common femoral artery 2–3 cm below the inguinal ligament in 17% of cases, or from a common origin with the superficial circumflex artery in 48% of cases. The artery is entirely absent in 35% of specimens. The artery is usually

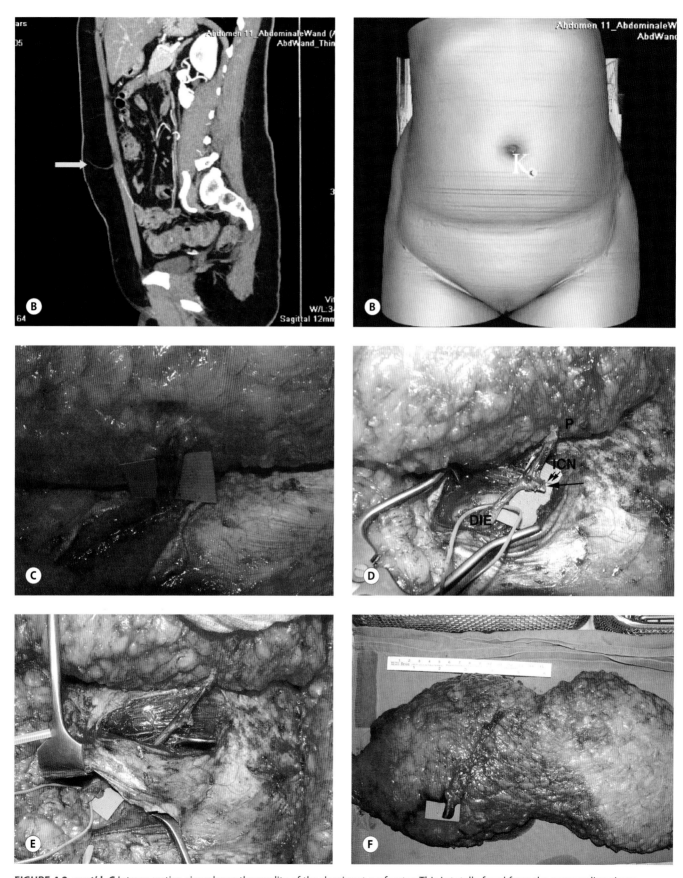

FIGURE 4.2, cont'd **C** Intraoperative view shows the quality of the dominant perforator. This is totally freed from the surrounding tissue.
D Intramuscular dissection of the perforator (P) into the main pedicle DIE (vessel loop). The rectus abdominis muscle fibers are split longitudinally,but the intercostal motor nerve (ICN) is preserved (two arrows). A large side branch (arrow) is clipped and left to use if an additional blood supply or venous drainage is required. **E** A separate incision is made obliquely at the lateral border of the rectus abdominis to give access to the main pedicle. **F** The DIEaP flap is completely harvested. **G** The internal mammary vessels are prepared.

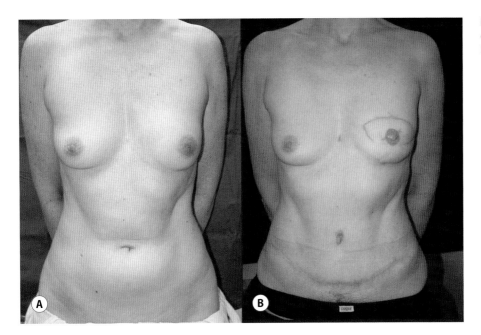

FIGURE 4.3 Pre- and post-operative views of a 48-year-old patient with an immediate breast reconstruction by a DIEaP flap.

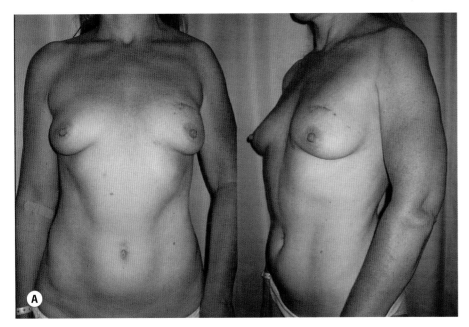

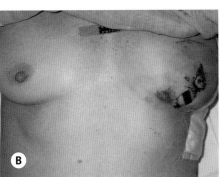

FIGURE 4.4 A 49-year-old patient who underwent left immediate breast reconstruction with a DIEaP and immediate nipple reconstruction.
A Preoperative view. **B** The flap on the 4th postoperative day. A skin paddle was left for flap control in the vertical incision which was excised under local anesthesia on the 5th postoperative day. **C** The results 9 months postoperatively.

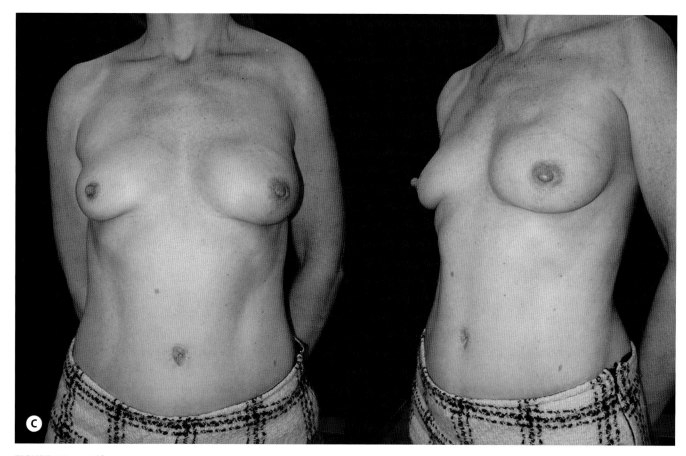

FIGURE 4.4, cont'd

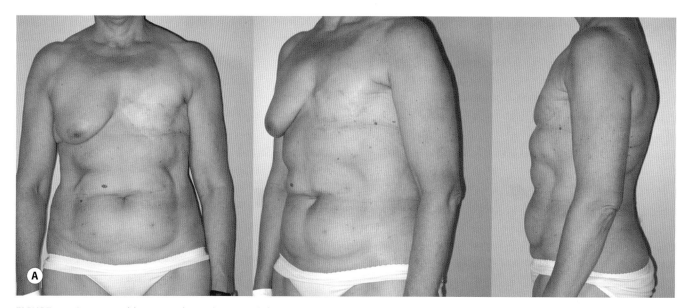

FIGURE 4.5 A 54-year-old patient who underwent a left secondary breast reconstruction using a DIEaP flap and contra lateral breast remodeling. **A** Preoperative views. **B** Postoperative views.

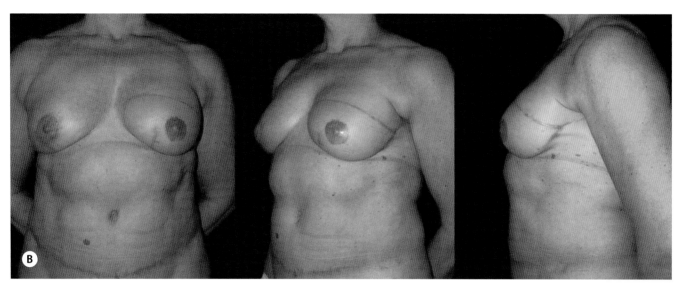

FIGURE 4.5, cont'd

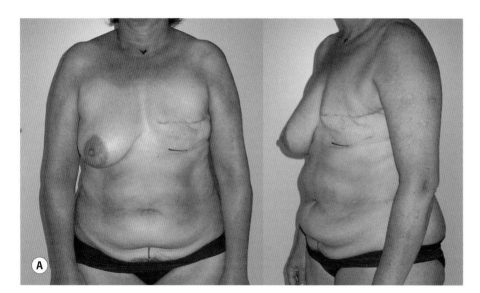

FIGURE 4.6 A 56-old-year patient who had a secondary left breast reconstruction with a DIEaP flap. **A** Preoperative views. **B** Postoperative views.

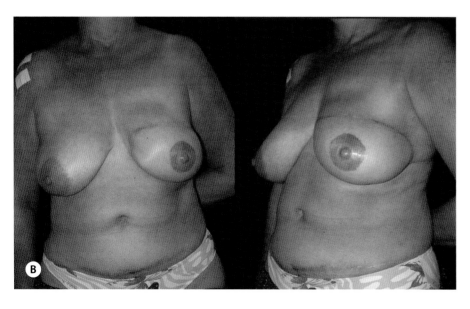

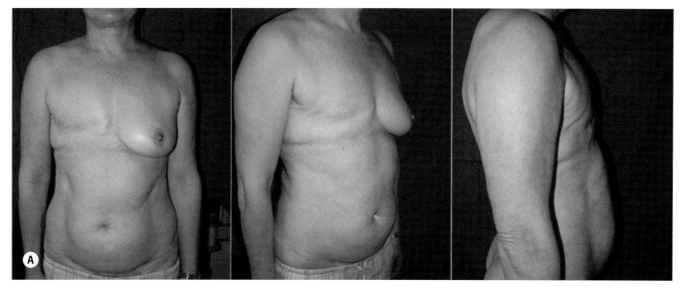

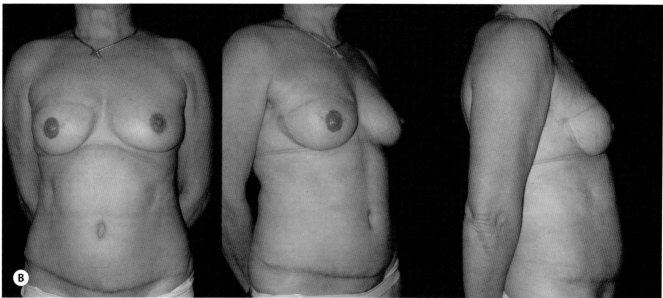

FIGURE 4.7 A 52-old-patient with a right secondary breast reconstruction using a SIEA flap. **A** Preoperative views. **B** Postoperative views.

accompanied by two venae comitantes, which drain into the deep femoral vein or occasionally into the saphenous bulb. In addition, there is a constant superficial inferior epigastric vein (SIEV) draining the lower abdominal skin and fat. The SIEV is a tributary of the greater saphenous vein close to the fossa ovale. The superficial inferior epigastric vessels pass superiorly and laterally in the femoral triangle, crossing the inguinal ligament at its midpoint, lying deep to Scarpa's fascia. The vessels continue to course cranially and superficially, penetrating Scarpa's fascia well above the inguinal ligament to lie in the superficial subcutaneous tissue. In a recent anatomical study Reardon et al.[24] identified the SIEA in 72% of specimens, with an average diameter of 1.6 mm (range 0.75–3.5 mm) at the level of the inguinal ligament. In 58% of cases the artery was present bilaterally. The SIEA lies lateral to the SIEV. The length of the pedicle ranged from 4 to 7 cm, with an average length of 4 cm.

Operative approach
Preoperative assessment of the perforators
The authors' current practice is to mark all available perforators, with the dominant perforators distinguished and clearly marked on the abdominal skin. Color Duplex imaging is a reliable and valuable method to assess the arterial and venous trees of the lower abdomen in addition to the internal mammary vessels.[18] However, we currently use preoperative multidetector row CT (MDCT) scans to determine the location of dominant perforators and have

done so for 2 years.[25,26] Unidirectional Doppler allows us to verify the exact location of the SIEA, generally midway between the anterior superior iliac spine (ASIS) and the pubis.

Flap marking

As is the case for all breast reconstructions using lower abdominal tissue, the amount of fat available is estimated by the 'pinch test.' The design of the DIEAP flap is an ellipse approximately 13 cm high and 35–40 cm wide, with the superior border of the flap at or just above the umbilicus. The upper edge of the flap is tapered laterally just above the ASIS to facilitate closure without dog-ears (Fig. 4.7B).

In the SIEA flap the vascular territory is limited to the ipsilateral lower abdomen, with some extension to half of the contralateral zone III (Fig. 4.7B, C). In our hands, the SIEA can support less tissue across the midline than a free TRAM or DIEP flap. Therefore, the flap is designed exclusively over zones I and II, any extension being laterally over the iliac region. Using this method, a flap of up to 32 × 13 cm can be harvested. The lower incision line is placed more inferiorly towards the pubic tubercle than with the DIEP flap in order to better visualize the vessels at this level.

DIEAP flap

Flap dissection

After marking the perforators and the flap (Fig. 4.8A), the patient is placed in a supine position. Depending on the MDCT findings, the dominant perforator is clearly marked (Fig. 4.8B). A solution of 1% lidocaine with epinephrine is used to infiltrate the entire superior edge and the inferior edge of the flap, except for the region of the superficial inferior epigastric veins, approximately midway between the ASIS and the pubis. The umbilicus is delivered by connecting three periumbilical stab incisions at 10 o'clock, 2 o'clock, and 6 o'clock. An orienting suture is placed at the 6 o'clock position.

The lower incision is made, taking care to identify and preserve the SIEV bilaterally. The SIEV is always dissected for approximately 3–5 cm toward the groin and clipped to allow for anastomosis should additional venous drainage be necessary later in the procedure. The upper incision is

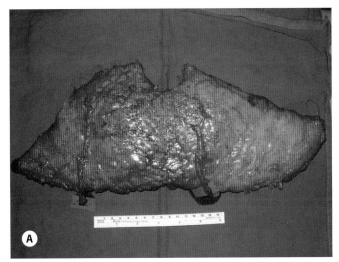

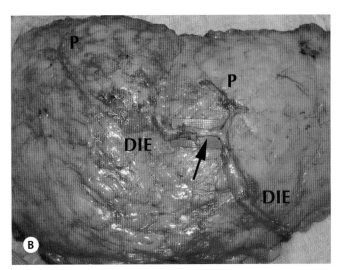

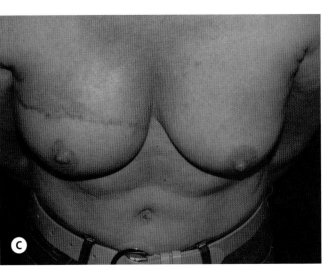

FIGURE 4.8 A case of double-pedicle DIEaP flap for unilateral breast reconstruction. **A** The DIEaP flap was harvested based on a two-pedicles DIE. **B** One DIE pedicle was anastomosed to a side branch of the second DIE pedicle to ensure blood supply to the required four zones (I–IV). **C** The results, with good symmetry and breast contour.

made with variable beveling (depending on the required flap volume) and carried down through skin and fat to the anterior rectus sheath. The flap is then elevated from lateral to medial, with electrocautery just above the anterior rectus sheath. As the dominant perforators are approached the cautery is reduced significantly to minimize thermal damage to the perforators. Once the perforator is visualized from its lateral aspect, it is carefully inspected to ensure that the artery is pulsatile and that the vein is of adequate caliber. Although MDCT has greatly facilitated and expedited flap harvesting, it has not replaced clinical judgment in perforator selection. The selected perforator is dissected free of surrounding connective tissue for 360° in a suprafascial plane. Care is taken on the medial aspect of the perforator to protect any branches that may not be directly visible from the surgeon's lateral perspective (Fig. 4.8C). The fascia is then opened from directly within the natural fascial opening for several centimeters in a cranial and caudal direction, and an elastic hook is used on the lateral edge of the opened fascia to expose the rectus muscle and begin the intramuscular portion of the dissection. Any loose connective tissue around the base of the perforator is dissected with a microbipolar cautery, allowing the surgeon to identify the cleavage plane in the rectus muscle through which the perforator traverses. Once this plane is identified it can be easily developed cranially and caudally with bipolar cautery and spreading maneuvers beginning the longitudinal splitting of the muscle. Dissection of the perforator is continued along its lateral aspect, 'unroofing the perforator' towards the main pedicle while splitting the muscle longitudinally. The medial aspect of the perforator is left undissected until the main pedicle is developed. As noted previously, when perforators traverse the rectus at the level of a tendinous inscription, they tend to be larger and to have a shorter, more direct intramuscular course to the main pedicle, which is convenient. Whether dissection through a tendinous inscription is easier than dissection through muscle is a matter of opinion. The natural cleavage plane in the rectus muscle is progressively developed until the main pedicle is visualized at the posterior aspect of the rectus. This is the point at which one encounters motor branches of the intercostal nerves passing superficial to the pedicle. These must be preserved.

Once the main pedicle is identified, self-retaining retractors are used to hold open the rectus muscle while muscular branches from the perforator and the main pedicle are ligated with either bipolar cautery or microvascular clips (Fig. 4.8D). As the pedicle is developed caudally, one eventually reaches the point at which the deep inferior epigastric vessels emerge from within the muscle into a submuscular plane. The pedicle is followed caudally, releasing it from surrounding fat until sufficient length is obtained, generally continuing dissection until the lateral edge of the rectus muscle is reached. In an effort to avoid later hernias or abdominal bulging, it is recommended to make a separate incision at the lateral inferior border of the rectus muscle near the inguinal ligament (Fig. 4.8E). This second incision avoids a continuous area of weakness, thereby avoiding the possibility of bulging, especially in obese patients. This

portion of the dissection is very similar to that in the free TRAM dissection. In many patients the point at which the DIEA bifurcates into its medial and lateral branches is evident. A valuable strategy we have employed in the past is to follow the largest side branch for 1–2 cm before ligating it to provide an additional vessel to which the SIEV can be anastomosed if the flap appears congested later in the procedure. For example, if the dominant perforator arises from the medial branch of the DIEA, the lateral branch of the DIEA can be dissected for 1–2 cm back in a cranial direction prior to ligating it. After microvascular transfer, this branch can serve as a recipient vein for the SIEV if additional venous drainage is required, as in the case of a flap found to have a dominant superficial venous drainage system. Once the pedicle is totally dissected to the desired length, the artery and vein(s) are separated in the groin or at the lateral edge of the rectus. Attention then returns to the perforator to dissect its medial aspect. A vessel loop with gentle lateral retraction facilitates this portion of the dissection. When the donor site is ready, the pedicle is transected and pulled through the longitudinal split in the rectus muscle and under the preserved motor nerves to deliver the flap while preserving the entire muscle and its innervation (Fig. 4.8F).

Preparing the recipient site

The major difference in delayed reconstruction is the need to determine and establish the level of the inframammary fold, taking into consideration the tendency of a fold marked at the start of the procedure to migrate caudally as the contracted mastectomy scar is opened and the abdominal donor site is closed. Therefore, in delayed reconstruction the level of the inframammary fold is marked more superiorly than the final desired position. The mastectomy flap skin below the level of the mastectomy scar is either entirely excised in full-thickness fashion or de-epithelialized over the area between the scar and the fold to increase the overall volume of the reconstructed breast. The medial portion of the pectoralis is still easily exposed.

Exposure of the recipient vessels

The ideal recipients for microvascular breast reconstruction using perforator flaps are the internal mammary vessels.[27,28] Although several other options exist, more than 98% of our reconstructions are accomplished using the internal mammary vessels as recipient vessels.[28]

On the left side of the chest the internal mammary bundle typically has only one vein and the vessels are smaller than those on the right. Therefore, on the left it is our preference to expose the vessels at the third intercostal space, whereas on the right the fourth intercostal space is used. This optimizes size match with the flap vessels. We have not found that removing the entire rib cartilage at either of these levels causes noticeable contour deformities, as the flap and pectoralis muscle cover this area. If present, medial mammary perforators, which typically emerge in the region of the second or third intercostal spaces, are preserved to provide additional sources of venous outflow if this is found to be necessary. This is particularly important on the left, where there tends to be only one internal mammary vein. Depending on their diameter, the internal mammary perforators can be used as an alternative to the main internal mammary vessels as recipients for free flap breast reconstruction.[28]

The pectoralis is split along its fibers to expose the entire length of the cartilaginous rib from the sternocostal junction to the costochondral junction. A combination of self-retaining retractors and elastic hooks is used to retract the pectoralis muscle and expose the entire cartilaginous portion of the selected rib, making it simple for a single surgeon to perform the exposure. A narrow rongeur is then used to progressively remove the cartilage from anterior to posterior and from lateral to medial. Every effort is made to leave the posterior perichondrium intact throughout this portion of the procedure, so that final exposure of the vessels is controlled and deliberate. Unintentional injury to the internal mammary vein when aggressively entering the posterior perichondrium can consume valuable time, as microsurgical repair is usually required, quite apart from the increased thrombogenicity of an injured recipient vessel. This is especially important in cases where the patient has been previously irradiated and the field is scarred, such as in cases of mastectomy following failed lumpectomy and radiation therapy. Once the cartilage has been removed, the posterior perichondrium is incised laterally and elevated in an avascular plane over the internal mammary vessels to expose them. Fixing a narrow-gauge pediatric feeding tube or drain on suction into the deepest portion of the microsurgical field helps remove any irrigation fluid or blood, thereby keeping the field clear (Fig. 4.8F). At this point the microscope is brought into the field to facilitate ligation of any branches arising from the midportion of the exposed vessels so that they are entirely free along their exposed length. The vessels are ligated immediately prior to flap transfer, with microvascular clamps placed at their proximal end and 'flashed' to ensure adequate inflow of the internal mammary artery (IMA).

Microvascular setup

Where two teams are available, the patient's legs can be raised to facilitate closure of the donor site during the microvascular anastomosis, thereby expediting the procedure. The flap is turned 180° and fixed to the chest with a moist laparotomy pad and staples. Because the internal mammary vein is more medial than the artery, the venous anastomosis is performed first, followed by the arterial anastomosis. The microvascular technique depends on the training and practice of the surgeon. It is our habit to perform end-to-end anastomoses in the vast majority of cases.

Additional venous drainage of the DIEAP flap

Once the microanastomosis of the DIEA/V with the IMA/V is complete, the flap is evaluated. If the flap appears totally congested despite a patent venous anastomosis, this is an indication that the lower abdominal tissue in that particular patient is drained predominantly by the SIEV (2% of our cases). Frequently, during the initial flap dissection an SIEV

is noted to be large. If the SIEV has been dissected for approximately 5 cm, it can usually reach the IM vessels directly and then the SIEV is anastomosed to either a second IMV (Fig. 4.9A,B) or a local medial mammary perforating vein (Fig. 4.10). Alternatively, the SIEV can be anastomosed to either the medial or the lateral branch of the DIEA/DIEV pedicle, as described above (Fig. 4.11). When the SIEV is insufficiently long, an arterial graft (usually the contralateral DIEA) is used to bypass the gap between the SIEV and the recipient vein.[29]

It is critical to evaluate the SIEV several minutes after re-establishing perfusion of the flap to determine whether or not it has adequate venous drainage through the deep inferior epigastric system alone (Box 4.1) An additional indication for using the SIEV is when a large flap is harvested including most of zone III or a part from zone IV (6% of our cases).[30]

Shaping the breast

In immediate reconstruction, shaping the breast begins by assessing the volume of the total flap transferred for

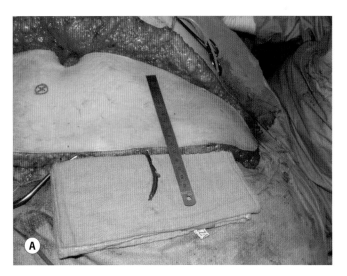

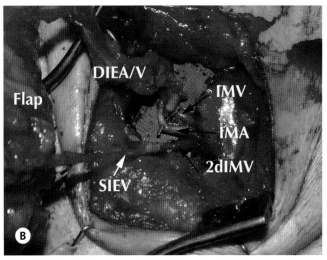

FIGURE 4.9 A DIEaP flap with additional venous drainage via the SIEV. **A** The SIEV was dissected as long as possible. **B** The SIEV was anastomosed directly to the second IMV.

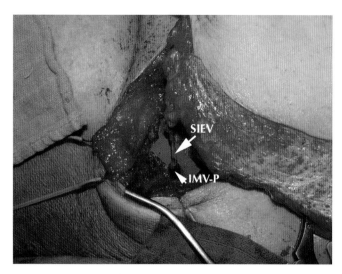

FIGURE 4.10 A DIEaP flap with additional venous drainage by the SIEV, which is anastomosed to an internal mammary vein perforator (IMV/P).

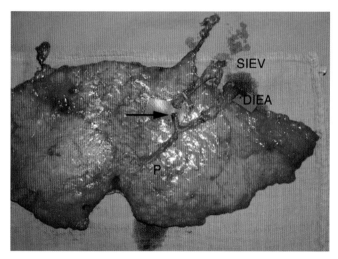

FIGURE 4.11 A DIEaP flap with additional venous drainage by the SIEV, which is anastomosed to a side branch of the DIE vessels.

BOX 4.1 Managing venous outflow

- Preserve medial mammary perforating veins as potential backup venous outflow sources when they are present.
- Always harvest 5 cm of SIEV when it is available.
- If the SIEV is large and becomes engorged during dissection of a DIEP flap, the flap most likely has a dominantly superficial venous drainage system and may require anastomosis of the SIEV.
- When harvesting a DIEA flap based on a medial row perforator, ligate the lateral row branch with sufficient length to provide an additional venous outflow source for the SIEV.

---

gross symmetry to the unoperated breast. In cases of bilateral reconstruction this will not be an issue, as the lower abdomen will simply be bisected. Excess volume is usually debrided from zone IV. The flap is oriented by placing its lateral tip on the side ipsilateral to the selected

perforator in a superolateral orientation, along the pectoralis tendon. One or two absorbable sutures can be placed to position the lateral tip of the flap along the pectoralis tendon, recreating the tail of Spence. A lateral suture is then placed to close off the lateral breast pocket if this has been violated during the ablative procedure. A single suture in the inferolateral flap can recreate the lateral border of the breast that lies inferior and slightly lateral to the anterior axillary fold. Breast projection can be augmented by gathering the flap towards the breast axis, or by folding the de-epithelialized medial edge of the flap, now positioned at the inferior pole of the reconstructed breast, under the bulk of the flap, holding this position by suturing the de-epithelialized dermis down to the pectoral fascia. The natural inframammary fold is preserved. Medial sutures are rarely required. Once this basic shaping is achieved, the flap is tucked under the native mastectomy flaps to determine the extent of de-epithelialization needed. It is then delivered back from under the mastectomy flaps and de-epithelialized. Before final suturing, the pedicle is always rechecked to ensure a natural lie that is free of any kinking or twisting of the pedicle.

Delayed reconstruction requires more time for preparation of the pocket. The inferior mastectomy flap, which lies in between the mastectomy scar and the inframammary fold, is usually de-epithelialized, leaving the attachments to the pectoral fascia intact. This adds significant volume to the reconstructed breast once the flap is positioned above this de-epithelialized dermis and subcutaneous fat. The superior mastectomy flap should be developed to provide an adequate pocket to accept the flap. Adequate debridement requires the excision of any scar or residual capsule in cases where implants or expanders have been used. Often, a tight band is present at the very edge of the superior mastectomy flap that should be scored sequentially to allow expansion of this often contracted tissue. In cases where the mastectomy flaps have been left with significant subcutaneous tissue, they should be thinned to allow an even and seamless transition between the skin paddle of the transferred lower abdomen and the mastectomy flap.

Donor site closure

An upper abdominal flap is developed to the level of the xiphoid centrally and the inferior costal margin laterally. This can be done before performing the microanastomosis to allow a two-team approach. Therefore, the abdomen should be prepared for closure before setting the flap on the thorax for the microanastomoses. This approach allows the donor site to be closed while the microvascular portion of the procedure is under way. Either the operating table is placed into a reflexed position (with appropriate Trendelenburg positioning at the discretion of the microvascular team), or the legs are elevated, keeping the back flat. The anterior rectus sheath is closed with a non-absorbable braided 0 suture (Fig. 4.12). It is absolutely critical that both layers of the anterior rectus sheath be visualized and included in the closure to minimize postoperative abdominal bulging, particularly below the arcuate line. In patients with risk factors such as major obesity or multiple previous

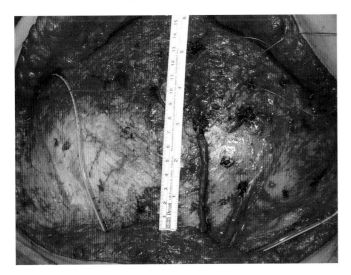

FIGURE 4.12 Careful closure of the two incisions in the deep fascia with non-absorbable stitches.

surgical incisions with weakness of the abdominal musculature, the addition of mesh to the abdominal closure should be considered.

Once the rectus sheath is closed, the abdominal wall superior to the umbilicus is evaluated for rectus diastasis. If this is present it is repaired using a 0 looped permanent suture, just as in cosmetic abdominoplasty. The umbilicus is then tacked to the anterior rectus sheath with a 4/0 absorbable suture. The suture is placed first into the anterior rectus sheath, then into the mid-dermis of the umbilicus at 10 o'clock, 2 o'clock, and 6 o'clock, and hemostats placed. Once the abdominal flap is closed and the position of the new umbilical aperture determined, these sutures are finally placed into the dermis of the umbilical aperture and tied.

Optimizing outcomes in DIEaP flap

The use of the DIEaP flap for breast reconstruction provides a breast with a natural appearance and texture. Like other perforator flaps, the DIEaP flap relies on specialized harvesting techniques. As with any new technique, for beginners or trainees the learning curve is obviously the main challenge (Boxes 4.2 and 4.3). Because of this, perforator flaps would ideally be included in every training program. Attending perforator flap courses and visiting centers where large numbers of perforator flaps are used will shorten the learning period and significantly reduce the rate of complications that may occur during early experience. Using imaging technology such as duplex ultrasound or MDCT scan in the preoperative planning is recommended to make the technique of perforator flaps more reliable in inexperienced hands.[25,26]

Precise preoperative mapping of perforators will significantly shorten the operative time and reduce complications related to poor choice of perforators. A unilateral DIEaP flap breast reconstruction takes 3 hours in our hands, thanks in part to the precise preoperative planning now possible using imaging technology in perforator mapping and a two-team approach. Moreover, partial flap failure and/or fat necrosis in DIEaP flaps can be reduced by correctly selecting the dominant perforator.

As noted above, MDCT can provide excellent preoperative information regarding the arterial diameter of a given perforator. However, the adequacy of draining veins is often not clear until they can be directly inspected during surgery. A perforator bundle that has a clearly pulsatile artery and a vein that is at least 0.5 mm in diameter is ideal. When no single perforator meets these guidelines, it may be necessary to dissect more than one perforator in a given row without sacrificing muscle or nerves (Fig. 4.13A). This is often a matter of continuing the longitudinal split in the muscle between two perforators. However, it may be necessary to cut a small piece of rectus abdominis muscle to allow the harvest of a flap having two perforators (Fig. 4.13B). It is also possible that the motor branch of an intercostal nerve passes between two perforators, requiring the nerve to be sectioned and then reanastomosed after flap harvesting (Fig. 4.13C).

Finally, there are situations where a lack of pulsatile perforator arteries or the presence of multiple very small perforators simply requires conversion to a muscle-sparing TRAM flap. Conversion of a DIEaP flap to a TRAM or muscle-sparing TRAM flap is often safer and easier than dissecting three or more perforators, which may cause similar damage to the rectus muscle as the use of a muscle-

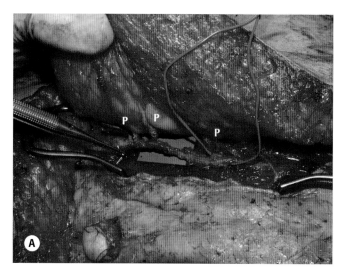

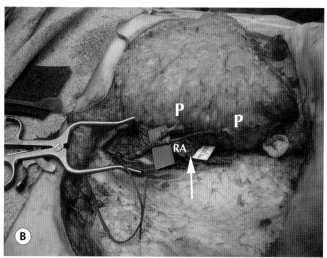

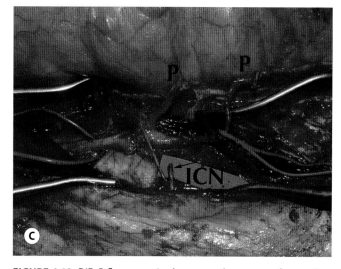

FIGURE 4.13 DIEaP flaps are raised on more than one perforator. P, perforator; ICN, intercostal nerve; RA, rectus abdominis. **A** A DIEaP flap is raised on three perforators on one row without sacrificing muscle or motor nerves. **B** A DIEaP flap is raised on two perforators with 1.5 cm sections of RA muscle (partial thickness). **C** A DIEaP flap is raised on two perforators, with cutting one ICN in between. The nerve is resutured after flap harvesting.

sparing free TRAM flap.[16] Fortunately, these situations are rarely encountered.

SIEA FLAP

Flap dissection

Because of anatomical variation in the SIE vessels, an algorithmic approach is taken when considering harvesting of the flap. We commonly select the contralateral abdomen to reconstruct a breast, as this facilitates a two-team approach and improves insetting of the flap. Dissection begins with surgical exploration of the SIE vessels: the initial incision is made along the inferior flap markings, but at this stage is not deepened to the subcutis. The SIE vessels are identified at a point between the pubic tubercle and the ipsilateral ASIS corresponding with the markings of the Doppler findings. The SIEA is found usually in association with two venae comitantes directly above Scarpa's fascia (Fig. 4.14A). The SIEV is usually located 2–3 cm medial to the SIEA. Side branches are meticulously coagulated or ligated. It is easier to dissect close to the vessels, and dissection includes a limited amount of the surrounding fatty tissue (Fig. 4.14B). The vessels cross the inguinal ligament, and at this point the artery descends vertically in the form of a loop towards its origin, whereas the venae comitantes continue distally to join the femoral or saphenous veins (Fig. 4.14C). In almost 50% of cases the venae comitantes join the SIEV before entering the deep venous system. If a larger skin territory is required the superficial circumflex vessels can be included with the SIEA flap. If the diameter of the SIEA is over 1 mm, the flap can be safely harvested based on these vessels. If not, the contralateral SIE vessels should be explored. The flap must remain attached to the deep fascia until the SIE vessels are explored and an appropriately sized artery located, so as to retain the possibility of converting it to a DIEaP flap. Pedicle length varies from 4 to 7 cm (Fig. 4.14D).

If no suitably sized arteries can be identified then the flap is converted to a conventional DIEaP flap and dissection of the perforators through the rectus abdominis performed.

Microanastomoses

The internal mammary (IM) vessels are dissected and prepared as described above. The IM vessels are dissected distally to obtain maximum recipient vessel length, which makes microanastomosis more comfortable and at a level above the pectoralis major (PM) muscle, thereby allowing the SIE vessels to lie on the PM without kinking. If a sizeable internal mammary artery (IMA) perforator is encountered above the pectoralis major (PM) muscle, these perforators are preferred, in keeping with our algorithm for choosing recipient vessels for breast reconstruction.[28] The IMA perforators are usually a better size match with the SIE vessels, and also create an ideal situation whereby recipient site morbidity is minimized as well as donor site morbidity.

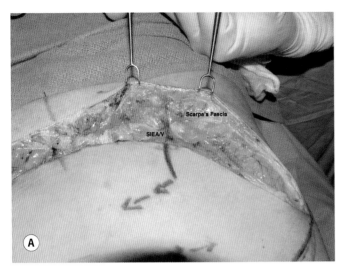

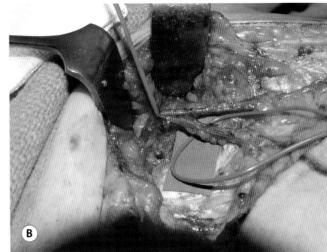

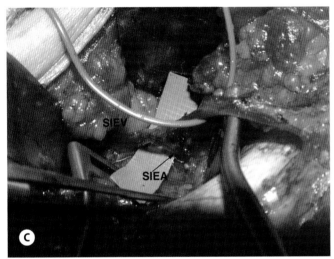

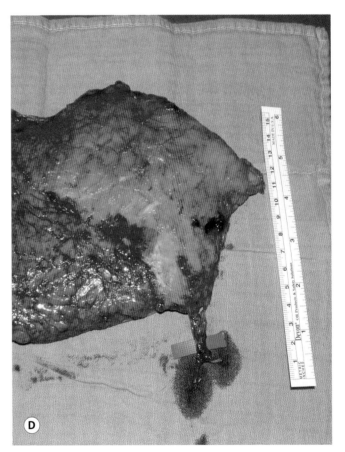

FIGURE 4.14 A 51-year-old patient who planned for a secondary breast reconstruction on the left side. **A** The DIEaP flap markings and the perforators are marked on the lower abdomen. **B** The MDCT findings in a different section and then transferred at the abdomen skin in a 3D image. The best perforator is (K) at the left side (ipsilateral) side. **C** Intraoperative view shows the quality of the dominant perforator. This is totally freed from the surrounding tissue. **D** Intramuscular dissection of the perforator (P) into the main pedicle DIE (vessel loop). The rectus abdominis muscle fibers are split longitudinally, but the intercostal motor nerve (ICN) is preserved (two arrows). A large side branch (arrow) is clipped and left to use if an additional blood supply or venous drainage is required.

SIEA flap insetting

The shorter SIE vessels make flap insetting somewhat more difficult than that of DIEaP or TRAM flaps. Also, the SIE vessels emerge from the subcutaneous level of the inferior border of the flap, rather than from its deep surface, as in the TRAM or DIEaP flaps. This can become a problem in breast reconstruction because the flap needs to be oriented in a suitable manner to achieve adequate shaping without kinking the pedicle. Positioning of the flap on the chest is critical and has to be undertaken with the utmost care. We have found that vertical orientation of the flap provides the safest positioning of the vessels, as they lie almost horizontally above the pectoralis muscle (Fig. 4.14E). In the case of ipsilateral SIEA flap harvest, the flap should be oriented in a more oblique direction, with folding of its lateral part to obtain maximal medial fullness (Fig. 4.14F). The final shape achieved on the operating table should have less lateral fullness and more tissue bulk medially. This pre-empts lateral sagging due to gravity, which can become apparent during follow-up.

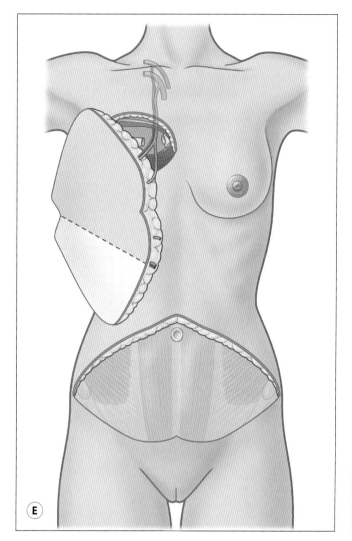

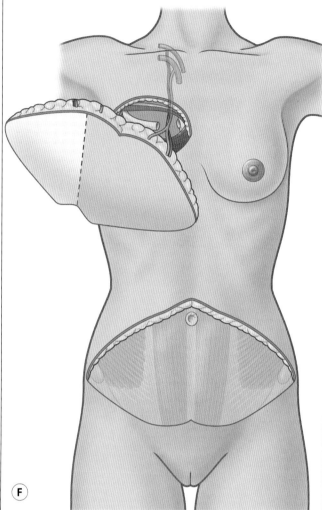

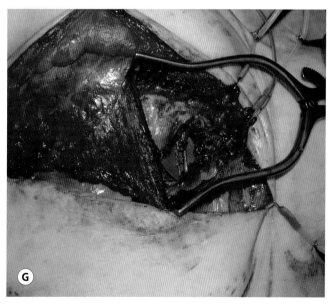

FIGURE 4.14, cont'd **E** A separate incision is made obliquely at the lateral border of the rectus abdominis to give access to the main pedicle. **F** The DIEaP flap is completely harvested. **G** The internal mammary vessels are prepared.

The flap is attached to the thoracic wall inferiorly with heavy absorbable stitches, especially in the lateral border. One or two stitches are placed between the superficial fascia and the PM fascia to ensure that there is no tension on the microanastomosis site due to the weight of the flap. The skin is closed using interrupted deep dermal 3/0 absorbable suture and subcuticular running monofilament absorbable suture. Two drains are inserted between the breast skin and the flap, far from the pedicle.

Donor site closure

The deep fascia is repaired at the level where the SIE vessels join the deep system, using strong interrupted sutures. The abdomen is closed as described above for a DIEaP flap, and two drains are inserted. These are removed only when drainage is less than 20 mL/24 hours.

Complications and side effects

In our center, the microanastomosis revision rate is estimated at 5%, with a total failure rate of 1%. DIEaP partial flap loss and/or fat necrosis is estimated at 8%. Limited partial necrosis can be easily managed by excision and closure or by local skin flap. Lipofilling techniques have allowed us to resolve many small to moderate contour defects resulting from the excision of areas of fat necrosis or partial flap necrosis. However, major partial flap necrosis usually requires a secondary flap surgery. Pedicled thoracodorsal artery perforator (TDAP) or lateral intercostal artery perforator (LICAP) flaps are mostly suitable for such problems.[35]

Regarding donor site morbidity, bulging still occurs in less than 1% of our patients. Patients who have factors that increase intra-abdominal pressure or weaken the abdominal wall, such as a high BMI, multiple abdominal operations, or an active smoking history, have a higher potential risk of developing abdominal bulging or asymmetry.[36]

The most common SIEA donor site complication is seroma formation, reported in up to 50% of patients because of disturbance to the lymphatic drainage during dissection of the SIE vessels in the groin.[11–13] The incidence of seroma formation in the groin may be reduced by skeletonizing the pedicle and not including the surrounding fatty tissue, which may disturb the inguinal lymphatic structures. A few patients (<4% in our series) report an area of paraesthesia over the inner thigh after harvesting of an ipsilateral SIEA flap.

POSTOPERATIVE CARE

All patients at our institution receive IV Nootropil (piracetam) 12 g/24 hours for 5 days and as a solution 20% orally 25 mL q.i.d. for another 5 days. This increases the viability of the distal portion of the skin flap by increasing capillary blood flow.

The flap is monitored using a combination of methods. Clinical evaluation of the color and capillary refill, temperature, handheld Doppler and implantable Doppler devices may all be used for monitoring. The patient's core temperature should be maintained with a warm room, a warming blanket, and warmed fluids as needed, and the use of vasoconstrictive agents should be avoided.

CONCLUSION

The DIEaP and SIEA flaps are excellent options for autologous breast reconstruction. Flap-related complications and aesthetic results are equivalent to those of the pedicled or free TRAM flaps, and donor site complications are significantly less common. Although the operation is contraindicated in patients who have had previous cosmetic abdominoplasty, there are few other absolute contraindications. The advent of MDCT has reduced operative times and facilitated reliable flap harvest even in the presence of multiple previous abdominal operations by confirming the presence of adequate perforators. Increasingly, hospital systems, third-party payers, and patients are demanding shorter hospital stays following surgery and more rapid at-home recovery. These goals need to be achieved with no sacrifice of aesthetic outcome. Both the DIEaP and SIEA flaps can reliably achieve all of these goals.

REFERENCES

1. Hartrampf CR, Scheflan M, Black PW. Breast reconstruction with a transverse abdominal island flap. Plast Reconstruct Surg 1982; 69: 216–225.
2. Grotting JC. The free abdominoplasty flap for immediate breast reconstruction. Ann Plast Surg 1991; 27: 351–354.
3. Feller AM. Free TRAM. Results and abdominal wall function. Clin Plast Surg 1994; 21: 223–232.
4. Nahabedian MY. Defining the 'gold standard' in breast reconstruction with abdominal tissue. Plast Reconstruct Surg 2004; 114: 804–806.
5. Koshima I, Soeda S. Inferior epigastric artery skin flaps without rectus abdominis muscle. Br J Plast Surg 1989; 42: 645–648.
6. Allen RJ, Treece P. Deep inferior epigastric perforator flap for breast reconstruction. Ann Plast Surg 1994; 32: 32–38.
7. Hamdi M, Weiler-Mithoff EM, Webster MH. Deep inferior epigastric perforator flap in breast reconstruction: experience with the first 50 flaps. Plast Reconstruct Surg 1999; 103: 86–95.
8. Blondeel P. One hundred free DIEP flap breast reconstructions: a personal experience. Br J Plast Surg 1999; 52: 104–111.
9. Hamdi M, Blondeel P, Van Landuyt K, et al. Bilateral autogenous breast reconstruction using perforator free flaps: a single center's experience. Plast Reconstruct Surg 2004; 114: 83–89.
10. Gill PS, Hunt JP, Guerra AB, et al. A 10-year retrospective review of 758 DIEP flaps for breast reconstruction. Plast Reconstruct Surg 2004; 113: 1153–1160.
11. Arnez ZM, Khan U, Pogorelec D, et al. Breast reconstruction using the free superficial inferior epigastric artery (SIEA) flap. Br J Plast Surg 1999; 52: 276–279.
12. Allen RJ, Heitland AS. Superficial inferior epigastric artery flap for breast reconstruction. Semin Plast Surg 2002; 16: 35–44.
13. Chevray PM. Breast reconstruction with superficial inferior epigastric artery flaps: a prospective comparison with TRAM and DIEP flaps. Plast Reconstruct Surg 2004; 114: 1077–1083.
14. Blondeel N, Vanderstraeten GG, Monstrey SJ, et al. The donor site morbidity of free DIEP flaps and free TRAM flaps for breast reconstruction. Br J Plast Surg 1997; 50: 322–330.
15. Futter CM, Webster MH, Hagen S, et al. A retrospective comparison of abdominal muscle strength following breast reconstruction with a free TRAM or DIEP flap. Br J Plast Surg 2000; 53: 578–583.

16. Nahabedian MY, Tsangaris T, Momen B. Breast reconstruction with the DIEP flap or the muscle-sparing (MS-2) free TRAM flap: is there a difference? Plast Reconstruct Surg 2005; 115: 436–444; discussion 445–446.
17. Holm C, Mayr M, Hofter E, Ninkovic M. Perfusion zones of the DIEP flap revisited: a clinical study. Plast Reconstruct Surg 2006; 117: 37–43.
18. Blondeel PN, Beyens G, Verhaeghe R, et al. Doppler flowmetry in the planning of perforator flaps. Br J Plast Surg 1998; 51: 202–209.
19. Heitmann C, Felmerer G, Durmus C, et al. Anatomical features of perforator blood vessels in the deep inferior epigastric perforator flap. Br J Plast Surg 2000; 53: 205–208.
20. Kikuchi N, Murakami G, Kashiwa H, et al. Morphometrical study of the arterial perforators of the deep inferior epigastric perforator flap. Surg Radiol Anat 2001; 23: 375–381.
21. El-Mrakby Hamdy H, Milner RH. The vascular anatomy of the lower anterior abdominal wall: A microdissection study on the deep inferior epigastric vessels and the perforator branches. Plast Reconstruct Surg 2002; 109: 539–543.
22. El-Mrakby Hamdy H, Milner RH. The suprafascial course of the direct paraumbillical perforator vessels. Plast Reconstruct Surg 2002; 109: 1766–1768.
23. Taylor GI, Daniel RK. The anatomy of several free flap donor sites. Plast Reconstruct Surg 1975; 56: 243–253.
24. Reardon CM, O'Ceallaigh S, O'Sullivan ST. An anatomical study of the superficial inferior epigastric vessels in humans. Br J Plast Surg 2004; 57: 515–519.
25. Hamdi M, Van Landuyt K, Van Hedent E, et al. Advances in autogenous breast reconstruction: the role of preoperative perforator mapping. Ann Plast Surg 2007; 58: 18–26.
26. Masia J, Clavero JA, Larrañaga JR, et al. Multidetector-row computed tomography in the planning of abdominal perforator flaps. J Plast Reconstr Aesthet Surg 2006; 59: 594–599.
27. Nahabedian MY. The internal mammary artery and vein as recipient vessels for microvascular breast reconstruction: are we burning a future bridge? Ann Plast Surg 2004; 53: 311–316.
28. Hamdi M, Blondeel P, Van Landuyt K, et al. Algorithm in choosing recipient vessels for perforator free flap in breast reconstruction: the role of the internal mammary perforators. Br J Plast Surg 2004; 57: 258–265.
29. Blondeel PN, Arnstein M, Verstraete K, et al. Venous congestion and blood flow in free transverse rectus abdominis myocutaneous and deep inferior epigastric perforator flaps. Plast Reconstruct Surg 2000; 106: 1295–1299.
30. Mehrara BJ, Santoro T, Smith A, et al. Alternative venous outflow vessels in microvascular breast reconstruction. Plast Reconstruct Surg 2003; 112: 448–455.
31. Nahabedian MY, Momem B, Galdino G, et al. Breast reconstruction with the free TRAM or DIEP flap: Patient selection, choice of flap, and outcome. Plast Reconstruct Surg 2002; 110: 466–475.
32. Chang DW, Reece GP, Wang B, et al. Effect of smoking on complications in patients undergoing free TRAM flap breast reconstruction. Plast Reconstruct Surg 2000; 105: 2374–2380.
33. Heller L, Feledy JA, Chang DW. Strategies and options for free TRAM flap breast reconstruction in patients with midline abdominal scars. Plast Reconstruct Surg 2005; 116: 753–759.
34. Hamdi M, Khuthaila D, Van Landuyt K, et al. Double-pedicle abdominal perforator free flaps for unilateral breast reconstruction: new horizons in microsurgical tissue transfer to the breast. J Plast Reconstr Aesthet Surg 2007; 9 April (e-pub).
35. Hamdi M, Wolfli J, Van Landuyt K. Partial mastectomy reconstruction. Clin Plast Surg 2007; 34: 51–62.
36. Nahabedian MY, Dooley W, Singh N, et al. Contour abnormalities of the abdomen after breast reconstruction with abdominal flaps: the role of muscle preservation. Plast Reconstruct Surg 2002; 109: 91–101.

Breast Reconstruction – Superior Gluteal Artery Perforator (SGAP) Flap

5

Matthew D. Goodwin and Bernard W. Chang

INTRODUCTION

The superior gluteal artery perforator (SGAP) free flap is a good alternative for autogenous breast reconstruction when abdominal tissue is not available (e.g., because of a paucity of tissue, previous abdominal surgery, including failed transverse rectus abdominis musculocutaneous (TRAM) or deep inferior epigastric artery perforator (DIEP) flap reconstruction, or incisions or scarring that have affected the blood supply to the abdomen). Sufficient gluteal tissue is usually present even in the very thin patient.

Gluteal tissue for autogenous breast reconstruction was first introduced by Fujino et al.[1] in 1975 for patients with congenital aplasia of the breast. Shaw,[2] Codner and Nahai[3] popularized the gluteal myocutaneous flaps (both superior and inferior gluteal), noting the disadvantage of a short pedicle necessitating vein grafts. Koshima et al.[4] described the superior gluteal artery perforator flap for pedicled reconstruction of sacral pressure sores. Allen and Tucker[5] first reported the technique of SGAP flap breast reconstruction in 1999, since when this flap has become an increasingly used method of microsurgical breast reconstruction. However, many breast microsurgeons still do not perform this procedure because of lack of experience with the technique and the availability of more familiar alternatives (e.g. TRAM, DIEP, and latissimus dorsi flaps).

Although the procedure is technically demanding, the anatomy of the superior gluteal donor site consistently has adequate tissue and vessels for microsurgical transfer. Plastic surgeons with good microsurgical experience should be able to perform this procedure both safely and consistently. Options for breast reconstruction from other autogenous donor sites (latissimus dorsi, anterolateral thigh (ALT)) usually require an implant to obtain enough volume for symmetry. SGAP breast reconstruction should be considered as an alternative method to complete a breast reconstructive surgeon's armamentarium.

INDICATIONS AND CONTRAINDICATIONS

Indications

Candidates for SGAP breast reconstruction may include patients electing autogenous breast reconstruction but who do not desire implant reconstruction. Implant reconstruction is less desirable in patients who have undergone previous chest wall radiation or failed previous reconstruction. In our practice, SGAP reconstruction may be offered to all patients choosing autogenous reconstruction; however, it is usually a secondary choice if DIEP flap reconstruction is available. The DIEP flap is usually more popular for donor site cosmetic reasons. Advantages of the SGAP flap include faster recovery than with the DIEP flap, no risk of hernia, good projection, sufficient tissue in thin patients, and a donor site that is relatively well hidden.

Contraindications

Relative contraindications typically include patients in poor general health for whom prolonged surgery and general anesthetic expose them to excess risk. In patients who are likely to require radiation the procedure is usually delayed until after treatment to avoid radiation damage to the flap and to replace recipient site radiation damage with healthy flap tissue. In our practice, obesity and tobacco use are usually not exclusionary criteria; however, the patient is counseled that the risk of flap failure, either complete or partial, or donor site complications is greater. We have found a significantly increased rate of flap failure in patients with body mass index (BMI) >30, the increased risk being related to the logistics of flap positioning during microsurgical anastomosis (i.e., increased flap thickness and a relatively short pedicle); therefore, we tend not to recommend SGAP reconstruction for this population The only absolute contraindication is if there is inadequate tissue or previous **67** surgery or trauma to either the donor or recipient sites that would make the operation too difficult or impossible to perform.

Disadvantages of the SGAP include slightly longer operative times (5–7 hours), the potential for vessel mismatch, shorter pedicle length, thinner donor site veins, more technical skills required for flap dissection and anastomoses, and a lower success rate than the DIEP flap. For these reasons, not as many reconstructive surgeons offer this technique, making it less widely available for patients.

BOX 5.1 Indications and contraindications

- Usually secondary choice to DIEP flap reconstruction
- Most patients are eligible candidates
- Avoid in obese patients because of shorter pedicle length and bulk of flap
- May be indicated for immediate or delayed reconstruction
- Consider expanding skin for delayed reconstruction if skin too tight or radiated
- Bilateral reconstruction can be performed at once or each side in two separate operations
- Avoid internal mammary recipient vessels in patients with cardiac history or a strong family history of cardiac disease

---

Patient selection

In the authors' practice, the lower abdominal perforators (DIEP and SIEA) and the SGAP are the workhorse flaps for autogenous breast reconstruction. All patients are carefully examined for sufficient donor site tissue in these locations, and for the possibility of implant reconstruction. Concomitant variables are assessed, including skin tightness, radiation changes, and other medical issues. Patient education is important, as well as assessing the patient's understanding of the processes involved in all types of reconstruction. The patients are presented with all reasonable options, along with associated risks and complications. Ultimately, patients may choose the method of reconstruction with which they feel most comfortable. Special consideration is given to bilateral reconstruction if SGAP breast reconstruction is chosen. If only one microsurgeon with experience is available, bilateral reconstruction is usually staged several months apart because of the complexity and length of the procedure. If two microsurgeons are available, bilateral SGAP reconstruction may be possible with only a minimal increase in operating room time, as flap harvest may be performed simultaneously.

PREOPERATIVE HISTORY AND CONSIDERATIONS

A thorough preoperative history and physical examination is necessary prior to surgery because of the duration of surgery and to minimize complications. In patients newly diagnosed with breast cancer the type of tumor is important as well as the potential for locoregional or distant spread. These factors may directly affect the outcome if radiation

therapy is needed, or if there is a high likelihood of local recurrence. Some patients may have already undergone preoperative adjuvant chemotherapy or previous radiation therapy as well. In patients having delayed reconstruction, prior radiation to the chest wall or tight, thin skin may necessitate pre-SGAP tissue expansion. Other risk factors requiring assessment include smoking history, age, diabetes, and other general health issues such as cardiac or pulmonary problems. Past medical history and physical examination pay close attention to the donor and recipient sites for evidence of previous surgery or trauma that may complicate the surgery.

In an effort to maximize postoperative breast symmetry, the patient is examined with regard to the donor site as well as the contralateral breast, assessing volume and skin quality. Ptotic or large contralateral breasts may require a mastopexy or reduction for balancing. In rare cases, the patient may have a smaller breast on the contralateral side that they wish to have augmented. This needs to be discussed carefully with the surgical oncologist and the patient before being pursued. The upper buttock region is assessed for adequate tissue by palpation. The tissue utilized is over the greater sciatic foramen, which can be palpated and is oriented in an oblique fashion (refer to technique section).

Patient education is very important and should employ numerous modalities (e.g., consultation, video, brochure, etc.). It is important to inform the patient fully so that they know what to expect and how they can help to avoid complications. This is especially important with regard to possible flap failure or the inability to perform reconstruction intraoperatively. Secondary options, if available, should be planned for and may be possible during the initial surgery if the SGAP is not feasible (e.g., because recipient vessels are inadequate). The timing for each stage of reconstruction as well as the expected hospital stay should be explained to the patient. They should be advised ahead of time to avoid positions in the postoperative period that may cause kinking or stretching of the vascular pedicle.

OPERATIVE APPROACH

There are numerous steps that should be anticipated by the operating room team to facilitate efficient use of time. The patient is prepared and draped after each repositioning. The microscope should be tested and prepared for use before starting flap ischemia time. Microsurgical instruments, clips, and sutures should be in the operative field at the time of flap harvest.

The operation begins with preparation of the recipient site and vessels with the patient supine, followed by repositioning the patient in the lateral decubitus position for donor site harvesting and pedicle dissection. The patient should be placed on a suction bean bag to secure this position, along with an axillary roll and Mayo stand for arm protection. After flap harvest, the flap vessels are prepared with microscope visualization on a side table while the donor site is closed. Again, the patient is repositioned supine for arterial and venous anastomosis, followed by closure.

Relevant surgical anatomy

Perforator flap reconstruction relies on the blood supply to skin and fat emanating from perforating vessels which travel between underlying muscle fibers. These vessels are dissected out as a pedicle through the muscle fibers down to their origin and terminate in the overlying skin and fat. This pedicle is divided and reanastomosed to recipient vessels at the site of reconstruction as a free tissue transfer.

The primary choice of recipient vessel for SGAP reconstruction is the internal mammary artery (IMA) and vein (Fig. 5.1). In the authors' practice the internal mammary vessels are almost always available, even after failed DIEP reconstruction, because the thoracodorsal vessels are our preferred recipient vessels for DIEP reconstruction. The second rib cartilage is easily palpated for reference, and the third cartilage is usually removed medially through a split in the pectoral muscle. The internal mammary vessels are located fairly medially. Each respective IMA originates from the first part of the subclavian artery and descends behind the costal cartilages 1–1.5 cm lateral to the sternum, with numerous branches to the intercostals and perforators to the overlying breast tissue and skin. The IMA ultimately splits to supply the musculophrenic and superior epigastric arteries at the level of the sixth costal cartilage. At the level of the third costal cartilage the IMA diameter is approximately 2–3 mm and is usually accompanied by one or two venae comitantes, which drain into the respective brachiocephalic veins. The diameter of the internal mammary vein typically ranges from 2.5 to 3.5 mm.

Alternative recipient vessels include the thoracodorsal vessels, but these are less ideal given the short flap pedicle length of the SGAP. Cephalic vein turndown from the

shoulder may be used as a venous backup or for additional venous drainage if necessary, and is identified between the clavicular and sternal heads of the pectoralis major muscle. It can be dissected distal into the upper arm through several small counter-incisions.

The superior and inferior gluteal arteries are the dominant blood supply to the gluteus muscle. They supply 20–25 cutaneous perforators overlying the muscle, with the superior gluteal artery perforators supplying the superolateral buttock region, and the inferior gluteal artery perforators supplying the inferior buttock region both medially and laterally. The superior gluteal artery and vein emanate from the pelvis through the greater sciatic foramen above the piriformis muscle just beneath the subgluteal fat pad. Several large branches exist at this level, traveling along the periosteum and into the overlying muscle. The main vessels and several small branches typically lie against the periosteum, making dissection difficult. Some surgeons have referred to this region as 'Medusa's head' owing to the number of branches and the risk of following the wrong vessel. Numerous perforating branches from the superior gluteal artery and venae comitantes supply the superior buttock tissue and skin, although usually one or two are dominant. The pedicle length typically ranges from 6 to 10 cm. Several cadaveric anatomic studies of the vascular anatomy for the SGAP flap have found perforator diameter to range from 0.9 to 1.5 mm.[6,7] At the level of the greater sciatic foramen, the point at which the superior gluteal vessels are divided, the superior gluteal artery diameter ranges from 2 to 3.5 mm and the venae comitantes from 2 to 4 mm.

Operative technique

Recipient site markings

The outline of the breast for immediate reconstruction should be marked in the standing upright position with special reference to the medial, lateral, and inframammary creases. These landmarks are especially important if these areas have been disrupted by the surgical oncologist, and need to be anchored at flap inset. If previous reconstruction or a mastectomy has been performed and a delayed reconstruction is planned, appropriate borders are marked based on judgment using the contralateral breast as a guide, if available. Previous scars are marked and appreciated to make safe skin flaps. The third costal cartilage is palpated and marked.

Donor site markings

The flap design should be centered over the main perforators of the superior gluteal artery (Fig. 5.2). These can be found by palpating the greater sciatic foramen (Figs 5.3 and 5.4) and are confirmed by a handheld Doppler with the patient prepared for surgery (Fig. 5.5). Often this will indicate that perforators are located slightly differently from the premarked greater sciatic foramen. The flap markings should then be adjusted with these Dopplered points as the central portion of the flap. The dominant perforators usually lie a few centimeters below the upper edge of the greater

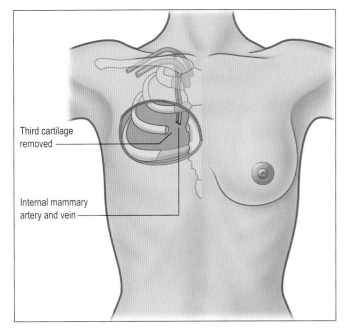

FIGURE 5.1 Illustration of recipient site demonstrating the location of the internal mammary vessels.

Third cartilage removed

Internal mammary artery and vein

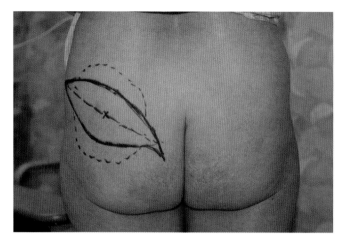

FIGURE 5.2 SGAP donor site markings.

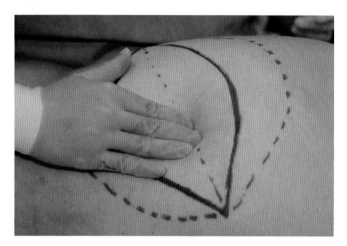

FIGURE 5.3 Palpating the greater sciatic foramen.

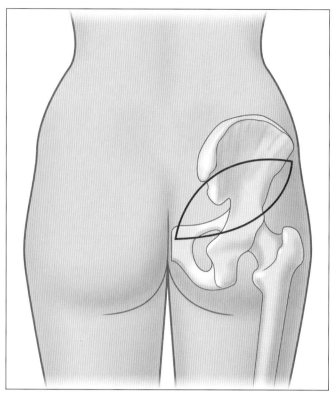

FIGURE 5.4 Relation of skin markings to the greater sciatic foramen.

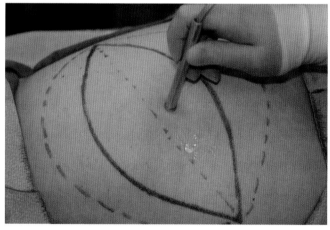

FIGURE 5.5 Locating cutaneous perforators with a handheld Doppler probe.

sciatic foramen. In an effort to hide the scars under the patient's panties or swimsuit, the axis of the flap is made slightly oblique or horizontal in orientation. The medial extension of the flap design is usually located several centimeters below the upper portion of the mid-gluteal crease, and may be curved down to avoid a dog-ear. The width of the flap is usually 8–12 cm, and may be closed with slight undermining.

Recipient site preparation

The patient is prepared and draped in the supine position. This may have been done prior to mastectomy by the oncologic breast surgeon. If a previous reconstruction had been performed, remaining tissue or implant material is removed. A capsulectomy is performed if capsular tissue is present. The recipient bed is assessed for areas where the breast borders may have been violated by the resection. These can be re-established using interrupted 3/0 Vicryl sutures. The third costal cartilage is then located by palpation in the upper medial quadrant. Dissection by electrocautery is used to split the pectoralis muscle along fibers and expose the costal cartilage. The perichondrium is dissected off using electrocautery and a Freer elevator. Great care must be

maintained when under the cartilage because the vessels and the parietal pleural are located immediately posteriorly. The cartilage is removed by use of a rib cutter and rongeur up to the edge of the sternum.

The posterior perichondrium is opened laterally with a #15 blade and a Freer elevator is passed beneath the perichondrium above the internal mammary vessels. The perichondrium is opened longitudinally with scissors and the vessels are exposed. Intercostal muscle is divided along the entire interspace between the second and fourth costal cartilages. There will often be some remaining fascia overlying the vessels that can be carefully removed with a Freer eleva-

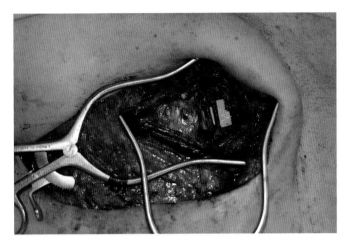

FIGURE 5.6 Internal mammary vessel exposure.

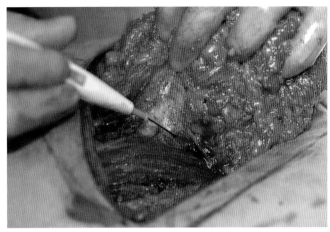

FIGURE 5.9 Elevating SGAP flap lateral to medial.

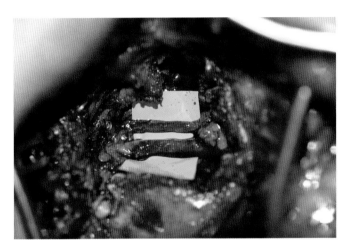

FIGURE 5.7 Separation of internal mammary artery and vein.

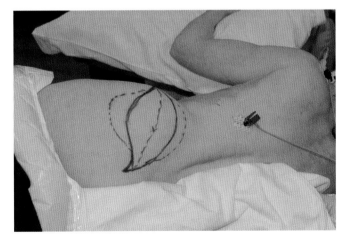

FIGURE 5.8 Patient positioning for flap harvest.

ent site is temporarily closed with staples and a bio-occlusive dressing.

Donor flap dissection

The patient is then repositioned in the lateral decubitus position with the bean bag for support (Fig. 5.8). Attention is paid to avoid brachial plexus stretch and joint injury (axillary roll, pillows, Mayo stand, etc.). The patient is re-prepared and draped. Using a handheld Doppler probe, several arterial perforators may be identified. These usually lie a few centimeters inferior to the marked site of the center of the greater sciatic foramen. If necessary, the flap marking is adjusted so that these perforators lie at the central portion of the flap. The skin is incised and dissection proceeds with electrocautery (power 30–40), beveling away from the flap for improved contour. Dissection continues directly down to the underlying muscle. Flap elevation is performed lateral to medial. Upon encountering the muscle at the lateral edge of the buttock, electrocautery is reduced to begin a careful search for perforators. The iliotibial band of the fascia lata is the most lateral structure. The gluteal fat is lifted off this fascia until the insertion of the gluteus maximus is encountered. This is noted when muscle fibers change from a cephalocaudal direction to an oblique-downward lateral direction. At this point, the fascia is incised and dissection proceeds directly on the muscle in the subfascial plane, taking care to identify and protect potential perforators (Fig. 5.9). The authors prefer to leave the deep dermis intact in the medial fourth of the flap so that the flap remains secure as the lateral side is dissected through.

Usually up to three potential perforators are discovered (Fig. 5.10). We typically use one perforator that has adequate caliber; however, we will occasionally use two perforators, especially if they are close together and are lined up in the same muscle split.

Dissection continues through the muscle adjacent to the perforator with the use of a long hemostatic forceps/clamp. Vessel clips are used liberally to divide the numerous muscular branches (Figs 5.11 and 5.12). Self-retaining

tor and Metzenbaum scissors. The vessels themselves are then separated along their extent to facilitate mobility upon ligation prior to anastomosis (Fig. 5.6). Note the quality and caliber of the vessels. A blue background is placed to assist with visualization of the vessels (Fig. 5.7). The recipi-

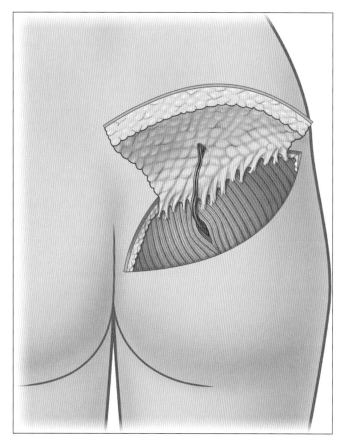

FIGURE 5.10 SGAP perforator.

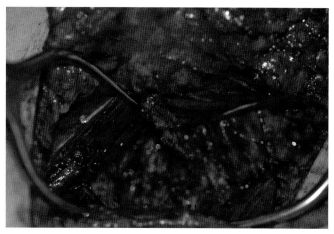

FIGURE 5.12 SGAP pedicle dissection.

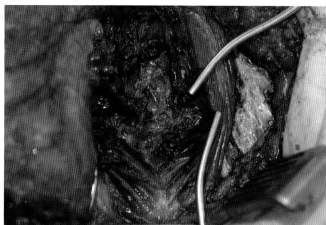

FIGURE 5.13 'Medusa's head.'

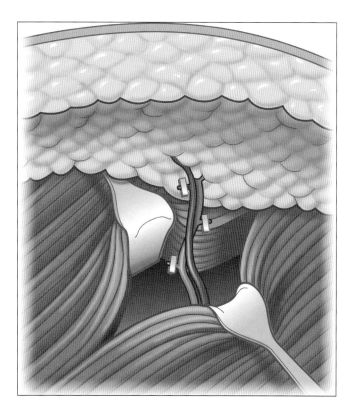

FIGURE 5.11 SGAP pedicle dissection.

retractors are placed, splitting the muscle along its fibers; they are frequently adjusted to enable sufficient visualization of the deep dissection. Depending on which perforator is selected, the pedicle dissection will usually lead to the fascial edges of the gluteus medius, minimus, or piriformis muscles. These must also be released for several centimeters to allow for adequate visualization. As the dissection proceeds deeper beneath these fascial planes, numerous large and small periosteal branches are encountered (Medusa's head) (Fig. 5.13). Care must be taken to examine each branch to avoid damaging the pedicle. It is important not to terminate dissection too early so as to preserve pedicle length and to have adequate arterial diameter for a good size match with the internal mammary artery. Pedicle length typically ranges between 6 and 10 cm. At the deepest extent of the dissection, the pedicle lies along the periosteum of the pelvis as it passes through the greater sciatic foramen. As it does so, numerous small branches exist and go under, in, and over the periosteum. Careful dissection is necessary here to avoid deep bleeding. Once the pedicle is free from the periosteum and branches are divided, the artery and vein are cleaned and separated if possible with a

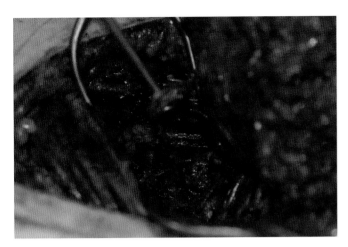

FIGURE 5.14 Pedicle dissection complete.

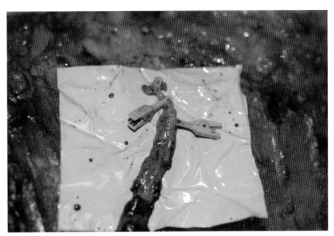

FIGURE 5.16 Separation of pedicle artery and vein.

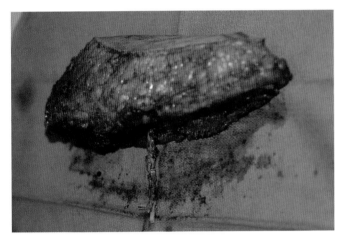

FIGURE 5.15 Flap divided.

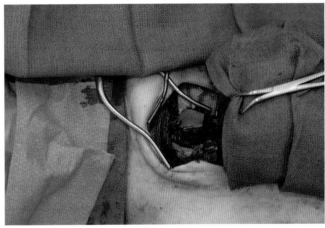

FIGURE 5.17 Flap positioning on chest for anastomosis.

right-angle clamp (Fig. 5.14). When preparing for pedicle division, it is our practice to give the patient 5000 units of intravenous heparin. Five minutes after this, the artery and vein are divided with vessel clips and ischemia time is noted. The medial portion of the flap that remains attached is dissected off with electrocautery.

The flap is then removed from the field and placed on a side table for microdissection and separation of the artery and vein within the pedicle using a sterile draped microscope (Fig. 5.15). The artery is cleaned first and a microclamp is applied to the vein (Fig. 5.16). Sterile saline is then infused antegradely to dilate the venous system. This facilitates preparation of the venous end, which normally is very thin, friable, and floppy. Furthermore, the inside of the vein must be assessed for nearby valves that could create an obstruction. If a valve is noted near the end of the vein, another site proximal to the valve should be selected and prepared.

The donor site is irrigated and assessed for hemostasis. The muscle is closed with interrupted 2/0 Vicryl sutures. A single fluted 15 Fr drain is placed, exiting at the superior lateral end of the wound. The deep fat and Scarpa's fascia

are closed with interrupted 2/0 Vicryl sutures. Extra sutures are often placed in the central portion because this is the area of greatest tension. The skin is closed with interrupted 3/0 Vicryl inverted dermal sutures, a running 4/0 Monocryl subcuticular suture, and Dermabond.

Anastomosis and flap inset

The team member who closed the donor site, together with operating room staff, re-prepares the patient, who is then returned to the supine position and the bean bag is removed. The recipient site is exposed with large retractors and sutures to retract the skin.

Once flap preparation on the side table is complete, the flap is brought into the surgical field. It is placed in a surgical towel and secured with towel clips in a manner that facilitates appropriate placement and exposure of the anastomosis (Fig. 5.17). Given the thickness of an SGAP flap, which can impede view of the anastomosis, we often elevate the patient's back to ease visualization. This is where optimized pedicle and recipient vessel length is valuable. The microscope is placed over the field in a position appropriate for both the microsurgeon and the assistant. The pedicle

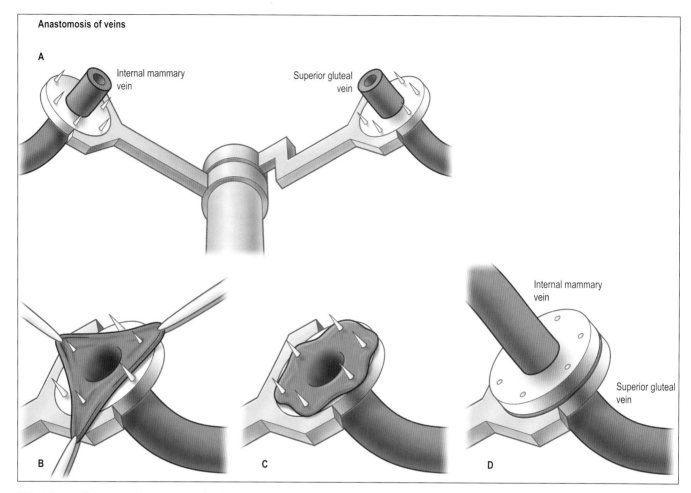

FIGURE 5.18 Illustration of venous coupler device.

and recipient sites are reassessed, further prepared, and approximated for anastomosis.

The arterial anastomosis proceeds first. The recipient artery is clipped distally. This is usually just above the fourth rib. A small double approximating vessel clamp is placed on the proximal side. The artery is divided just proximal to the clip with microscissors. The artery is then assessed for patency and adequate blood pressure by quickly and carefully releasing and then replacing the vessel clamp. The recipient arterial end is then cleaned, dilated, and freshened. The flap side artery is then placed in the other side of the double approximating vessel clamp, approximating the two arterial sides. Using an 8/0 nylon microsuture in an interrupted fashion, the arterial ends are anastomosed.

The venous anastomosis is next performed with a venous coupler device (Synovis Micro Companies Alliance, Birmingham, AL), using a vessel sizer to choose the appropriate size of coupler. We usually use coupler sizes ranging from 2.0 to 3.5 mm. A small vessel clip is placed on the distal end of the recipient vein, usually just above the fourth rib. A single small vessel clamp is placed on the proximal side. The vein is divided just proximal to the clip with microscissors. The recipient side vein end is then cleaned,

dilated, and freshened. The flap side vein is placed in a single vessel clamp. The two venous ends are placed within the coupler holes and secured to the prongs (Fig. 5.18). When ready, the coupler device is activated for anastomosis.

The vessel clamps are removed in the following order: distal vein, proximal vein, distal artery, proximal artery. End of ischemia time is noted. The anastomoses are assessed for patency and leaks. Occasionally, additional sutures are needed to stop arterial leaks. Mild oozing is monitored for several minutes; this will usually stop. Continued oozing from the venous side will usually require removal and revision of the coupler device.

Once the anastomoses are deemed patent and intact, the path of the pedicle is assessed for hemostasis and potential sites of compression or kinking. We will often divide some pectoralis muscle on the edges to prevent compression on the pedicle. This is also a good point to ensure recipient site hemostasis.

The retractors are then removed and the flap is inset. Take care to avoid over-rotation and stretching of the pedicle. Occasionally, we will place several deep absorbable sutures securing the Scarpa's fascia layer of the flap to the chest wall to prevent the flap sliding, which may damage

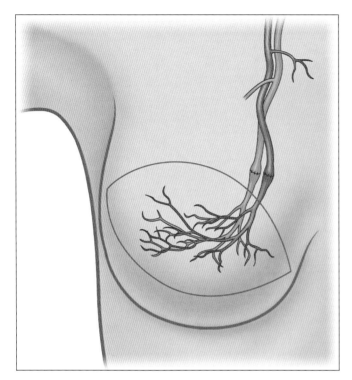

FIGURE 5.19 Flap inset.

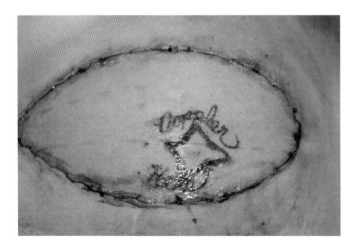

FIGURE 5.20 Flap inset with percutaneous Doppler marking.

the pedicle. Most often, however, we simply use the skin envelope with dermal sutures to secure the flap. A fluted 15 Fr drain is placed, exiting through the skin in the axilla. The drain should be positioned away from the pedicle.

The mastectomy skin flaps are trimmed and the SGAP skin de-epithelialized as necessary for appropriate inset. Care must be taken to avoid an overly tight skin envelope that can compress the flap. A handheld Doppler probe is used to re-identify the cutaneous arterial perforators. These are marked and the SGAP skin paddle designed around them for postoperative monitoring. The skin is closed with interrupted 3/0 Vicryl deep dermal sutures, a running 4/0 Monocryl subcuticular suture, and Dermabond (Figs 5.19 and 5.20). The patient is undraped, cleansed, and anesthesia terminated. This marks the end of the operation.

Revisions

Complete reconstruction with the SGAP flap usually requires three or four procedures on separate occasions. These include an initial free flap as described above, and staged revision.

SGAP flap and mastectomy flap reshaping usually is performed at least 3 months after the initial free flap operation. This usually involves trimming or removing the remaining skin paddle and contouring the edges of the flap to improve breast shape. Occasionally some liposuction is necessary for shaping and softening areas of fat necrosis. Often this is combined with a contralateral breast reduction, mastopexy, or augmentation as necessary to improve symmetry.

The donor site scar is often revised at this point, with trimming of dog-ears and liposuction of irregularities to improve upper buttock contour. The contralateral buttock is also sometimes treated with liposuction for symmetry.

Nipple reconstruction

Reconstruction of the nipple–areolar complex (NAC) can sometimes be performed in the second stage when there is adequate symmetry between the breasts. If a procedure for symmetry is required beforehand, however, NAC reconstruction should be delayed until a third stage, often performed in the office setting. There are numerous techniques in the literature adequate for NAC reconstruction. Attention should be paid to skin perfusion of the NAC.

NAC tattooing

This is the final procedure performed after all shaping and symmetry procedures have healed.

Alternatives
Inferior gluteal artery perforator (IGAP) flap reconstruction

Based on the other major blood supply to the gluteal muscle (as stated in the surgical anatomy section), IGAP flap is another alternative in breast reconstruction ideal for those few patients with insufficient bulk in the upper buttock region. It is designed over the inferior portion of the buttock, with the resulting scar located just above the infragluteal fold. The dissection and volume this flap provides are similar to that of the SGAP flap. It is our preference not to use this flap much because of the scar location and occasional sciatic nerve irritation due to swelling around the nerve from adjacent dissection of the inferior gluteal pedicle.

Bilateral SGAP reconstruction

When the surgical team includes two microsurgeons, simultaneous bilateral SGAP reconstruction can be performed safely and with reasonable operating times.[8,9] Each side can be operated on simultaneously for most of the procedure, except for when using the microscope for anastomosis. Ideally, each side has its own separate team, including assistant, surgical scrub technician, and surgical instruments.

IMA perforators for recipient vessels

Occasionally, IMA perforators can be found that are adequate for recipient vessel anastomosis. This requires their having been left following the mastectomy and having sufficient caliber. This technique, however, can spare the patient morbidity from harvesting of the rib cartilage, and spares the vessels for potential future procedures, such as coronary artery bypass.

Sensate SGAP flap

The inclusion of nerve repair in SGAP reconstruction has been described in order to create a sensate breast reconstruction.[10] Typically, one or two nerve perforators are repaired to the T4 thoracic nerve branch. The success of this maneuver is variable.

Implantable Doppler flap monitoring

Some surgeons elect to use an implantable venous Doppler probe (Cook Vascular, Inc., Leechburg, PA) to assist with postoperative flap monitoring. This can provide an early warning of venous or arterial occlusion before skin paddle changes are apparent. In our practice, this device is typically used in breast reconstruction to the thoracodorsal vessels, such as the deep inferior epigastric artery perforator (DIEP) flap. We feel that the pedicle in SGAP flap to the IMV is too short, and the cuff on the probe can possibly contribute to kinking of the vessels.

BOX 5.2 Optimizing outcomes

- Choose patients carefully prior to surgery
- Avoid performing SGAP reconstruction in obese patients
- Gain experience in other microsurgical breast reconstruction procedures and then advance to SGAP reconstruction
- Optimize exposure of donor and recipient vessels
- Be careful when dissecting near the origin of the superior gluteal vessels; make sure you are following the pedicle and not side branches
- Do not retract too much on the flap pedicle during dissection, especially near branch points, as this may lead to thrombosis
- Check for rotational defects in the pedicle after anastomosis or kinking in the pedicle
- Do not inset flap too tightly. If need be, leave some of the wound open and allow to close by secondary intention or delayed primary closure
- Re-explore in the OR early if necessary

Implantable Doppler flap monitoring
- Long complex procedure requires anticipation by operating room team members to avoid excess OR time
- Beware of Medusa's head and of small periosteal branches during dissection of donor flap
- Vessel length in the pedicle and the recipient site will facilitate visualization during anastomosis and flap positioning for inset

---

OPTIMIZING OUTCOMES

Outcomes are generally optimized by proper patient selection, meticulous operative technique, and attention to detail. The SGAP flap is generally considered one of the more difficult to harvest and the anastomosis can be difficult because of the short pedicle length or a small vessel caliber. The arterial and venous anastomoses can be facilitated by selecting a perforating branch of the internal mammary vessels in order to equalize vessel caliber. It is sometimes necessary to perform an end-to-side arterial anastomosis to the internal mammary artery when a perforating branch is not available.

COMPLICATIONS AND SIDE EFFECTS

Common and serious

The most serious complications of SGAP reconstruction are similar to those of all operations requiring general anesthesia: myocardial infarction, deep venous thrombosis, pulmonary embolism, possibly even death. SGAP surgery, especially when combined with mastectomy, is prolonged – usually more than 6 hours, which increases these risks. Patient selection based on medical history, physical examination, and preoperative testing is paramount for avoiding these disasters.

Flap failure, either partial or complete, is the most serious complication specific to free flap reconstruction, and can be a result of a multitude of factors, including microsurgical technique, patient anatomy, patient risk factors, and postoperative care. For published series of more than 10 SGAP reconstructions, flap failure rates range from 0% to 7.7%.[10,11] In our unpublished data of 106 flaps on 90 patients over 7 years, the success rate has increased yearly with experience, from 88.7% to 96.5%, with an overall success rate of 92.5%.[12]

Even with these listed factors, surgical technique is usually a component of every flap failure, especially complete loss. Meticulous microsurgical technique will avoid anastomotic obstruction. Details of technique are beyond the scope of this chapter. Venous occlusion is responsible for the vast majority of flap failures.[13] The pedicle can be compromised by kinking, stretching, a tight skin closure, or an expanding hematoma or seroma. The importance of attention to detail cannot be overemphasized.

Occasionally patient anatomy prohibits SGAP reconstruction. Patients having had radiation may have scarred or shrunken IMA vessels. Very rarely patients simply have vessels that are too small for free flap reconstruction.

Patient risk factors, including smoking, atherosclerosis, obesity, hypertension, and hypercholesterolemia, often negatively affect outcome, most often these contributing to partial flap loss. Various blood clotting disorders can also lead to clotted venous pedicles or excessive bleeding.

Postoperative care is important in preserving the integrity of the flap and its perfusion. Excessive motion or inappropriate patient positioning can compromise the flap pedicle. Frequent monitoring by those knowledgeable on the signs of flap compromise can potentially lead to a failing flap being saved. Other complications include bleeding and hematoma; seroma formation; infection; wound breakdown; scarring; pain; and pneumothorax.

How to prevent and manage complications

Bleeding and hematoma are prevented by meticulous hemostasis. An enlarging hematoma can potentially lead to a venous clot when it compresses the pedicle. An expanding flap pocket, change in the color of the flap or mastectomy skin, tachycardia, and anemia are all signs that should raise suspicion. There should be a low threshold for returning to the operating room for evacuation when these are present in the immediate postoperative period.

Seroma is a long-term sequela that most often presents at the donor site (>80% SGAP patients). Drains are left in the reconstruction and donor sites until daily drainage drops to consistently less than 30 mL/day. This is usually 1 week at the reconstruction site and 2–3 weeks at the donor site. Despite this, seromas often form at the donor

site, requiring percutaneous aspiration during follow-up visits. Seromas should not be left to expand without treatment to avoid potential wound breakdown.

Wound infections at either surgical site are rare. Pre- and intraoperative antibiotics should be given routinely. The authors typically give a short course of postoperative antibiotics as well. Erythema, swelling, and purulent drainage are signs of infection that should be aggressively treated with antibiotics and/or surgical drainage as necessary. Incisional dehiscence typically results from the aforementioned complications and should be treated with standard local wound care.

As with any surgery, scars are a sequela of every incision. Therefore, the surgeon must balance the need for surgical exposure with the development of scarring. Patients should be educated preoperatively about these scars in order to have a realistic expectation of the final cosmetic result. Scar revision and the treatment of deeper fibrotic scars and fat necrosis are usually performed in the revision stages.

The most acutely painful site in this surgery is typically where the rib cartilage is removed. Patient-controlled anal-

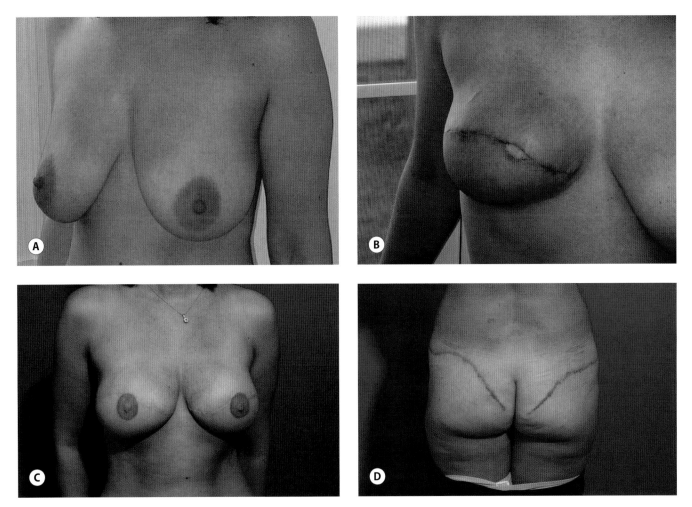

FIGURE 5.21 Images of patient with bilateral staged SGAP flap breast reconstruction. **A** Prior to mastectomy. **B** Following right mastectomy with immediate right SGAP flap reconstruction; 2 weeks postoperatively. **C** Final post-reconstruction results following left SGAP flap reconstruction, revision stages with nipple reconstruction, and areolar tattooing. **D** Bilateral donor site scars.

gesic (PCA) usually provides adequate pain relief. We prefer to avoid the use of non-steroidal anti-inflammatory drugs (e.g., ketorolac) in the immediate postoperative period for fear of bleeding complications. Patients will most often have some degree of splinting; therefore, an incentive spirometer should be routinely used to relieve atelectasis. Long-term pain from scarring or pinched nerves is rare but possible, and should be treated appropriately.

It is uncommon for patients to develop a symptomatic pneumothorax from the rib cartilage resection. Careful dissection and rib removal should avoid damaging the parietal pleura. If a pneumothorax is suspected, the diagnosis can be confirmed with radiographs. A small pneumothorax can often be treated with a small suction tube and closed immediately.

POSTOPERATIVE CARE

Immediate

Upon completion of the operation patients are extubated in the operating room and may be transferred to the recovery room or directly to the observation/intensive care unit. Typically they will spend the first postoperative night in this unit, as the level of care required necessitates hourly monitoring of both patient and flap. Nursing staff should

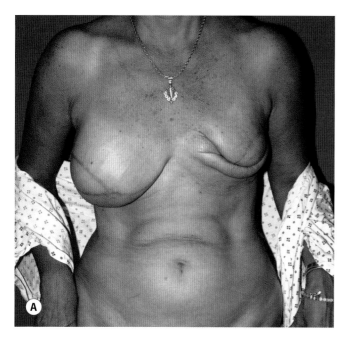

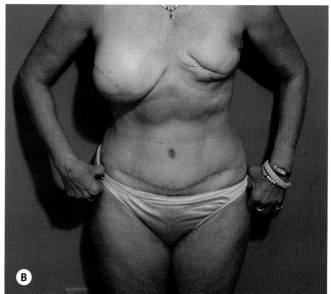

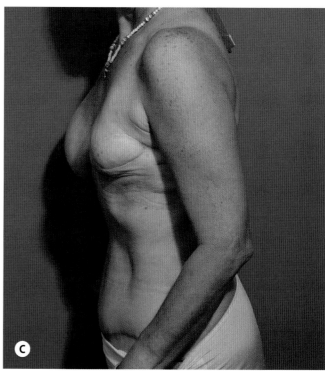

FIGURE 5.22 Images of patient with history of bilateral mastectomy with bilateral latissimus dorsi flap reconstruction and implant placement with postoperative left-sided radiation and implant failure. **A** Preoperatively. **B, C** After right implant removal and DIEP flap.

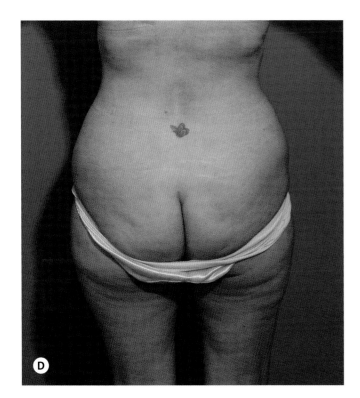

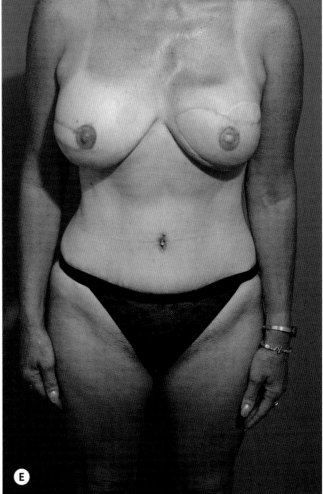

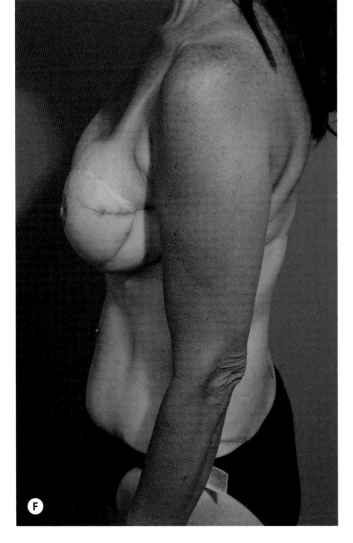

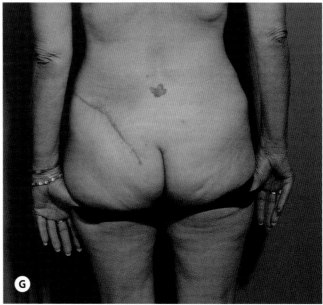

FIGURE 5.22, cont'd D Upper buttock shows ample tissue for a potential SGAP donor site. **E, F** Final post-reconstruction results following left SGAP flap reconstruction, bilateral revisions with nipple reconstruction, and areolar tattooing; anterior and lateral views. **G** SGAP donor scar.

be aware of the signs of flap compromise, including color changes, flap temperature, capillary refill times, loss of Doppler pulse, and expanding hematoma. Patients remain on bed rest and nil by mouth for the first night, and receive IV fluid, antibiotics, and pain control by PCA. Postoperative deep venous thrombosis (DVT) prophylaxis should be used routinely with sequential compression devices. Adjuvant DVT prophylaxis (e.g., subcutaneous heparin, enoxaparin, etc.) should be considered, especially in overweight or obese patients.

On postoperative day 1 the patient is transferred to the surgical floor if the flap is judged successful. They are begun on a clear diet and advanced as tolerated. Activity may also include transferring to a reclining chair.

On postoperative day 2 the patient's Foley catheter is removed and she may begin ambulating. Pain control is changed to oral medication. Occupational therapy and drain care are taught to prepare the patient for discharge.

On postoperative day 3, if the patient is tolerating food, oral pain control, ambulation, and voiding spontaneously, she may be discharged with instructions for follow-up in clinic 1 week later. Prescriptions for pain control and antibiotics are provided, but the patient is instructed to limit activity, although she may shower. We often prescribe some home nursing care to assist with drain care.

The first week's follow-up appointment usually consists of drain removal from the breast pocket. The patient returns for further follow-up appointments as necessary for removal of the donor site drain and revision planning. As previously stated, percutaneous aspiration of seromas is often required.

Long-term

The interval between steps is usually 3 months, hence the process can take 6 months to 1 year, or longer if complications occur. Upon completion the patient should return for yearly follow-up for cancer surveillance. The SGAP flap will enlarge and shrink with weight fluctuations and develop progressive ptosis, similar to the contralateral breast. Unlike with implant reconstruction, further surgery is usually unnecessary.

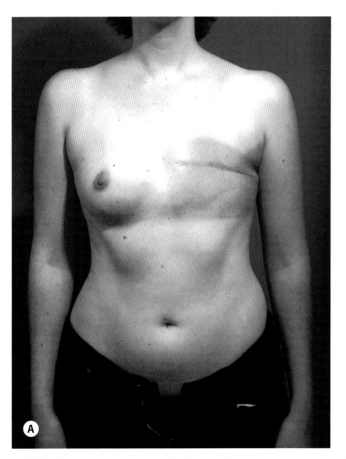
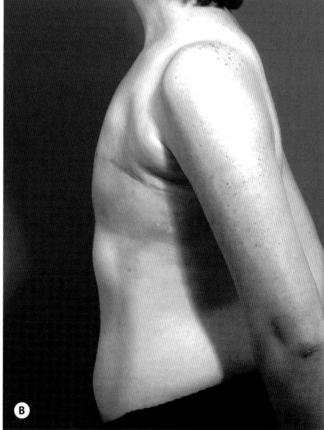

FIGURE 5.23 Images of patient with history of left-sided mastectomy with postoperative radiation. Right-sided prophylactic mastectomy with bilateral reconstruction is planned. **A, B, C** Left-sided mastectomy site demonstrating post-radiation skin changes; anterior, left, and right lateral views.

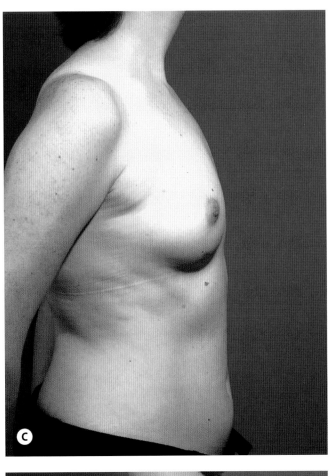

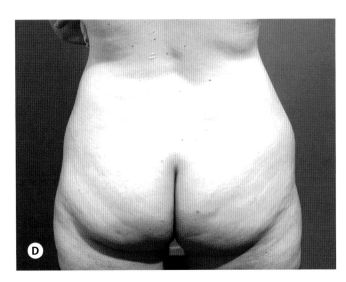

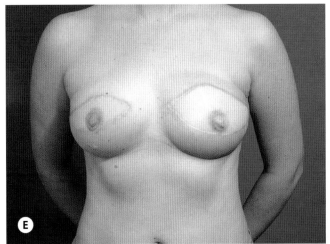

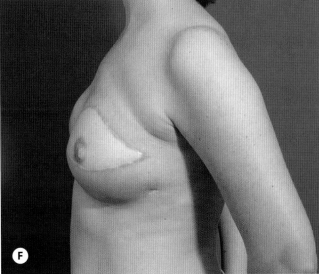

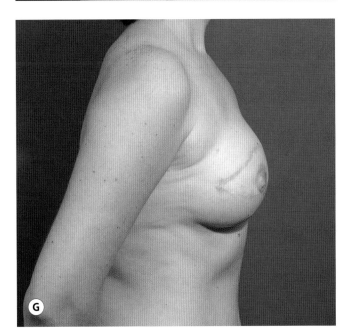

FIGURE 5.23, cont'd D The buttock shows ample tissue for potential bilateral SGAP donor sites. **E, F, G** Final post-reconstruction results following bilateral stage SGAP flap reconstruction, bilateral revisions with nipple reconstruction, and areolar tattooing; anterior, left, and right-sided views.

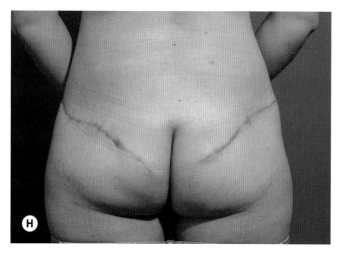

FIGURE 5.23, cont'd H Final bilateral donor site scars.

CONCLUSIONS

As autogenous tissue has become increasingly utilized for breast reconstruction surgical techniques have evolved, setting new standards and raising patient expectations. Traditional donor sites for breast reconstruction may not be available, yet the same outcome is still expected. SGAP reconstruction is a valuable option for patients who are not candidates for reconstruction using their abdominal tissue. Although this is challenging procedure, it has consistent anatomy and provides excellent results, which makes it an important part of the breast reconstructive surgeon's repertoire.

REFERENCES

1. Fujino T, Harashina T, Aoyagi F. Reconstruction for aplasia of the breast and pectoral region by microvascular transfer of a free flap from the buttock. Plast Reconstruct Surg 1975; 56: 178.
2. Shaw WW. Superior gluteal free flap breast reconstruction. Clin Plast Surg 1998; 25: 267.
3. Codner MA, Nahai F. The gluteal free flap breast reconstruction: making it work. Clin Plast Surg 1994; 21: 289.
4. Koshima I, Moriguchi T, Soeda S, et al. The gluteal perforator-based flap for repair of sacral pressure sores. Plast Reconstruct Surg 1993; 91: 678.
5. Allen RJ, Tucker C. Superior gluteal artery perforator free flap for breast reconstruction. Plast Reconstruct Surg 1995; 95: 1207.
6. Mu LH, Yan YP, Luan J, et al. Anatomy study of superior and inferior gluteal artery perforator flap. Zhonghua Zheng Xing Wai Ke Za Zhi 2005; 21: 278–280.
7. Kankaya Y, Ulusoy MG, Oruç M, et. al. Perforating arteries of the gluteal region. Ann Plast Surg 2006; 56: 409–412.
8. Guerra AB, Soueid N, Metzinger SE, et al. Simultaneous bilateral breast reconstruction with superior gluteal artery perforator (SGAP) flaps. Ann Plast Surg 2004; 53: 305–310.
9. Della Croce FJ, Sullivan SK. Application of the superior gluteal artery perforator free flap for bilateral simultaneous breast reconstruction. Plast Reconstruct Surg 2005; 116: 87–104.
10. Blondeel PN. The sensate free superior gluteal artery perforator (SGAP) flap: a valuable alternative in autologous breast reconstruction. Br J Plast Surg 1999; 52: 185–193.
11. Feller AM, Richter-Heine I, Rudolf KD. The superior gluteal artery perforator flap (S-GAP flap). Handchir Mikrochir Plast Chir 2002; 34: 257–261.
12. Huang K, Chang B. 106 Consecutive superior gluteal artery perforator (SGAP) flaps in a community hospital: A single surgeon's experience. Presented at the World Society of Reconstructive Microsurgery meeting, Athens, Greece, June 2007.
13. Nahabedian MY, Momen B, Manson PN. Factors associated with anastomotic failure after microvascular reconstruction of the breast. Plast Reconstruct Surg 2004; 114: 74–82.

6

Latissimus Dorsi Breast Reconstruction

Colleen M. McCarthy and Joseph J. Disa

INTRODUCTION

The latissimus dorsi myocutaneous (LDM) flap has evolved over time to incorporate a wide range of applications in breast reconstruction. For example, the LDM flap can be used to transfer a large volume of well-vascularized soft tissue to the anterior chest wall. Because of this, the LDM flap is particularly useful in patients with a history of prior chest wall irradiation who may not otherwise tolerate expander/implant reconstruction. The LDM flap may be similarly useful in women who are not candidates for an abdominally based, autogenous tissue reconstruction (i.e., patients with a history of multiple abdominal operations, a prior abdominoplasty, and/or thin patients with limited infraumbilical fat). Because of the robust blood supply of the latissimus dorsi muscle, the LDM flap may also be used in women who are at high risk of wound complications following either implant-based reconstruction and/or pedicled transverse rectus abdominis (TRAM) flap reconstruction, including those who are diabetic, heavy smokers, and/or morbidly obese. Finally, the latissimus dorsi muscle may be used to reconstruct defects following lumpectomy and/or quadrantectomy of the breast.

Most patients will be candidates for latissimus breast reconstruction. The LDM flap can provide a skin island up to 8 cm wide, a variable amount of fat, and a large surface area of well-vascularized muscle.[1] However, although the anatomy of the flap is consistent, the volume of soft tissue available to reconstruct a mastectomy defect often falls short of that required to obtain adequate projection and/or symmetry with the opposite breast. The most favorable results following latissimus dorsi flap reconstruction alone will be achieved in patients who have a small breast volume and minimal ptosis. In fact, moderate- to large-volume breasts will generally require the additional volume provided by the use of a prosthesis. Furthermore, in patients with large or markedly ptotic breasts, some type of match-

ing procedure may be required in order to obtain symmetry.

In cases where the latissimus dorsi flap adds sufficient skin to fully reconstruct the cutaneous envelope, it is possible to perform a single-stage procedure whereby a permanent prosthesis is placed underneath the LDM flap. Although our experience suggests that satisfactory results can be obtained with single-stage reconstruction, in the vast majority of patients a more reliable approach appears to involve two-stage, combined LDM flap–expander/implant reconstruction.[2] A tissue expander is placed under the LDM flap at the primary procedure. Postoperatively, tissue expansion is performed over a period of weeks or months. This allows the volume of the reconstructed breast to be adjusted postoperatively to correct for an expected 20–30% shrinkage in flap size. The temporary expander is exchanged for a permanent implant at a subsequent operation. By performing a capsulotomy and/or 'fine tuning' the implant pocket at the time of exchange, the procedure allows for the creation of a breast with greater ptosis and more natural contours.

ANATOMY

The latissimus dorsi is a broad, fan-shaped muscle that originates on the lower thoracic vertebra, lumbar sacral processes, and iliac crest and inserts on the lesser tubercle of the humerus. Contraction of the latissimus dorsi results in the extension, adduction, and medial rotation of the humerus. When contraction is compromised, the teres major and subscapularis muscles compensate these actions. The innervation of the latissimus dorsi muscle is through the thoracodorsal nerve, from the posterior cord of the brachial plexus. The thoracodorsal nerve joins the thoracodorsal artery and vein 3–4 cm before entering the lateral edge of the muscle.[3]

The blood supply to the latissimus dorsi arises from one dominant pedicle and is supported by many segmental vessels (type V pattern of circulation). The thoracodorsal artery branches from the subscapular artery just distal to the circumflex scapular artery and enters the muscle in the posterior axilla, 10–11 cm inferior to the origin of its insertion. Just proximal to the entrance of the thoracodorsal artery into the muscle, it gives one or two branches to the serratus anterior. This vascular architecture allows continued perfusion if the proximal portion of the artery is damaged through collateral connections with the lateral thoracic artery. The segmental arterial contribution is separated into medial and lateral rows. The medial row originates from several segmental branches of the lumbar artery and supplies the muscle origin around the lumbar spine. The posterior intercostal arteries contribute four to six perforators to feed the inferior lateral muscle fibers. Venous drainage is accomplished by venae comitantes of the corresponding arteries.[1,3]

INDICATIONS AND CONTRAINDICATIONS

Use of the LDM flap is indicated in patients who elect not to undergo a TRAM or related flap, or in whom abdominally based reconstruction is contraindicated. This includes patients in whom the infraumbilical soft tissues are limited, those who previously have undergone abdominoplasty, and/or those who have abdominal scars that may complicate healing at the donor site. The latissimus dorsi flap can also be used in patients who may have already undergone a TRAM or related flap procedure. Finally, latissimus dorsi reconstruction does not compromise the abdominal wall, which may be important in patients desiring a future pregnancy, or those whose lifestyle does not allow for the potential diminution of truncal strength.

Autogenous latissimus dorsi reconstruction

Satisfactory results can be achieved with an LDM flap alone in some patients (i.e., obese patients with small breasts, or thin patients with very small breasts). Instead, most LDM flap reconstructions require the use of an implant to obtain adequate projection.

Immediate latissimus dorsi–expander/implant reconstruction

In patients who require the additional volume provided by the addition of a prosthesis to the latissimus reconstruction, two-stage expander/implant reconstruction is an extremely reliable approach. A tissue expander is placed at the time of the LDM flap harvest and inset. Postoperatively, tissue expansion is performed over a period of weeks or months. The expander is exchanged for a permanent implant during the secondary procedure. By performing a capsulotomy and/or 'fine tuning' the implant pocket at the time of exchange, the procedure allows for the creation of a breast with greater ptosis and more natural contours.

A large skin excision at the time of mastectomy, due to previous biopsies or locally advanced disease, may preclude primary coverage of a tissue expander. The absence of an adequate skin envelope is an absolute contraindication to expander/implant reconstruction alone. Thus, in patients without the volume of soft tissue required to permit a tension-free closure over an expander, the ipsilateral LDM flap can be used to provide additional soft tissue.

LDM flap reconstruction may also facilitate immediate expander/implant reconstruction in patients with a history of prior chest wall irradiation. Ipsilateral breast tumor recurrence occurs in approximately 8–20% of women 10 years after the treatment of breast cancer with lumpectomy and postoperative radiotherapy.[4-6] The standard surgical treatment after a local recurrence is a 'salvage mastectomy'. Immediate post-mastectomy reconstruction in a patient who has received prior chest wall irradiation is, however, considered by many to be a contraindication to implant-based reconstruction.[7-9] Not only is tissue expansion difficult in previously irradiated tissues, but the risks of infection, expander exposure, and subsequent extrusion are increased. Although autogenous tissue alone remains our method of choice in the setting of prior chest wall irradiation, many women are neither willing nor are candidates for this form of reconstruction. Thus, the use of combined LDMF–expander/implant reconstruction is a reliable option for those who wish to undergo post-mastectomy reconstruction yet are candidates neither for autogenous tissue reconstruction alone nor for expander–implant reconstruction alone. Based on our experience, it appears that the use of autogenous tissue flaps provides pliable, well-vascularized soft tissue which can facilitate both wound healing and the process of tissue expansion in the setting of prior irradiation.

Delayed post-mastectomy latissimus dorsi reconstruction

For those who may not have access to or are unable to decide on primary reconstruction while adjusting to their cancer diagnosis, delayed expander–implant reconstruction is an option. Similarly, those who have failed implant and/or autogenous tissue reconstruction may elect to pursue breast reconstruction in a delayed fashion.

In the setting of delayed post-mastectomy reconstruction, the amount of remaining mastectomy skin is often greatly reduced because it comes from non-skin-sparing mastectomies. Therefore, expansion may achieve less volume, making the creation of breast ptosis more difficult. The combination of a latissimus dorsi flap and tissue expansion may thus be appropriate in cases in which the remaining mastectomy skin is of insufficient quality to tolerate tissue expansion. This is typically the case in the insetting of delayed reconstruction after mastectomy and postoperative radiation therapy (see immediate latissimus dorsi–expander/implant reconstruction).

Reconstruction of the lumpectomy defect

As breast conservation is pushed further in terms of larger resections in smaller patients, increasing distortion of the breast is predictable. In addition, breast aesthetics may deteriorate progressively with time as side effects of radiation affect the final shape of the breast. Although the theoretical benefit of breast conservation therapy is the maintenance of cosmesis by preservation of breast form, residual deformity and asymmetry are not uncommon. Thus, despite surgical conservatism in these patients, reconstruction of these defects is often necessary.

Several controversies exist with regard to the appropriate management of a lumpectomy defect. A major concern is the timing of the reconstruction with respect to tumor resection.[10] Other points of contention include the effectiveness of postoperative cancer surveillance and the management of a recurrence. For example, if a local cancer recurrence develops following reconstruction of a lumpectomy defect, a potential reconstructive option has already been used. Total mastectomy is currently the standard of care for the surgical treatment of local recurrence. One of the best reasons not to use autogenous tissue in the reconstruction of lumpectomy defects is therefore its great utility in reconstruction of the total mastectomy defect. For example, if the latissimus flap is used for a partial defect and a recurrence develops, the subsequent mastectomy defect must be reconstructed from other remaining donor sites. Critics suggest that the aesthetic outcome following post-mastectomy reconstruction is similar or even superior to outcomes following reconstruction of the lumpectomy defect; thus, potentially subjecting a patient to multiple procedures and multiple donor-site harvests increases morbidity without substantial gain. Many would instead elect to perform a completion mastectomy and post-mastectomy reconstruction for a patient who presents with a lumpectomy defect.

For those who elect to pursue reconstruction of a lumpectomy defect the use of autogenous tissue is preferred, as the majority of these patients will have a history of prior radiotherapy. Smaller defects, particularly those in the superolateral portion of the breast, can be treated with a pedicled latissimus dorsi muscle flap. A portion of the latissimus dorsi muscle can be harvested through a transverse or oblique incision, or with the assistance of an endoscope. As the inframammary fold, nipple, and overall breast shape generally remain intact, their anatomy should be preserved. Anteriorly, an incision is made by incorporating pre-existing breast scars where possible. The latissimus flap then is transferred into the defect and inset, either superficial to the pectoralis major beneath remaining breast tissue, or deep to the elevated skin surrounding the defect.

RELATIVE CONTRAINDICATIONS (Boxes 6.1–6.4)

The loss of latissimus dorsi muscle function is generally well tolerated and does not result in significant upper-extremity weakness.[11] Latissimus harvest should be avoided, however, in patients with lower-extremity weakness, where the muscle plays an important role in gait by elevating the hemipelvis and facilitating circumabduction. Latissimus dorsi muscle function is also important for wheelchair transfer.

BOX 6.1 Indications

- Patients desiring immediate or delayed post-mastectomy reconstruction
- Patients with mastectomy skin flaps of insufficient quality to tolerate expansion, i.e. delayed reconstruction after chest wall irradiation
- Failed tissue expansion, failed implant, or failed abdominally based reconstruction
- Patients in whom microsurgical tissue transfer is not an option
- Patients wishing to avoid large abdominal scars or the risk of reducing abdominal/truncal strength; patients desiring future pregnancy
- Women with considerable prior abdominal surgery or abdominal radiation
- Reconstruction of segmental or lumpectomy defects

BOX 6.2 Relative contraindications

- Prior posterior thoracotomy with sacrifice/division of the latissimus dorsi muscle
- Patients who need functional latissimus dorsi, i.e., elite athletes, wheelchair users

BOX 6.3 Advantages

- Provision of additional vascularized skin and muscle to the breast mound in a single operative procedure
- Consistent neurovascular anatomy; highly reliable flap
- Provides adequate volume for small-volume breasts without the use of a prosthesis
- Quicker convalescence than with abdominally based flaps
- No abdominal weakness after surgery

BOX 6.4 Disadvantages

- Patient repositioning may be necessary after flap harvest
- Slight cosmetic deformity from loss of posterior axillary fold
- Propensity for donor-site seroma formation
- Potential for functional loss in patients who may rely on upper-body strength (wheelchair users, swimmers, rock climbers, golfers, tennis players, etc.)
- The need for an implant is not often eliminated, despite the transfer of autogenous tissue
- Permanent dependency on prosthesis can also lead to long-term complications, such as implant leak or deflation and capsular contracture

The latissimus muscle and/or its blood supply is usually damaged by a posterolateral thoracotomy, and occasionally during an axillary lymph node biopsy. Because of the relative approximation of the thoracodorsal vasculature to the nerve, in patients in whom the thoracodorsal nerve is damaged it may be safest to assume that the vessels are injured. In patients with a history of prior chest and/or axillary surgery, the function of the latissimus muscle should therefore be assessed preoperatively.

Innervation of the latissimus dorsi can be tested indirectly by evaluation of isometric contraction of the muscle. With the patient's hands positioned on her waist, she should be instructed to push her elbows downwards. Contraction of viable muscle can then be assessed by palpation of the lateral edge of the latissimus dorsi. In ambiguous cases, electrical stimulation or electromyography may be used to further evaluate function. If muscular contraction is not elicited by any of the above techniques, however, it must be assumed that the muscle has been denervated and is atrophic. During such a harvest, the muscle layer will appear extremely thin and pale. Although success has been achieved under these conditions, acceptable aesthetic results may be difficult to achieve because of the delicacy of the atrophied muscle.

Significant compromise of the thoracodorsal vessels can similarly reduce the bulk of the proposed flap, warranting the consideration of alternative reconstruction options. However, if the thoracodorsal vessels alone have been damaged, the latissimus dorsi flap can often still be used owing to retrograde flow through the serratus branches. In patients who have undergone a previous axillary lymph node dissection, care must be taken not to ligate the serratus branches until the patency of the thoracodorsal artery and vein has been demonstrated.

PREOPERATIVE CONSIDERATIONS

Preoperative planning is critical to achieving a successful outcome. The following issues must be considered when individualizing the reconstructive procedure.

Mastectomy skin flaps

The goal of post-mastectomy reconstruction is to recreate a breast that looks and feels like the removed breast. Placement of the latissimus dorsi flap into the mastectomy defect requires attention to the preservation of ptosis and the breast's natural contours. If the skin island of the LDM flap is positioned too high on the chest wall, the bulk of the muscle will be out of position to accomplish this goal. Instead, by sacrificing the inferior mastectomy skin flaps down to the level of the inframammary fold, the skin island of the LDM flap may be positioned more inferiorly. This arrangement allows the bulk of the flap to provide ptosis and a gives a more natural contour to the reconstructed breast.

Similarly, in the setting of prior chest wall irradiation expansion of mastectomy skin flaps may be limited. By excising the mastectomy flaps in the inferior pole of the

breast at the time of expander placement, the skin island of the LDM flap can be placed inferiorly. Overexpansion of the native back skin in the lower pole of the breast can then be performed. Ultimately, this serves to create a looser skin envelope and a greater potential for breast ptosis.

Posterior scar location

If a skin paddle is required for reconstruction, it is usually oriented either horizontally or obliquely, depending on reconstructive requirements. The maximum width of the skin paddle is usually 7–8 cm and depends on skin laxity. Wider skin islands tend to be difficult to close primarily. The scar resulting from a horizontal skin-paddle harvest can usually be covered by the bra strap. By contrast, the scar resulting from an obliquely oriented skin paddle may be designed along the relaxed skin tension lines of the back, thereby reducing the potential for hypertrophic scarring.

Creating a submuscular pocket

In the setting of implant-based reconstruction, both infectious complications and wound healing problems can have negative consequences. Not only can these outcomes necessitate the explantation of a permanent prosthesis, thereby delaying the reconstructive process, but more importantly, they can delay the administration of adjuvant therapy for breast cancer. By placing a prosthesis in a completely submuscular position, the risk of expander exposure and contamination in the setting of mastectomy flap necrosis is minimized.

Placement of an expander beneath the pectoralis major muscle allows for muscle coverage of the superomedial portion only. In this setting, the inferolateral portion of the device sits directly underneath the latissimus muscle. If the pectoralis major is insufficient to cover the superior portion of the implant, or is scarred and/or fibrotic secondary to prior radiation treatment, the implant can be placed in the mastectomy space and covered in its entirety with the latissimus flap.

Selecting an expander

Generally, textured, anatomic expanders are used. Textured expanders may reduce the amount of device migration, whereas anatomical expanders preferentially expand the lower pole of the breast. Together, these improvements result in improved breast shape. Low, medium and full/tall height expanders are available for use. Generally, the authors prefer a medium height expander. Intraoperatively, the mastectomy weight is recorded and the width of the expander pocket is then measured. An appropriate expander is then selected based on its base dimensions and volume capability.

Selecting a permanent implant

Before the exchange procedure patients must consider the type of permanent implant (saline or silicone) to be used in the reconstruction. Both types are currently available. The use of silicone gel implants generally allows for a softer, more natural-feeling breast. Although controversy surrounding the use of silicone-filled implants still exists, issues of silicone safety have been carefully investigated,[12–14] and there is currently no definitive evidence linking breast implants to cancer, immunologic diseases, neurologic problems, or other systemic diseases. Patients should, however, be counseled regarding the recommendation that silicone implants be changed approximately every 10 years to minimize the risk of a silent leak.[15]

OPERATIVE APPROACH

Delayed latissimus dorsi–expander/implant reconstruction

Patient positioning
The LDM flap is created with the patient in the lateral decubitus position. The ipsilateral arm is completely prepared so that it remains in the operative field. For most of the procedure it is kept flexed to 90°, partially abducted, and can be stabilized using a Mayo stand. This configuration gives maximal exposure of both the axilla and the adjacent thorax.

Preoperative markings
The patient can be marked preoperatively in the upright sitting position or on the operating table in the lateral decubitus position. The origin and insertion of the latissimus dorsi muscle, as well as its relation to the scapula, are outlined. A transverse or oblique skin paddle may be planned as described above (Fig. 6.1).

Flap harvest
The incisions are created around the skin island. Skin flaps are elevated at the level of the subcutaneous fat both anteriorly and posteriorly above the latissimus dorsi muscle. The incisions are beveled to maintain a layer of fat over the latissimus muscle to provide extra bulk and improve contouring. The insertions of the latissimus muscle are incised circumferentially and the flap is elevated. The plane of dissection is then identified beneath the latissimus muscle yet superficial to the remaining musculature of the posterior thorax. The latissimus muscle is then elevated from its origins, proceeding distally to proximally. Medially, caution must be exercised to identify the medial and lateral rows of the segmental arteries that feed the muscle. These perforators that arise from the lumbar and intercostal arteries must be ligated or cauterized to ensure hemostasis and to prevent postoperative hematoma.

In this area of the tip of the scapula, the teres major, serratus anterior, and rhomboids meet the connective tissue of the superior origin of the latissimus dorsi. The space between the latissimus dorsi and serratus anterior muscles is enlarged with blunt dissection. Caution must be observed not to dissect under the serratus muscle, but between the serratus and latissimus.

Once the latissimus is separated from the serratus, the pedicle will become visible as the flap is elevated towards the axilla. Flap dissection continues proximally to the level of the branches from the serratus anterior muscle. If the dissection is being performed in a previously undissected axilla and the patency of the thoracodorsal vessels is certain, then the serratus branches may be divided to gain additional anterior rotation of the flap. In addition, some surgeons will prefer to divide the thoracodorsal nerve in order to eliminate the potential for muscle contraction, despite the fact that the latissimus muscle will atrophy over time. Once the flap is completely elevated, attention is turned anteriorly.

Insetting of the flap and expander placement
The mastectomy incision is re-excised. Electrocautery is used to elevate both the superior and inferior mastectomy skin flaps off the pectoralis major muscle. Superolaterally, a subcutaneous tunnel is dissected in order to connect the back incision with the mastectomy defect. The tunnel must be wide enough to allow transfer of the flap without tension, but not so wide that the implant can migrate posteriorly.

The LDM flap is then transferred to the mastectomy defect via the subcutaneous tunnel. Care is taken to avoid avulsion of the nutrient vessels originating from the serratus anterior. Maintaining the insertion of the muscle and limiting dissection to the level of the serratus branches is a safe way to avoid excessive tension on the pedicle, and is usually adequate for mobilization of the flap. In some patients, particularly thin patients, it may be necessary to transpose the muscle origin to the chest to avoid excessive fullness in the axilla. In fact, some surgeons will routinely divide the muscle insertion to facilitate reconstruction of the anterior axillary fold.

The flap can be placed into the anterior breast pocket and tacked in place to avoid tension on the pedicle while the donor defect is closed in layers. One or more closed suction drains should be placed to prevent postoperative seroma formation.

The inferior mastectomy skin flaps are then excised. When an acceptable position is attained, the flap is sutured to the inferior, medial, and lateral mastectomy flaps with absorbable sutures. The width of the expander pocket is then measured and the appropriate expander selected based on its base dimensions and volume capability. Textured, anatomic expanders are used in an attempt to limit the amount of device migration. Anatomical expanders preferentially expand the lower pole of the breast.

The expander is then placed in the pocket with its inferior edge at the lower limit of the pocket. In the setting of bilateral expansion, care must be taken to achieve symmetry with respect to the height of expander placement. The superior border of the latissimus flap is then inset to provide complete muscular coverage of the expander. One or two suction drains are placed in the mastectomy space. After wound closure, intraoperative expansion is performed to tissue tolerance. Up to 50% of the tissue expander volume

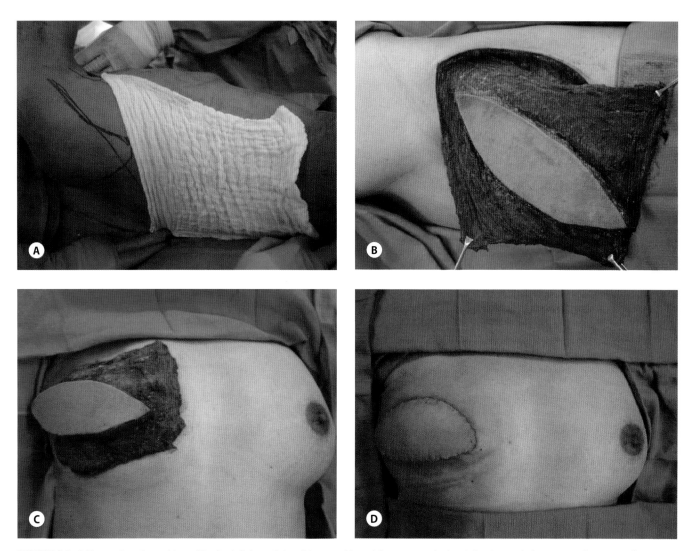

FIGURE 6.1 A The patient is positioned in the left lateral decubitus position. A lap sponge is the right size and shape to make an excellent latissimus dorsi pattern. **B** Back view. The latissimus myocutaneous flap is elevated in a distal to proximal direction. **C** Anterior view. The latissimus myocutaneous flap is transferred to the mastectomy defect anteriorly and used to cover a temporary expander. **D** Anterior view. Wound closure obtained.

is generally placed, which helps to fill the submuscular cavity and prevent skin contracture.

Postoperative expansion

Drains are removed when output is less than 30 mL in 24 hours. In the absence of skin flap necrosis or infection, postoperative expansion generally begins 10–14 days after surgery. Expansion is performed weekly or biweekly, depending on patient comfort and skin tolerance. Approximately 60–100 mL of normal saline are injected percutaneously through the integrated, expander port at each visit. The final expander volume is usually 20–30% greater than the planned implant volume, or 20% greater than the recommended volume of the expander. This overexpansion ultimately creates a looser skin envelope and a greater potential for ptosis.

Exchange procedure

The exchange procedure is performed a minimum of 4–6 weeks after the last expansion and/or 4–6 weeks after the completion of postoperative chemotherapy. The patient is positioned on the operating table such that it is made possible intraoperatively to position the table with the patient sitting upright. The patient's arms are placed across the abdomen, appropriately padded and taped to the table. The forehead is similarly padded and taped to prevent movement during flexion of the table. Perioperative antibiotics are administered. The patient is prepared and draped so that both breasts are in the operative field. The mastectomy incision is re-excised and sent for pathologic review. The mastectomy flaps are elevated in the subcutaneous plane, to a point where an 8–10 cm incision parallel to the fibers of the latissimus muscle can be made in order to gain access to the expander pocket. The expander is removed.

A circumferential capsulotomy and/or radial capsulotomies are performed as needed to maximize breast ptosis and inferior pole projection. Evaluation of the height and width of the contralateral native breast facilitates the appropriate selection of a permanent implant. Various implant sizers are trialed with the patient in the upright sitting position, and the final prosthesis is selected. The patient is returned to the supine position, the pocket is irrigated with normal saline, and hemostasis is obtained. The chest is re-prepared and draped and the surgeon's gloves are changed to minimize the risk of contamination. The permanent device is then placed in the pocket and carefully positioned. The muscle layer is closed using a running, absorbable suture. Double-layer skin closure is performed.

Immediate latissimus dorsi–expander/implant reconstruction

Patient positioning
The mastectomy (and axillary lymph node dissection) may be performed with the patient in the supine position, followed by repositioning into the lateral decubitus position, or with the patient in the lateral decubitus position, thereby decreasing operative time.

Mastectomy
Perioperative antibiotics are administered. The mastectomy is performed by the oncologic surgeon. At the conclusion of the operation the entire field is redraped over the mastectomy drapes, and a separate set of sterile instruments is used. Hemostasis within the mastectomy pocket is assured and the viability of the mastectomy flaps evaluated. Any non-viable soft tissue is excised. The pectoralis muscle may be elevated off the chest wall. The most inferomedial attachments of the pectoralis major muscle are released, but care is taken to leave the sternal attachments intact to prevent medial displacement of the tissue expander. If the pectoralis major muscle is insufficient to cover the expander completely, or is too scarred or fibrotic, the device can be placed instead in the mastectomy space and covered with the latissimus flap. Neither the rectus abdominis fascia nor the serratus muscle/fascia is elevated. The mastectomy wound is then temporarily closed and a sterile occlusive dressing applied (Figs 6.2, 6.3).

Harvesting of the LDM flap and placement of the expander is undertaken as in a delayed procedure. Postoperative expansion and exchange of the temporary expander for a permanent implant is similarly performed.

OPTIMIZING OUTCOMES (Box 6.5; Figs 6.4, 6.5)

Complications
Latissimus dorsi breast reconstruction is a relatively simple technique that is generally well tolerated. The flap has a vigorous blood supply and can be used with minimal risk of necrosis, even in smokers, diabetics, and those who are morbidly obese. Thus, LDM flap reconstruction can often be performed on patients who might not be suitable candidates for the more complex and lengthy autologous tissue procedures.

Complications are generally minor, with few systemic health implications and minimal overall morbidity. By far, the most common complication is a donor-site seroma.[11,16,17] Quilting sutures have been used in an attempt to reduce the formation of a postoperative fluid collection.[18] Whether or not quilting sutures are used, closed-suction drains should be used and left in the donor site until their output is less than 30 mL in 24 hours. Significant LDM flap necrosis is rare. Partial necrosis may occur in up to 10% of cases.[17,19]

Early complications following combined latissimus flap–expander insertion are significantly more common than following the exchange procedure. Early complications include mastectomy skin flap necrosis, hematoma, seroma, infection, and implant exposure/extrusion.[20] Late complications include device malfunction, such as implant leak or deflation, and capsular contracture.[21] Whereas capsular contracture occurs to some extent around all implants, in some the degree of contracture will worsen over time. It is similarly understood that patients who have undergone postoperative radiotherapy have a significantly higher incidence of capsular contracture than controls.[9,22] In patients with significant capsular contracture resulting in size or shape distortions and/or symptomatology, revision procedures are performed. At this stage, circumferential capsulotomy and/or capsulectomy may be carried out.

CONCLUSIONS
For patients who undergo mastectomy for the treatment of breast cancer, the restoration of a normal breast form through reconstruction is important to body image and quality of life. The use of an LDM flap has the capability of producing excellent results in the well-selected patient. Individualizing the selection of a reconstructive technique will be the predominant factor in achieving reconstructive success.

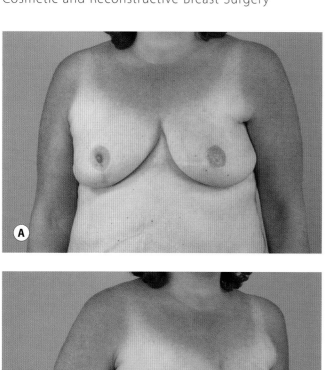

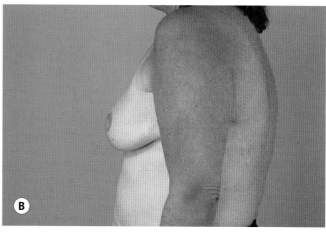

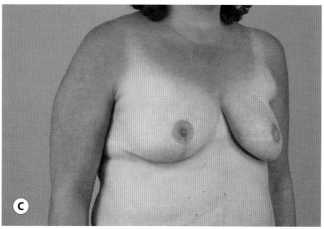

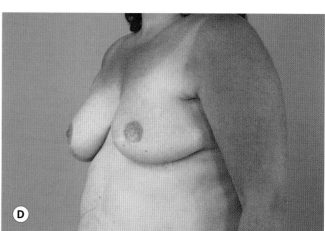

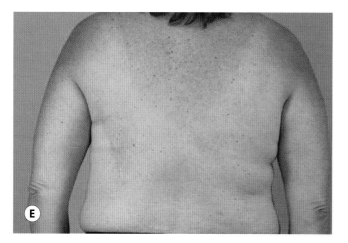

FIGURE 6.2 Recurrent breast cancer 4 years after prior lumpectomy/radiation to the left breast. Left salvage mastectomy with immediate latissimus dorsi/tissue expander-implant (TE-I) reconstruction using a 360 mL silicone gel implant. Right reduction mammoplasty performed. **A** Three years postoperatively. AP view. Breast with natural contours and ptosis achieved. Excellent symmetry. Excellent result. **B** Lateral view. Note well-healed donor-site scar. **C** Oblique view. **D** Oblique view. **E** Donor site scar.

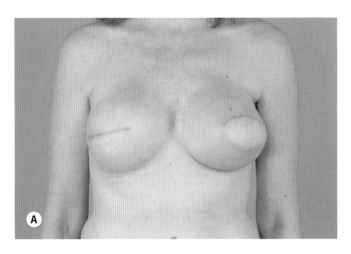
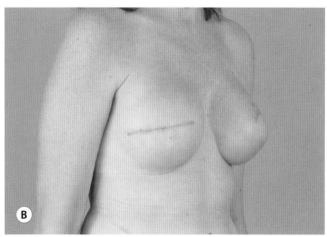

FIGURE 6.3 History of prior left lumpectomy/radiation. Salvage mastectomy left breast for recurrent breast cancer; prophylactic mastectomy right breast. Immediate latissimus dorsi/TE-I reconstruction left; immediate TE-I reconstruction right. **A** AP view. Note radiation tattoos midline. Excellent symmetry. Very good overall result. **B** Oblique view.

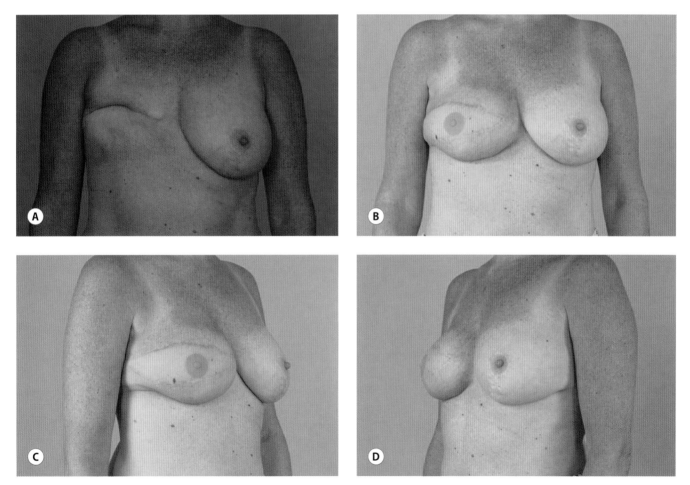

FIGURE 6.4 History of prior mastectomy and radiation right breast. Delayed, expander/implant reconstruction performed right; contralateral augmentation/mastopexy left for symmetry. Failed reconstruction right breast secondary to exposure of permanent implant. Patient presents for secondary reconstruction of right failed reconstruction. **A** Preoperative photo. **B** AP view. Postoperative photo. Right, two-stage combined latissimus-expander/implant reconstruction performed. **C** Right oblique view. **D** Left oblique view.

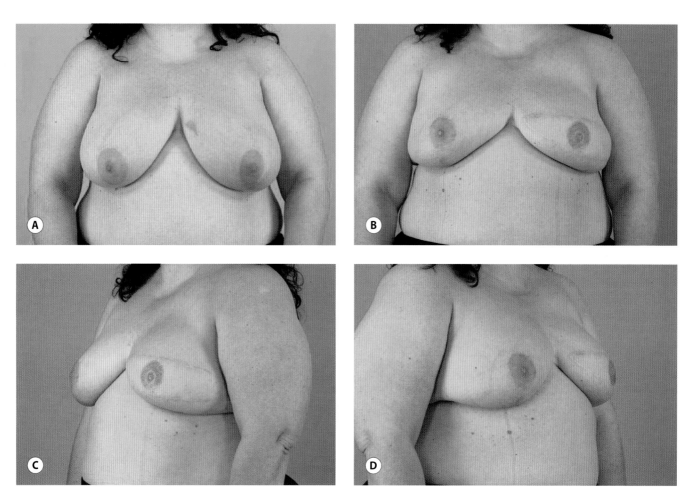

FIGURE 6.5 Immediate combined latissimus dorsi-expander/implant reconstruction performed left breast. Contralateral symmetry procedure performed right breast. **A** Preoperative photo. **B** AP view. Postoperative result. Note latissimus dorsi skin paddle and reconstructed nipple–areolar complex. **C** Left oblique view. **D** Right oblique view.

REFERENCES

1. Hammond DC. Latissimus dorsi flap breast reconstruction. Clin Plast Surg 2007; 34: 75–82; abstract vi–vii.
2. Disa JJ, Cordeiro PG, Heerdt AH, et al. Skin-sparing mastectomy and immediate autologous tissue reconstruction after whole-breast irradiation. Plast Reconstruct Surg 2003; 111: 118–124.
3. Mathes SJ, Nahai F. Reconstructive surgery: principles, anatomy and technique. New York: Churchill Livingstone, 1997.
4. McIntosh A, Freedman G, Eisenberg D, et al. Recurrence rates and analysis of close or positive margins in patients treated without re-excision before radiation for breast cancer. Am J Clin Oncol 2007; 30: 146–151.
5. McIntosh SA, Ogston KN, Payne S, et al. Local recurrence in patients with large and locally advanced breast cancer treated with primary chemotherapy. Am J Surg 2003; 185: 525–531.
6. Voogd AC, van Tienhoven G, Peterse HL, et al. Local recurrence after breast conservation therapy for early stage breast carcinoma: detection, treatment, and outcome in 266 patients. Dutch Study Group on Local Recurrence after Breast Conservation (BORST). Cancer 1999; 85: 437–446.
7. Forman DL, Chiu J, Restifo RJ, et al. Breast reconstruction in previously irradiated patients using tissue expanders and implants: a potentially unfavorable result. Ann Plast Surg 1998; 40: 360–363; discussion 363–364.
8. Krueger EA, Wilkins EG, Strawderman M, et al. Complications and patient satisfaction following expander/implant breast reconstruction with and without radiotherapy. Int J Radiat Oncol Biol Phys 2001; 49: 713–721.
9. Spear SL, Boehmler JH, Taylor NS, et al. The role of the latissimus dorsi flap in reconstruction of the irradiated breast. Plast Reconstruct Surg 2007; 119: 1–9; discussion 10–11.
10. McCarthy CM, Pusic AL, Disa JJ, et al. Breast cancer in the previously augmented breast. Plast Reconstruct Surg 2007; 119: 49–58.
11. Clough KB, Louis-Sylvestre C, Fitoussi A, et al. Donor site sequelae after autologous breast reconstruction with an extended latissimus dorsi flap. Plast Reconstruct Surg 2002; 109: 1904–1911.
12. Eggertson L. Breast implant advisory panel: more study on silicone leakage. CMAJ 2006; 174: 443–444.
13. Palley HA, Palley ML. The regulatory process, the Food and Drug Administration, and the silicone breast implant controversy. J Health Social Policy 1999; 11: 1–20.
14. Ault A. US Institute of Medicine panel deliberates on breast-implant safety. Lancet 1998; 352: 380.
15. Heden P, Bone B, Murphy DK, et al. Style 410 cohesive silicone breast implants: safety and effectiveness at 5 to 9 years after implantation. Plast Reconstruct Surg 2006; 118: 1281–1287.
16. Adams WP Jr, Lipschitz AH, Ansari M, et al. Functional donor site morbidity following latissimus dorsi muscle flap transfer. Ann Plast Surg 2004; 53: 6–11.
17. Apffelstaedt J. Indications and complications of LDM flaps in oncologic breast surgery. World J Surg 2002; 26: 1088–1093.
18. Daltrey I, Thomson H, Hussien M, et al. Randomized clinical trial of the effect of quilting latissimus dorsi flap donor site on seroma formation. Br J Surg 2006; 93: 825–830.

19. Roy MK, Shrotia S, Holcombe C, et al. Complications of LDM flap breast reconstruction. Eur J Surg Oncol 1998; 24: 162–165.

20. Cordeiro PG, McCarthy CM. A single surgeon's 12-year experience with tissue expander/implant breast reconstruction: part I. A prospective analysis of early complications. Plast Reconstruct Surg 2006; 118: 825–831.

21. Cordeiro PG, McCarthy CM. A single surgeon's 12-year experience with tissue expander/implant breast reconstruction: part II. An analysis of long-term complications, aesthetic outcomes, and patient satisfaction. Plast Reconstruct Surg 2006; 118: 832–839.

22. Spear SL, Onyewu C. Staged breast reconstruction with saline-filled implants in the irradiated breast: recent trends and therapeutic implications. Plast Reconstruct Surg 2000; 105: 930–942.

Breast Reconstruction: Repair of the Partial Mastectomy Defect

7

Steven J. Kronowitz

INTRODUCTION

In recent years there has been an increase in the proportion of breast cancer patients treated with partial mastectomy followed by radiation therapy (XRT), referred to as breast conservation therapy (BCT). This trend is partly due to increased mammographic screening with detection of early breast cancers, but also to the increasing use of preoperative chemotherapy in patients with locally advanced breast cancer.[1–3] Following BCT, 20–30% of patients are reported to have a poor cosmetic result, with deformities of the treated breast.[4–7] Poor outcomes following BCT are likely to be underestimated in the literature because many patients are reluctant to seek additional surgical treatment.

Although patients treated with total mastectomy often request breast reconstruction, those treated with partial mastectomy usually do not. There are several reasons for this. For some, the enhancement of body image through breast preservation provides sufficient psychological satisfaction. Others may fear additional operations or may simply not be aware of the reconstructive options.[8] These factors, along with the desire of many patients to preserve their breast regardless of their perceived cosmetic outcome, have led to a more aggressive use of partial mastectomy, with more extensive local resections being classified in the category of partial mastectomy.[8] As partial mastectomies become more extensive, the risk of suboptimal cosmetic results will most likely increase.[9] The importance of incorporating immediate reparative techniques in the multidisciplinary care of these patients has never been so critical.

Besides an obvious improvement in cosmetic outcome, immediate repair of partial mastectomy defects offers many other potential advantages. It can facilitate the breast surgeon's ability to resect wider margins around the tumor, which in turn has the potential to lower the rates of local recurrence of breast cancer.[9] Immediate repair of partial mastectomy defects can also increase the eligibility of large-breasted patients for BCT. Some radiation oncologists are reluctant to treat large-breasted patients because of poor aesthetic outcomes. Radiation delivered to a large breast can lead to increased fibrosis owing to difficulties with daily set-up and the increased fat content of the breast.[10] A reduced breast size allows for a more uniform radiation dose at a lower level, reducing unacceptable late radiation reactions.[11,12] Immediate repair of a partial mastectomy defect using breast reduction techniques represents an alternative for patients who would not otherwise be considered candidates for conservation therapy.

Immediate repair does not pose a problem with postoperative cancer surveillance.[11] It also may provide some medical benefits. Even though a contralateral breast reduction for symmetry is often required in patients who undergo repair of a partial mastectomy defect, and although contralateral breast reduction does increase the potential for complications, a benefit of this procedure is that it allows for sampling of tissue from the contralateral breast. Occult carcinomas have been found in approximately 4.5% of contralateral breast reduction specimens in patients undergoing a symmetry procedure for breast reconstruction.[10] Although the detection of occult carcinoma is not a reason to perform a contralateral breast reduction, it may provide a benefit for high-risk patients. Breast reduction surgery has also been shown to significantly reduce the risk of breast cancer, especially among women over the age of 40.[13]

The purpose of this chapter is to highlight the benefits of immediate reparative approaches using local tissue techniques to repair partial breast defects prior to the delivery of radiation therapy because such techniques maintain the color and texture of the breast. Patients who choose to undergo BCT often do so to limit the extent of surgery, and are therefore not eager to undergo a major secondary reconstructive procedure that is usually required after radiotherapy. Although the details of the operative approach will focus only on performing immediate repair using the remaining breast tissue, other techniques will be mentioned in the decision-making sections of the chapter, so that the clinician can determine the best approach for each individual patient given a variety of presenting circumstances.

INDICATIONS AND CONTRAINDICATIONS
(Box 7.1)

Timing of repair

Waiting to repair a large partial mastectomy deformity until after XRT usually necessitates a complex transfer of a large volume of autologous tissue, which many patients are unwilling to pursue. In addition, after XRT, the difficulties associated with secondary repair within an irradiated surgical field limit the use of the adjacent irradiated breast tissue, and breast implants are not a preferred option. In the case of severe deformities after BCT, the only option may be to abandon BCT and offer the patient a completion mastectomy with total breast reconstruction. However, the cosmetic outcomes of total breast reconstruction after BCT are less than optimal, owing to the inelasticity of the irradiated breast skin envelope and the increased risk of mastectomy skin flap necrosis.

BOX 7.1 Indications and contraindications

Indications
- Large-sized breast: D-cup bra or larger
- Ptotic-shaped breast
- Immediate repair before XRT
- Only required breast skin resection: (1) re-excision of a previous biopsy site or (2) anticipated skin resection is located within the Wise skin resection pattern
- Sufficient amount of breast tissue remaining after the partial mastectomy to result in a reconstructed breast with an adequate volume and a natural contour
- Low risk of having a positive margin on the permanent sections, even if the intraoperative tumor margin was negative

Relative contraindications
- Small-sized breast: C-cup bra or smaller
  - Medium or large tumor
  - Inner quadrant tumor
- Non-ptotic-shaped breast
- Delayed repair after XRT
- Insufficient volume of remaining breast tissue after partial mastectomy to reconstruct a breast with an adequate volume and a natural-appearing contour
- Concern that a negative intraoperative tumor margin may be positive on the permanent sections
- Extensive resection of breast skin located outside the Wise skin resection pattern

---

In the case of immediate repair, we prefer the use of local breast tissue because of the simplicity of these approaches and because such techniques maintain the color and texture of the breast. Although breast reduction is generally favored over local tissue rearrangement, the breast reduction technique is usually limited to patients with large breasts (D-cup bra size or larger). Local tissue rearrangement can be a good alternative for patients with moderate-sized breasts (B- or C-cup) who have minimal or no nipple ptosis, especially when the partial defect is located in the lower outer quadrant of the breast and involves minimal or no skin resection. Although we usually prefer immediate repair, if an unexpected deformity results after partial mastectomy or the tumor margin status is unclear at the time of the partial mastectomy, consideration should still be given to performing the repair prior to XRT. In these circumstances, we also prefer to use the remaining breast tissue.

Immediate reparative techniques also allow the plastic surgeon to participate in the planning of the incisions and the surgical approach to tumor resection. Even if reconstruction is not required (because the defect is smaller than anticipated, or the cancer is more extensive than anticipated and precludes partial mastectomy), the involvement of the plastic surgeon in preoperative planning simplifies any subsequent breast reconstruction that may be required.

Often, there is no choice but to perform a delayed reconstruction. Delayed reconstruction after XRT usually requires a latissimus dorsi musculocutaneous flap or thoracodorsal artery perforator flap; however, use of these flaps may increase the likelihood of lymphedema and may limit future reconstructive options. In some patients following XRT a contralateral breast reduction alone, without repair of the involved breast, will allow them to improve their symmetry while limiting the extent of the surgical procedure.

Impact of breast size on repair

As the role of BCT continues to expand, it is important to remember that most patients with an A-cup breast size, and even some patients with B- or C-cup sizes, are not candidates for BCT because of poor cosmetic outcomes. In these patients there is usually inadequate remaining breast tissue following BCT to perform a repair, thus necessitating the use of a vascularized tissue flap to correct the deformity. In small-breasted patients it may be preferable to perform a mastectomy with immediate total breast reconstruction to avoid the adverse effects of XRT on the breast skin envelope and the resultant abnormal position of the nipple–areola complex, which make these deformities so difficult to correct. However, in large-breasted patients in whom the partial mastectomy is predicted to result in a significant deformity, surgeons should consider incorporating immediate reparative techniques into the multidisciplinary care of patients with breast cancer who undergo BCT.

Following breast augmentation, women who have been diagnosed with breast cancer are sometimes considered for BCT. Although these women appear to have large breast volumes, most had A- or B-cup bra sizes prior to augmentation and should therefore be considered as small-volume. The fact is that patients with A- and B-cup size breasts are not good candidates for BCT because the resultant cosmetic outcome is poor. Unfortunately, some women in this category will have BCT and later present to a plastic surgeon because of infection, deformity, pain or implant displacement, requiring secondary operations. Subsequent reconstruction for these patients can be difficult because of the XRT; thus, the use of autologous tissue is necessary. Many of these patients will often require a complex microsurgical procedure, such as a gluteal flap, because small-breasted patients tend to have minimal adipose tissue in their lower abdominal regions. Better preoperative planning can potentially obviate these problems. For some, consideration of total mastectomy with immediate reconstruction may reduce the incidence of poor outcomes.

Women with moderate breast volume, especially those without breast ptosis, can also be a difficult management problem. Usually, these women are not considered good candidates for breast reduction because of insufficient residual breast tissue following the partial mastectomy, and because their lack of breast ptosis does not require any modification to the position of their nipple–areola complex. However, relatively small defects in these patients can be repaired with satisfactory outcomes using the local tissue rearrangement technique.

Influence of tumor margin status

Attention to tumor margin status prior to rearrangement of the breast parenchyma is of the utmost importance. If at the time of partial mastectomy the tumor margin status is unclear, or an unexpected deformity occurs after the partial mastectomy, consideration should still be given to performing the repair prior to XRT. In these circumstances, the use of the breast reduction technique is preferred.

Where there is preoperative or intraoperative concern regarding the ability to determine the adequacy of the tumor margins, the partial mastectomy wound is closed primarily without tissue rearrangement. After confirmation of negative margins, the repair is performed within several weeks of the partial mastectomy, and the start of XRT is not usually delayed. Good decisions regarding the approach to unexpected deformities after partial mastectomy require good communication between the breast surgeon and the plastic surgeon.

In the MD Anderson experience[14] only 5% of patients had a positive tumor margin after undergoing immediate repair after partial mastectomy. This relatively low rate of positive tumor margins reflects the large defect sizes that are usually encountered in patients who undergo partial mastectomy and require repair. This is lower than rates for positive margins in patients who do not undergo repair[15] because the defect sizes reported in such patients are usually smaller.

Given the low incidence of a positive tumor margin, immediate repair of the partial mastectomy defect can be considered. The experience at the MD Anderson Cancer Center has demonstrated that many of these women who are scheduled for delayed repair because of larger anticipated defects usually will proceed to completion mastectomy with immediate breast reconstruction and not additional re-excision.[14] The relatively low (5%) incidence of local recurrence of breast cancer[14] is further evidence of its safety, and should support the role of immediate repair of partial mastectomy defects using the breast reduction technique as a definitive method of breast reconstruction.

PREOPERATIVE HISTORY AND CONSIDERATIONS

A number of considerations regarding the repair of a partial mastectomy defect can be highlighted. To determine the optimal technique for each patient, consideration should be given to the following: the anticipated size and location of the breast skin defect, the proximity of the anticipated breast parenchymal defect to the nipple–areola complex, and whether the patient may require a lower abdominal flap (i.e., transverse rectus abdominis myocutaneous (TRAM) flap, deep inferior epigastric perforator (DIEP) flap, or superficial inferior epigastric artery (SIEA) flap) to repair the partial mastectomy defect.

Size and location of the skin defect

The anticipated size and location of the skin defect are essential factors in the decision regarding the most appropriate repair technique. When the breast skin resection (tumor extirpation) is located within the boundaries of the Wise pattern, the situation is ideal. When this skin to be resected is located outside the Wise pattern, it can be problematic. In such situations, consideration can be given to modifying the Wise skin pattern to incorporate the resected skin. If the skin to be resected involves only the re-excision of an existing biopsy site, and if there is an adequate skin bridge between the biopsy site and the Wise pattern, the biopsy site can be re-excised separately and the tumor extirpation performed through an access incision located along the superior or inferior limb of the Wise pattern. Although the appropriateness of a separate access incision for tumor resection is up to the breast surgeon, this approach can result in an optimal cosmetic outcome with minimal distortion of the breast shape.

Several options are available when an extensive skin resection is required outside the Wise pattern. The Wise pattern can be rotated in either a clockwise or a counterclockwise direction to encompass the skin resection. However, the resultant position of the vertical limb of the Wise pattern closure (not located in the inferior aspect of the breast) can result in a scar contracture, especially when the tumor is located in the medial aspect of the breast, resulting in a flattened contour and distortion of the breast shape. Another alternative, which has been described by Kroll and Singletary,[16] is a laterally based rotation–advancement flap of redundant axillary skin and subcutaneous tissue. Although excellent cosmetic results can be obtained with this local tissue rearrangement technique, especially with lateral defects, it may impair the ability to use lymphatic mapping to perform sentinel node biopsy and may further increase the potential for lymphedema. Axillary incisions can also decrease the blood supply to the mastectomy skin flaps, result in axillary contracture that can limit shoulder motion and increase shoulder pain, as well as adding additional scars to the reconstruction.

When a large amount of skin needs to be resected, many of the advantages of BCT are lost. When breast skin defects are so extensive that they must be repaired using a flap, further consideration should be given to whether BCT is the best option with respect to breast reconstruction. Although a latissimus dorsi flap can replace a large region of skin, its skin island has a different color and texture from the breast skin, which can lead to a less than ideal cosmetic outcome. Consideration should also be given to whether a latissimus dorsi flap alone will be able to provide an adequate tissue volume for the repair. If a breast implant will also be required, it may be preferable to perform a mastectomy with total breast reconstruction, as implants are not recommended in patients who have had or will have XRT.[17] In patients who are not candidates for a lower abdominal (TRAM, DIEP, or SIEA) flap breast reconstruction because of inadequate or excessive abdominal pannus, or abdominal scarring, a latissimus dorsi flap may use the only available autologous tissue source should the patient develop a local recurrence of breast cancer or a contour deformity after XRT.

Proximity of the breast parenchymal defect to the nipple–areola complex

Another important consideration in the decision regarding reconstructive technique is the proximity of the anticipated breast parenchymal defect to the nipple–areola complex. When the anticipated defect is centrally located (sub-areolar) within the breast, patients are advised preoperatively of the possibility that the only remaining blood supply to the nipple–areola complex after resection will be from the skin attachments, which may preclude the use of the breast reduction technique. Preoperatively the options are discussed, including the breast reduction technique using a free nipple graft and local rearrangement of the surrounding breast parenchyma without repositioning the nipple–areola complex (local tissue rearrangement). Patients are advised that when the local tissue rearrangement technique is used in such circumstances, the contralateral breast is not reduced at the time of repair because further recommendations are based on the cosmetic outcome.

Lower abdominal (TRAM, DIEP, or SIEA) flap is required to repair partial breast defect

The use of lower abdominal flaps to repair partial breast defects is generally discouraged. If the patient requires a lower abdominal flap for partial reconstruction it is usually better to complete the mastectomy and reconstruct the entire breast with the flap than to discard healthy lower abdominal tissue, especially as the remaining breast tissue

is still at risk for the subsequent development of malignancy. In case of a severe cosmetic deformity after partial mastectomy and XRT with a contracted breast skin envelope and malposition of the nipple–areola complex, it may also be preferable to perform a completion mastectomy with total breast reconstruction using an abdominal flap. The use of an abdominal flap to repair the partial mastectomy defect can result in discarding more tissue than is used. When repair of a complex breast deformity is necessary and is beyond the capacity of a latissimus dorsi musculocutaneous flap, alternative donor sites such as the abdomen are considered.

Women requiring complex reconstruction using microvascular techniques will require the use of recipient vessels. The internal mammary and the thoracodorsal arteries are usually considered. The use of the internal mammary blood vessels may preclude their use if further reconstruction is required in the future. However, it is often possible to reuse the internal mammary vessels as recipients in the event that an additional free flap is required. In addition, it has been shown that the thoracodorsal vessels are less often usable than the internal mammary vessels for delayed reconstruction after chest wall and axillary XRT.[18] Furthermore, the use of the thoracodorsal dorsal vessels as recipients for immediate reconstruction may prevent the use of an ipsilateral pedicled latissimus dorsi flap if a contour deformity were to occur as a consequence of XRT. As the practice of reconstruction after partial mastectomy continues to increase with the increasing potential that patients may require multiple flaps because of either adverse outcomes or local recurrence, we may need to increase our use of secondary recipient vessels, such as the retrograde internal mammary blood vessels.

Another option for immediate reconstruction after partial mastectomy that would preserve the ipsilateral internal mammary vessels in the event of a subsequent microvascular breast reconstruction would be a pedicled hemi-TRAM flap. This option would also preserve the latissimus dorsi flap in the event that it be needed to correct a subsequent deformity following the radiation. An ipsilateral pedicled TRAM flap (only prograde internal mammary vessels remain available) could be considered if a reasonable amount of time accrued for establishment of a local blood supply to the TRAM flap prior to further reconstruction. The amount of fatty tissue usually required for reconstruction after partial mastectomy can be provided reliably by a pedicled hemi-TRAM flap because it requires less tissue than for a total breast reconstruction. However, in women who have had delayed reconstruction of a partial mastectomy defect with a TRAM flap and subsequently require the division of the internal mammary vessels to perform a microvascular total breast reconstruction, the establishment of a local blood supply to the TRAM flap may not be as reliable and may compromise the blood supply and jeopardize the viability of the flap. Ultimately, the use of a TRAM flap may not be the best option for repair of the partial mastectomy defect because it is most suitable for total breast reconstruction. In addition, the TRAM flap can also easily reconstruct both breasts if a contralateral breast cancer were to develop, and provides adequate tissue for even large-breasted patients.

OPERATIVE APPROACH

As emphasized throughout this chapter, we prefer immediate repair of partial mastectomy defects using local breast tissue (local tissue rearrangement or breast reduction techniques) because of the simplicity of these approaches and because techniques using local tissue maintain the color and texture of the breast. Although breast reduction is generally favored over local tissue rearrangement, this technique can be a good alternative for defects that are small relative to the breast size, especially when there is minimal or no skin resection.

Local tissue rearrangement

Although there are many methods of local tissue rearrangement, it may be preferable to avoid additional skin incisions and perform a 'remodeling of the breast' with complete freeing and release of the breast skin envelope from the underlying breast parenchyma. The attached parenchyma, with its preserved blood supply, is plicated together to recreate the contour of the breast mound. Fatty tissue from the axillary region can also be mobilized into the breast to supplement any volume deficiency. The previously freed skin envelope is then redraped over the recontoured breast mound. This approach does not require the position of the nipple–areola complex to be changed (ideal for non-ptotic breast shapes). If excision of the breast skin is not required, the partial mastectomy can be performed through a circumferential incision around the nipple–areola complex. Using this approach, most tumors are easily accessible for resection. The avoidance of additional incisions on the breast skin can improve the cosmetic outcome if a completion mastectomy with immediate total reconstruction is subsequently found to be required because of positive margins on the permanent pathology.

Breast reduction technique

At the MD Anderson Cancer Center, the majority of partial mastectomy defect repairs use the breast reduction technique. Probably the most important consideration in the decision regarding the design of the dermoglandular pedicle to perform the repair is the location of the tumor. In order to design the dermoglandular pedicle, we have formulated 'zone designations' based on tumor location (Fig. 7.1).

Most commonly, we use an inferiorly based dermoglandular pedicle. It is likely that the widespread use of the inferior pedicle in standard reduction mammoplasty has made our surgeons more familiar with use of this pedicle design and more comfortable with modifying it, which is often required with repair of partial mastectomy defects. We also tend to find more favorable cosmetic outcomes with an inferior pedicle[14] because it maintains inferior pole projection and incorporates into the Wise skin resection pattern, which we have found to be particularly useful with

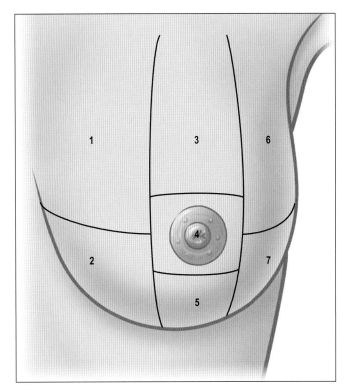

FIGURE 7.1 Zone designations of the breast based on tumor location used to determine the optimal design for the dermoglandular pedicle to repair a partial mastectomy defect.

repair of partial mastectomy defects; and, if required, the inferior pedicle can easily be modified to accommodate a free nipple graft.

When the inferiorly based dermoglandular pedicle is used to repair a partial mastectomy defect, we have begun to modify the standard design (Fig. 7.2). The most common modification is the inferomedial pedicle, which, when compared with a standard inferior pedicle, may provide an enhanced blood supply to the nipple–areola complex because it retains the medial wedge of breast tissue that is usually discarded with a standard inferior pedicle design. When a standard inferior pedicle is impinged upon by the tumor resection, the pedicle is extended medially (the least frequent location for breast cancer) to increase the blood supply (intercostals and internal mammary perforating blood vessels) and the volume of breast tissue available for repair.

Most likely, the additional medial wedge of breast tissue retained with the inferomedial pedicle reduces the incidence of complications by reducing dead space, especially in the repair of upper inner quadrant (zone 1) defects, which we have found to be associated with a relatively high incidence of complications when the medial wedge is not retained. In addition, in patients with very large breasts having a long distance between the nipple–areola complex and the inframammary fold, the additional blood supply provided by the inferomedial pedicle may improve the viability of the nipple–areola complex and reduce the need for conversion to a free nipple graft.

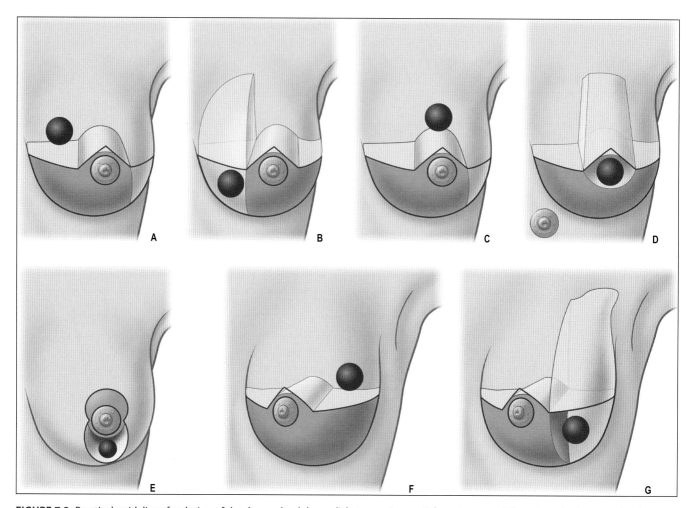

FIGURE 7.2 Practical guidelines for design of the dermoglandular pedicle to repair a partial mastectomy defect using the breast reduction technique, by tumor location. **A** Upper inner quadrant (zone 1). Inferomedial pedicle. Retained medial component fills the defect upon closure of the Wise skin pattern and maintains the cleavage of the breast. **B** Lower inner quadrant (zone 2). Inferolateral pedicle. Retained lateral component provides additional blood supply to the nipple–areola complex if tumor resection encroaches on the inferior pedicle. A thick layer of subcutaneous tissue is maintained on the medial aspect of the Wise skin pattern flap to fill the defect upon closure of the Wise pattern and maintain cleavage of the breast. **C** Upper central quadrant (zone 3). Inferomedial pedicle. Retained medial component provides a cosmetic advantage and additional blood supply to the nipple–areola complex in patients with very large ptotic breasts, possibly obviating the need for a free nipple graft. **D** Middle central quadrant (zone 4). Amputative design with free nipple graft and maintenance of a thick layer of subcutaneous tissue on the central aspect of the Wise skin pattern flap to fill the defect and improve contour. **E** Lower central quadrant (zone 5). Vertical scar reduction mammoplasty. **F** Upper outer quadrant (zone 6). Inferomediolateral pedicle. Retained lateral component fills the defect upon closure of the Wise skin pattern and retained medial component provides cosmetic advantage. **G** Lower outer quadrant (zone 7). Inferomedial pedicle. Retained medial component provides a cosmetic advantage and additional blood supply to the nipple–areola complex if lateral resection encroaches on the blood supply to the complex. A thick layer of subcutaneous tissue is maintained on the lateral aspect of the Wise skin pattern flap to fill the defect.

The wedge of medial breast tissue retained with the inferomedial pedicle can also provide significant cosmetic benefits, especially for repairs after resection of tumors located in the upper inner quadrant (zone 1), a notoriously difficult location in which to provide an adequate volume of tissue for repair (Figs 7.3 and 7.4). Compared to other dermoglandular pedicles, we have found that the inferomedial pedicle also enhances the cosmetic outcomes of most repairs that use the breast reduction technique in the lower outer (zone 7) (Fig. 7.5) and upper central (zone 3) (Fig. 7.6) quadrants of the breast. For defects in zone 7, the cosmetic result can be improved further by retaining the thickness

of breast tissue on the lateral Wise pattern skin flap. The retained medial wedge of breast tissue increases the fullness in the medial aspect of the repaired breast, which improves the flattened appearance that tends to occur with the use of a standard inferior pedicle. It also augments the cleavage of the breast, which improves the cosmetic outcomes in large-breasted patients, in whom we perform the majority of partial mastectomy repairs.

However, there are several quadrants of the breast in which an inferomedial pedicle is not preferred. For defects located in the lower inner quadrant (zone 2), we usually use an inferolateral pedicle and compensate for the loss of

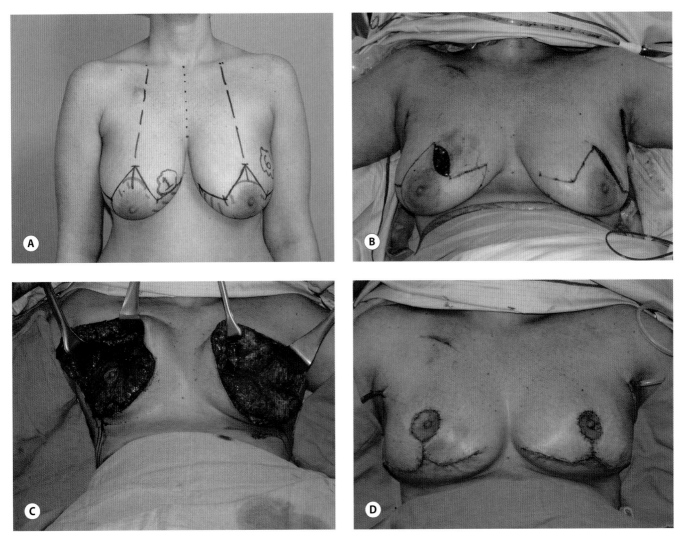

FIGURE 7.3 A 39-year-old woman with D-cup size breasts who presented with a T2N3 tumor in the left breast and a T2N0 tumor in the right breast. She had neoadjuvant chemotherapy with an excellent response and desired BCT. Preoperative markings for a tumor in right breast (zone 1) and a tumor in left breast (zone 6). **B** Access incisions to perform the tumor resections as well as for the right axillary sentinel lymph node biopsy and the left level I and II axillary lymph node dissection. **C** Intraoperative view after tumor resection showing extirpative defects and dermoglandular pedicle designs. The defect in the right breast was repaired using an inferomedial pedicle, and an inferomediolateral pedicle was used to repair the left breast. **D** Intraoperative view after repairs. Notice how the retained medial wedge of breast tissue filled the defect (zone 1) in the right breast and how the retained lateral wedge of breast tissue filled the defect (zone 6) in the left breast.

tissue by retaining the thickness of breast tissue on the medial Wise pattern skin flap. For defects located in the upper outer quadrant (zone 6) (Fig. 7.3), we often use an inferomediolateral pedicle. The lateral component fills the defect and the medial component provides the previously mentioned cosmetic advantages and enhances the blood supply to the nipple–areola complex. For defects located in the direct vicinity of the inferior pedicle along the breast meridian (lower central quadrant: zone 5) (Fig. 7.7), we often use a superior pedicle with a vertical skin reduction pattern. This tends to be the only circumstance in which a Wise skin resection pattern is not preferred.

When the anticipated defect is centrally located in the breast underlying the nipple–areola complex, we advise patients preoperatively that the only remaining blood supply to the complex after tumor resection may be from the skin attachments, which may preclude the use of the standard breast reduction technique. In this setting, the surgical options, including the breast reduction technique (inferomediolateral pedicle) with a free nipple graft or local rearrangement of the surrounding remaining breast parenchyma without repositioning of the nipple–areola complex, are discussed with the patient preoperatively. In the circumstance of local tissue rearrangement, the contralateral breast is not reduced at the time of the repair. Rather, if the cosmetic outcome is unacceptable, consideration is given to proceeding with a completion mastectomy and total breast reconstruction, thereby avoiding the adverse effects of XRT.

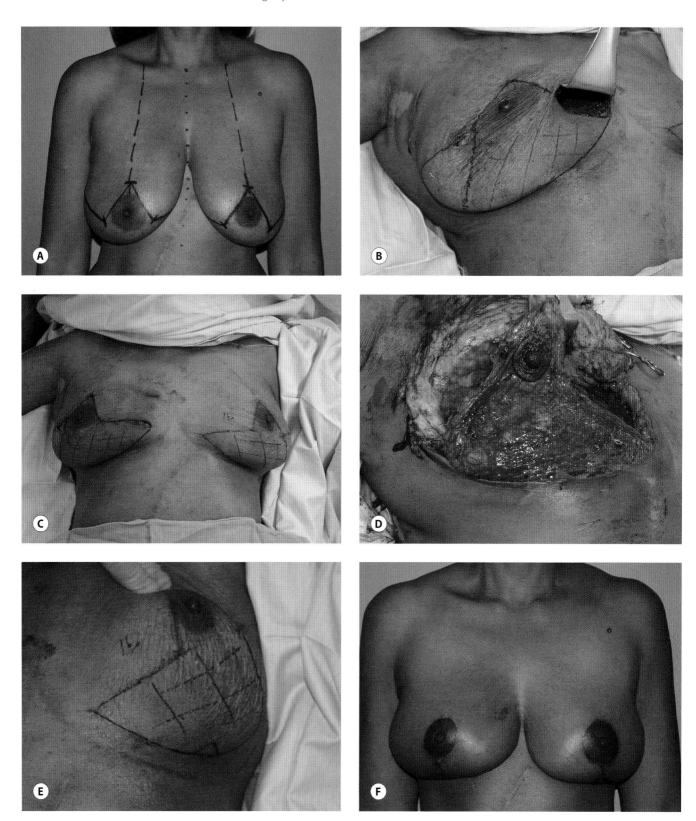

FIGURE 7.4 Breast repair after partial mastectomy in a 46-year-old woman with a 38D bra size who presented with a T1N0 (stage I) invasive ductal carcinoma in the upper inner quadrant of the right breast. **A** Preoperative view. Wise skin pattern markings in preparation for reconstruction with the breast reduction technique. **B, C** Intraoperative views after partial mastectomy (resection weight of 80 g) showing the defect (7% of the initial breast volume) (zone 1) of the breast. Re-excision at the previous biopsy site was performed separately from the tumor resection, which was performed through an access incision along the superior limb of the Wise pattern. **D** Immediate repair of the defect was performed using an inferomedial pedicle (additional tissue resected in performing the reconstruction weighed 60 g). **E** A contralateral breast reduction was also performed to achieve symmetry (weight of tissue resected from the contralateral breast was 110 g). **F** Postoperative view 6 weeks after repair showing how the retained medial wedge of breast tissue filled the defect in zone 1. In addition, the re-excised biopsy site was barely noticeable and did not detract from the appearance of the breast.

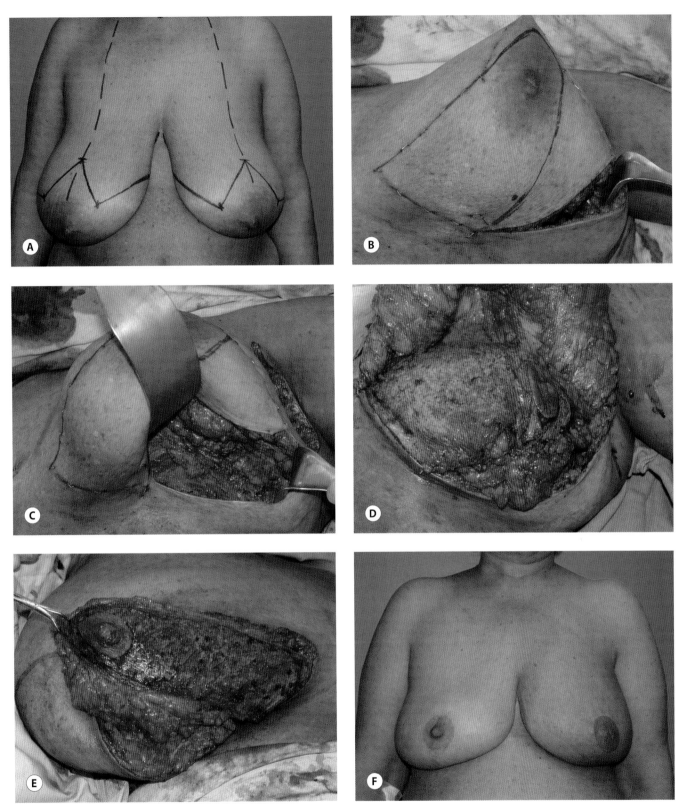

FIGURE 7.5 Breast reconstruction after partial mastectomy and radiation therapy in a 57-year-old woman with a 38DD bra size who presented with a T3N1 (stage III) invasive ductal carcinoma of the left breast (zone 7). **A** Preoperative view. The patient received neoadjuvant chemotherapy and the tumor responded well to the treatment. **B, C** Intraoperative views after a partial mastectomy (resection weight of 252 g) and a left level I and II axillary node dissection. The tumor resection was performed through an access incision along the inferior limb of the Wise pattern. **D** The resultant defect, which corresponded to 18% of the initial breast volume, was immediately repaired with an inferomedial pedicle (additional tissue resected in performing the repair was 325 g). Although the tumor resection encroached on the inferior component of the pedicle, it preserved the blood supply to the medial aspect. **E** Although not currently practiced, the right breast reduction was performed after the left breast reconstruction but at the same surgery, also using an inferomedial pedicle (weight of tissue resected from the right breast was 635 g). **F** Postoperative views 10 months after repair and 8 months after radiation therapy. Note the fullness in the medial aspect of the breasts and the smooth contour of the reconstructed lower outer quadrant of the left breast. (**A** and **F** reproduced with permission from Boice JD Jr, Persson I, Brinton LA, et al. Breast cancer following breast reduction surgery in Sweden. Plast Reconstruct Surg 2000; 106: 755.)

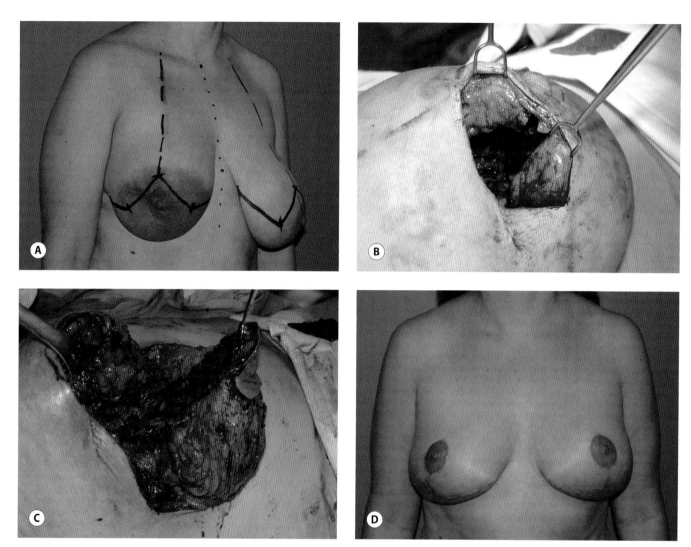

FIGURE 7.6 Unexpected deformity after partial mastectomy requiring delayed repair prior to radiation therapy. This 41-year-old woman presented 2 weeks after undergoing a partial mastectomy for a central quadrant tumor. The patient was very dissatisfied with the result and understood that the cosmetic outcome would be further adversely affected by the radiation therapy. **A** Preoperative view. Wise skin pattern markings in preparation for partial mastectomy repair with the breast reduction technique. **B** Because the extent and exact location of central resection (presumed zone 3) could not be determined preoperatively, the nipple–areola complex was explored to determine whether there was an adequate blood supply before the breast reduction technique was begun. **C** Intraoperative view demonstrates that the blood supply retained to the nipple–areola complex was adequate for repair with an inferomedial pedicle. **D** Postoperative views 3 months after repair. The patient was happy with the result, as was the breast surgeon.

Our results indicate that contralateral breast reduction for symmetry is necessary in 95% of women following repair of a partial mastectomy defect.[14] Our practice is to delay the contralateral reduction until the ipsilateral radiation therapy has been completed. When the contralateral breast reduction for symmetry is performed prior to the XRT, the ipsilateral repaired breast may become larger (chronically edematous due to impaired lymphatic drainage) or smaller (radiation-induced fat necrosis with subsequent atrophy) than the contralateral breast when it is reduced at the same time as the repair of the ipsilateral breast. However, the optimal timing to perform the contralateral breast reduction for symmetry will probably vary for each patient, and will be indicated when the size of the repaired breast remains unchanged.

OPTIMIZING OUTCOMES OF THE BREAST REDUCTION TECHNIQUE (Box 7.2)

Complications and side effects

Probably the two most important factors in reducing the potential for complications during repair of partial mastectomy defects are timing and technique (Fig. 7.8). Immediate repair of partial mastectomy defects before XRT is safer than delayed repair after XRT, and is the authors' preferred option. In our experience,[14] complication rates were 30% for the repair of partial mastectomy defects overall, 26% for immediate repair, and 42% for delayed repair. The higher risk of complications with delayed repair was mainly related to the fact that irradiated tissues have a reduced capacity for wound healing and respond poorly to surgery.

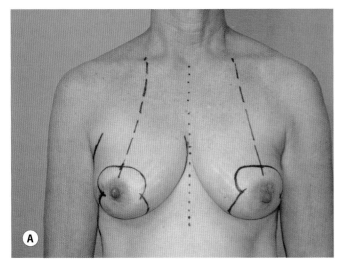

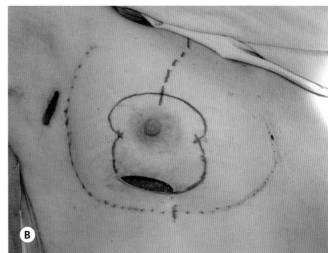

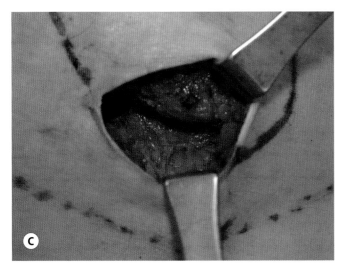

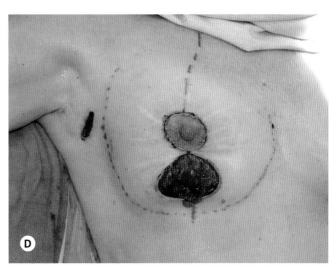

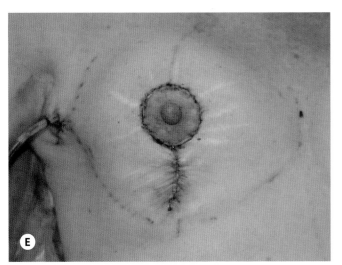

FIGURE 7.7 Repair of a partial mastectomy defect in a 52-year-old woman with a T2 tumor (zone 5) of the right breast. **A** Preoperative markings with a vertical skin reduction pattern. **B** Intraoperative view of the access incision used by the breast surgeon to perform the tumor resection. **C** Intraoperative view of the defect (zone 5). **D** Intraoperative view during the repair with a superior dermoglandular pedicle. **E** Intraoperative view after completion of the repair. Over the next several months the fullness in the superior aspect of the repaired breast is expected to descend inferiorly to fill the lower poles.

BOX 7.2 Optimizing outcomes of the breast reduction technique

- Important to include either the medial or lateral wedge of breast tissue as part of the dermoglandular pedicle to ensure an adequate blood supply to the nipple–areola complex
- Whenever feasible, include the medial wedge with the dermoglandular pedicle (excluding zone 2 defects), in order to optimize the cosmetic outcome by retaining the fullness in the medial aspect of the repaired breast
- To prevent delayed wound healing, avoid positioning of the Wise skin resection pattern within the inframammary fold
- In order to optimize breast symmetry:
  - Defer the contralateral breast reduction for symmetry until after the completion of XRT, to allow adequate time for the repaired ipsilateral breast to assume its final size (radiation-induced fat necrosis with subsequent atrophy)
  - Perform the same dermoglandular pedicle design for the contralateral breast symmetry procedure as was used for the repair of the partial mastectomy defect of the ipsilateral breast
- Preoperatively, coordinate skin incision placement with the breast surgeon:
  - Prefer to access the tumor for resection using a skin incision along or within the Wise skin pattern
  - Prefer to only re-excise a previous biopsy site if it is located outside the Wise skin pattern
- To reduce the occurrence of wound dehiscence and delayed wound healing at the T-junction upon closure of the Wise skin pattern, consider including a triangular piece of breast skin located within the Wise pattern along the inferior edge, located centrally within the breast meridian

Reparative technique	Timing of reconstruction		
	All reconstruction	Immediate reconstruction	Delayed reconstruction
LTR	30%	21%	50%
BR	29%	24%	50%
FLAP	38%	67%	20%

FIGURE 7.8 Complication rates of various reparative techniques associated with the repair of partial mastectomy defects. LTR, local tissue rearrangement; BR, breast reduction; FLAP, latissimus dorsi myocutaneous flap.

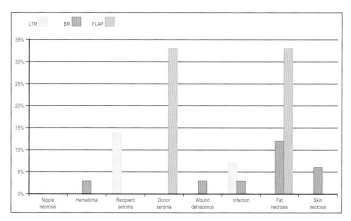

FIGURE 7.9 Specific complications observed with immediate repair after partial mastectomy with various reparative techniques. LTR, local tissue rearrangement; BR, breast reduction; FLAP, latissimus dorsi myocutaneous flap.

In the setting of immediate repair before XRT, the use of the breast reduction technique was associated with reasonable rates of complications and minimal side effects;[14] however, it is imperative to select the dermoglandular pedicle design with the lowest risk for complications, while still optimizing the cosmetic outcome. Complications observed with immediate repair after partial mastectomy using local tissue or the breast reduction technique were similar to those commonly seen with standard reduction mammoplasty (Fig. 7.9).[14] On the other hand, delayed repair resulted in a high incidence of complications, often associated with poor wound healing in previously irradiated tissues (Fig. 7.10).[14] These complications were especially evident with the local tissue rearrangement and breast reduction techniques.

When performing the breast reduction technique, it is imperative to limit the amount of undermining of the remaining breast tissue to avoid fat necrosis. Seroma formation and infection can be reduced by limiting the formation of dead space within the repaired breast. Upon closure of the Wise skin pattern, dead space is filled by advancing the breast tissue adjacent to the defect. Closed-suction drains can also reduce the potential for seroma formation, especially as many of these patients will also have removal of axillary lymph nodes.

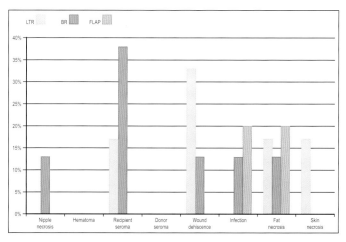

FIGURE 7.10 Specific complications observed with delayed repair after partial mastectomy with various reparative techniques. LTR, local tissue rearrangement; BR, breast reduction; FLAP, latissimus dorsi myocutaneous flap.

A preoperative discussion between the plastic and breast surgeon to determine the location for the skin incisions will not only improve the cosmetic outcome but also reduce the potential for complications. Often, the breast surgeon can access the tumor through a skin incision located along the

Clinical Pearls

- Discourage the use of breast implants to repair partial mastectomy defects after XRT

- Latissimus dorsi flaps are most commonly used to repair partial mastectomy defects located in the outer quadrants of the breast

- The increasing presence of ambulatory care surgery centers may be the ideal setting to perform immediate repair of partial mastectomy defects

- The participation of a plastic surgeon in planning for partial mastectomy is crucial: the plastic surgeon can indicate to patients and referring breast surgeons which patients, from a cosmetic point of view, would benefit from a total mastectomy with immediate reconstruction rather than from a partial mastectomy

- Often, the breast surgeon can use a skin incision located along or within the Wise pattern to perform the tumor resection

- If there is concern regarding the adequacy of the intraoperative tumor margin, the wound can be closed primarily and the defect repaired subsequently (within several weeks) after obtaining a negative margin on the permanent sections

- Immediate reparative techniques allow the plastic surgeon to participate in the planning of the incisions and the surgical approach to tumor resection:
  - Even if a repair is not required at the time of the partial mastectomy (because the defect is smaller than anticipated, or the cancer is more extensive than anticipated and precludes partial mastectomy), the involvement of the plastic surgeon in preoperative planning simplifies any subsequent breast reconstruction that may be required

- In small-breasted patients, consider total instead of a partial mastectomy to avoid the adverse effects of XRT on the breast skin envelope

Potential Complications/Pitfalls

- Caution is advised in performing revision procedures on the repaired breast after XRT

- In order to preserve reconstructive options in the event that a mastectomy will be required, because of either a positive margin on the permanent sections a local recurrence, avoid the use of a lower abdominal flap (TRAM, DIEP, or SIEA) to repair a partial mastectomy defect

- When a large amount of breast skin needs to be resected with the partial mastectomy, many of the advantages of BCT are lost

- When the anticipated defect is centrally located (directly underlying the nipple–areola complex), patients are advised preoperatively of the possibility that the only remaining blood supply to the nipple–areola complex after resection will be from the skin attachments, which may preclude the use of the breast reduction technique

- In patients who are not candidates for a lower abdominal flap (TRAM, DIEP, or SIEA) breast reconstruction (because of inadequate or excessive abdominal pannus, or abdominal scarring), use of a latissimus dorsi flap may remove the only available autologous tissue option should the patient develop a local recurrence of breast cancer or a contour deformity after XRT

- Patients who choose to undergo BCT often do so to limit the extent of surgery, and therefore are not eager to undergo a major reconstructive secondary procedure after completion of BCT

- Performing a delayed repair of a partial mastectomy defect after XRT with a latissimus dorsi flap may increase the propensity for or worsen lymphedema owing to the need to dissect the vascular pedicle with the irradiated axilla

- When performing the breast reduction technique to repair the ipsilateral breast, avoid performing the contralateral breast reduction for symmetry until after XRT, to allow adequate time for the repaired breast to attain its final size (radiation-induced fat necrosis with subsequent atrophy)

- Encourage the use of a separate axillary incision to perform the lymphadenectomy (axillary sentinel lymph node biopsy or complete axillary lymph node dissection) to avoid the need to undermine and subsequently decrease the blood supply to the lateral Wise skin flap

Wise pattern. This approach, along with the use of separate axillary incision to perform a sentinel lymph biopsy or a complete axillary node dissection, can minimize the need to undermine the lateral Wise skin flap, which can reduce its blood supply. In marking the Wise pattern, the inclusion of a triangular piece of breast skin located along the inferior edge of the Wise pattern and centrally within the breast meridian can also reduce the potential for delayed wound healing. The triangular piece of skin allows for the leading edges of the medial and lateral Wise skin flaps to be trimmed prior to inset, and also reduces the tension at the T-junction closure.

not removed for several weeks because of the associated axillary lymph node dissection that accompanies many of these procedures. Any healing problems are usually managed with local wound care and are allowed to heal secondarily. Any revision procedures to the repaired breast after XRT are usually discouraged.

POSTOPERATIVE CARE

Postoperatively, the patient is instructed to use a non-underwired support bra. The closed-suction drain is usually

CONCLUSION

There are no exact measures to determine which patients will or will not benefit from partial mastectomy reconstruction. Most patients with medium-sized or large breasts will probably benefit from immediate repair, but some patients with small breasts may not. The participation of a plastic surgeon in planning for partial mastectomy is crucial: the plastic surgeon can indicate to patients and referring breast surgeons which patients, from a cosmetic point of view, would benefit more from a total mastectomy with breast reconstruction than from a partial mastectomy. Although these considerations should prove useful in the decision-making process, ultimately it is up to the multidisciplinary breast team who, along with the patient, should determine which is the best approach.

Ultimately, until we consider the repair of partial mastectomy defects as a 'routine' method of immediate breast reconstruction we will not make a significant impact on preventing these deformities and improving the quality of life of our patients. These objectives can be best accomplished by continuing to educate and referring physicians to the benefits that repair of partial mastectomy defects prior to XRT can provide. The increasing provision of ambulatory care surgery centers may be the ideal setting to perform immediate repair of partial mastectomy defects in order to ease the scheduling burden that often discourages its use.

REFERENCES

1. Cance WG, Carey LA, Calvo BF, et al. Long-term outcome of neoadjuvant therapy for locally advanced breast cancer. Ann Surg 2002; 236: 295.
2. Shen J, Valero V, Buchholz T, et al. Effective local control and long-term survival in patients with T4 locally advanced breast cancer treated with breast conversation therapy. Ann Surg Oncol 2004; 11: 854.
3. Chen AM, Meric-Bernstam F, Hunt KK, et al. Breast conservation after neoadjuvant chemotherapy: the MD Anderson Cancer Center Experience. J Clin Oncol 2004; 22: 2303.
4. Bajaj AK, Kon PS, Oberg KC, et al. Aesthetic outcomes in patients undergoing breast conservation therapy for the treatment of localized breast cancer. Plast Reconstruct Surg 2004; 114: 1442.
5. Clough KB, Kroll SS, Audretsch W. An approach to repair of partial mastectomy defects. Plast Reconstruct Surg 1999; 104: 409.
6. Clough KB, Nos C, Salomon RJ, et al. Conservative treatment of breast cancers by mammaplasty and irradiation: a new approach to lower quadrant tumors. Plast Reconstruct Surg 1995; 96: 363.
7. Matory WE, Werthheimer M, Fitzgerald TJ, et al. Aesthetic results following partial mastectomy and radiation therapy. Plast Reconstruct Surg 1990; 85: 739.
8. Slavin SA, Love SM, Sadowsky NL. Reconstruction of the radiated partial mastectomy defect with autogenous tissues. Plast Reconstruct Surg 1992; 90: 854.
9. Clough KB, Cuminet J, Fitoussi A, et al. Cosmetic sequelae after conservative treatment for breast cancer: classification and results of surgical correction. Ann Plast Surg 1998; 41: 471.
10. Rietjends M, Petit JY, Contesso G. The role of reduction mammaplasty in oncology. Eur J Plast Surg 1997; 20: 246.
11. Losken A, Elwood ET, Styblo TM, et al. The role of reduction mammaplasty in reconstructing partial mastectomy defects. Plast Reconstruct Surg 2002; 109: 968.
12. Smith ML, Evans GR, Gurlek A, et al. Reduction mammaplasty: its role in breast conservation surgery for early-stage breast cancer. Ann Plast Surg 1998; 41: 234.
13. Boice JD Jr, Persson I, Brinton LA, et al. Breast cancer following breast reduction surgery in Sweden. Plast Reconstruct Surg 2000; 106: 755.
14. Kronowitz SJ, Feledy JA, Hunt KK, et al. Determining the optimal approach to breast reconstruction after partial mastectomy. Plast Reconstruct Surg 2006; 117: 1.
15. Pawlik TM, Perry A, Strom EA, et al. Potential applicability of balloon catheter-based accelerated partial breast irradiation after conservative surgery for breast carcinoma. Cancer 2004; 100: 490.
16. Kroll SS, Singletary SE. Repair of partial mastectomy defects. Clin Plast Surg 1998; 25: 303.
17. Spear SL, Onyewu C. Staged breast reconstruction with saline-filled implants in the irradiated breast: recent trends and therapeutic implications. Plast Reconstruct Surg 2000; 105: 930.
18. Temple CL, Strom EA, Youssef A, et al. Choice of recipient vessels in delayed TRAM flap breast reconstruction after radiotherapy. Plast Reconstruct Surg 2005; 115: 105.

Mastopexy

Kristin A. Boehm and Foad Nahai

Throughout time, the female breast has been an organ of functional as well as aesthetic significance. Composed of connective tissue, adipose, and glandular elements, the breast is exposed to almost constant physiologic alterations in a woman's lifecycle, extending from puberty to late adulthood. Factors such as pregnancy, lactation, weight fluctuation, and gravity inevitably lead to diminished elasticity, changes in fat content, and elongation of connective tissue supporting elements, thereby altering breast form and contour. The result is mammary ptosis.

Ptosis refers to the relative descent of the nipple–areolar complex in relation to the breast mound and inframammary fold. Although there is some degree of variability as to the numeric measurements that constitute the aesthetically ideal breast,[1–3] it is almost universally accepted that such a breast has minimal ptosis and a nipple–areolar complex centrally located at the most projecting part of the breast mound. This desire to recreate a youthful, non-ptotic breast has fueled ongoing research and surgical refinement of mastopexy procedures. A mastopexy reconstructs a ptotic breast by repositioning the nipple–areolar complex and creating an aesthetically pleasing breast mound. Statistical evidence points to the fact that surgical correction of mammary ptosis has become an increasingly popular procedure. According to the American Society for Aesthetic Plastic Surgery, 125 896 mastopexies were performed in 2006, representing a 4% increase from the previous year and a 533% increase since 1997.[4] Such clinical relevance has prompted innovators in plastic surgery to reconsider ways to safely and successfully optimize postoperative breast form.[5–7] The result has been numerous published mastopexy techniques, all of which strive to elevate the nipple–areolar complex, restore superior pole breast fullness, and minimize scarring.

ANATOMY

At maturity, the female breast extends from the level of the second or third rib inferiorly to the inframammary fold, which is typically located at the level of the sixth or seventh rib. Along the transverse axis, it extends from the lateral border of the sternum to the anterior axillary line. The glandular elements take on a protuberant, conical form, the base of which ranges from 10 to 12 cm. The nipple is usually located at the level of the fourth intercostal space, with a natural nipple–areola to breast proportion of approximately 1 : 3.[8]

The breast itself is a combination of adipose tissue and lobes of glandular tissue surrounded by fibrous connective tissue. Its posterior surface is defined by a layer of superficial fascia which interdigitates with the pectoral fascia of the chest wall. The suspensory ligaments of Cooper pass between lobules of breast tissue and extend from the superficial fascia to the dermis of the breast skin envelope. These bands provide structural support for the glandular elements of the breast while simultaneously permitting mobility. The density of adipose tissue and glandular tissue can vary significantly in response to several factors and ultimately cause elongation of the breast's supportive structural network. Hormonal changes inherent in pregnancy and lactation engorge a woman's breast tissue and invariably expand the skin and underlying breast architecture. In a number of women, particularly those who are larger-breasted to begin with, tissue elasticity and recoil are not sufficient to reverse these changes once the pregnancy is complete, leaving a permanent change in breast contour and position. Over time, breast implants can have a similar effect in terms of stressing the breast's supportive network and contributing to mammary ptosis. Body weight fluctuation can also alter breast volume and cause elongation of the supportive network. If significant enough, the tissues may not accommodate even with weight loss, leaving stretched skin and connective tissues that do little to maintain breast shape. This is perhaps most clearly demonstrated in the bariatric patient population, who in the course of their weight loss typically experience significant breast volume involution and develop rather severe grades of ptosis and skin excess. Age too can diminish the amount of glandular tissue, leaving overstretched supportive elements and loose skin that cannot counteract the constant effects of gravity pulling the breast downward on the chest wall.

INDICATIONS FOR MASTOPEXY

Although ptosis may have several etiologies, it is nonetheless the common underlying denominator in women undergoing mastopexy procedures. Various degrees of ptosis have been well described, and the resultant classification system can help surgeons to choose the surgical technique that will optimize results. Probably the oldest and most commonly used description is that of Regnault.[9] Regnault's system relies upon the position of the nipple–areolar complex relative to the inframammary fold to define the severity of ptosis. First-degree ptosis is characterized by a nipple situated 1 cm from the inframammary fold, above the lower contour of the breast. In second-degree ptosis the nipple is 1–3 cm below the inframammary fold but not yet at the lowest contour of the breast. Third-degree ptosis is defined by a nipple more than 3 cm below the inframammary fold and at the lowest contour of the breast gland. A fourth condition, called glandular ptosis or pseudoptosis, occurs when the breast tissue falls below the inframammary crease but the nipple itself is at or above the level of the fold (Fig. 8.1).

PREOPERATIVE CONSIDERATIONS

In evaluating potential mastopexy patients it is important to not only quantify the degree of ptosis, but also to assess skin quality and breast parenchyma volume. Characteristics such as skin thickness and the presence of striae can be indicators of skin elasticity and the potential to contribute to postoperative shape control. In patients with an excess of glandular tissue the additional weight may actually be contributing to the ptosis, and some parenchymal resection should be considered. By contrast, patients with a relative paucity of breast tissue may have significant upper pole hollowing, which may be difficult to correct without simultaneous implant placement.

Many surgeons find mastopexy procedures somewhat problematic and unsatisfying because any improvement achieved is at best temporary. Gravity and the aging process begin almost immediately to counteract the newly uplifted breast position. In contrast, the resultant scars are permanent even if the ptosis correction is not. It is therefore imperative to have an in-depth conversation with patients considering mastopexy about realistic expectations and potential complications. Patients need to consider whether the visible scars justify the improvement in shape. They need to understand that the shape and upper pole fullness so easily recreated with manual repositioning of the breast on the chest wall are very challenging to achieve surgically, and some degree of superior flattening or skin excess may persist postoperatively. Breasts may appear somewhat smaller following a mastopexy, and the only way to add volume, particularly for upper-pole fullness, is with an implant, which has its own set of attendant complications. Risks of asymmetry, altered sensation and nipple–areolar necrosis bear mentioning.

TECHNIQUES

The ideal mastopexy achieves long-standing correction of breast ptosis with minimal scarring. There is no shortage of published techniques that strive to meet this goal. A recent study of mastopexy preferences among board-certified plastic surgeons categorized these techniques according to the location of the incision: inverted T, short

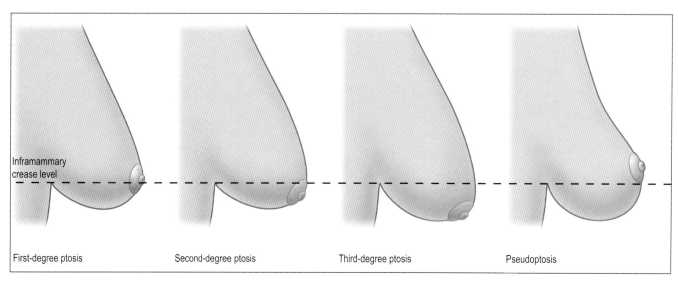

Inframammary crease level

First-degree ptosis   Second-degree ptosis   Third-degree ptosis   Pseudoptosis

FIGURE 8.1 Classification of breast ptosis.

scar, and periareolar.[10] Study data revealed that whereas inverted-T procedures remain the most popular, there is an increase in the number of surgeons performing short-scar techniques, which incidentally had the highest patient and physician satisfaction rate.

Author's preferred technique: vertical scar mastopexy

The vertical mastopexy procedures as popularized by Lassus[11,12] and Lejour[5,13] elevate the nipple–areolar complex based on a superior pedicle. This relies on the creation of lower-pole medial and lateral pillars which, when sutured together, provide support, elevation, and narrowing of the breast width. The superior pedicle is invaginated in such a way as to create retroareolar projection and superior pole fill.

The new nipple position is marked preoperatively by placing a finger in the inframammary crease and transposing this level anteriorly on to the breast along the marked breast meridian (Fig. 8.2). This new nipple site ranges between 10 and 14 cm from the midline and 18–22 cm from the suprasternal notch. These distances can be compared between the two sides and adjusted to achieve optimal symmetry. The vertical axis of the breast should be marked from the inframammary crease on to the abdomen somewhere between 10 and 14 cm from the midline. This is then used to determine the medial and lateral markings. The medial marking is made by pushing the breast laterally and then continuing the vertical axis located beneath the inframammary fold superiorly up on to the breast. The lateral mark is made in the same manner but by pushing the breast medially. A curve located 1–3 cm above the existing inframammary crease is used to connect these medial and lateral lines. Another curved line around the nipple–areolar complex joins these lines superiorly up to the previously

ously made point, rendering a mosque dome marking around the areola (Fig. 8.3A–C). Hidalgo[14] feels that this design puts unnecessary tension on the periareolar closure which can lead to scar hypertrophy, areolar widening, and malposition. He recommends a variation in which a line is designed from the desired new position along the areolar border and down to the superior points of the medial and lateral lines that were drawn.

Intraoperatively, the areola is marked with a 38–42 mm cookie cutter. The skin between the areola to be preserved and the preoperative markings is de-epithelialized (Fig. 8.4). The de-epithelialized inferior portion of the breast is then incised both along the medial and lateral edges down to the level of the pectoralis fascia (Fig. 8.5). Lejour[15] emphasizes that the skin edges now on each side should be elevated from the underlying glandular tissue with a thickness of 0.5 cm in an effort to promote postoperative skin retraction and reduced scarring. Others feel this jeopardizes blood supply to these tissues and increases the risk of fat necrosis and potential skin loss, and is unnecessary to achieve good results.[14,16] This now isolated portion of lower-pole breast tissue is elevated at the level of the pectoralis fascia from the inframammary crease to the upper pole. In this manner, a superiorly based flap of breast tissue incorporating the nipple–areolar complex is mobilized (Fig. 8.6). This flap of tissue is then tucked into the retroareolar space that has been created and sutured to the pectoralis muscle fascia in this region (Figs 8.7, 8.8). This maneuver places additional parenchymal bulk behind the nipple–areolar complex and recreates central projection. Lejour in particular emphasizes tacking the tissues high on the fascia in an overcorrected fashion to compensate for inevitable postoperative settling.[15] The remaining medial and lateral pillars of skin and underlying breast tissue are then reapproximated in a vertical fashion extending from the inferior border of the areola to the lowermost skin edge, followed by closure of the deep dermis and skin (Fig. 8.9). Bringing these two pillars together provides support to maintain the areola in its newly elevated position and prevent descent. Reapproximating the pillars in several layers extending from the chest wall anteriorly creates a reinforced central column which will maintain this tissue support.[14] If additional volume or upper pole fill is desired, an implant can be placed in either the subglandular or the subpectoral space before sewing the pillars together. Placement of a drain aids in the evacuation of fluid and obliteration of dead space behind the pillars. Purse-string closure of the skin along the lower end of the vertical scar and the areola can accommodate the loose skin that is invariably present in these two areas.

One obvious advantage of this technique is its ability to reshape the breast through a vertical scar only. It is essential that the lower extent of the new vertical scar be placed well above the existing inframammary fold so that it does not extend on to the abdomen. In marking the breast, the curved inferior line connecting the medial and lateral pillars should be several centimeters above the crease in order to eventually finish with a vertical scar above this level.

Joining the medial and lateral pillars establishes a column of breast tissue that maintains the newly elevated

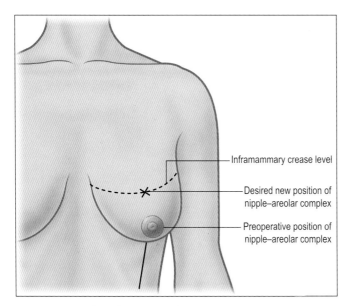

FIGURE 8.2 Marking the new nipple position.

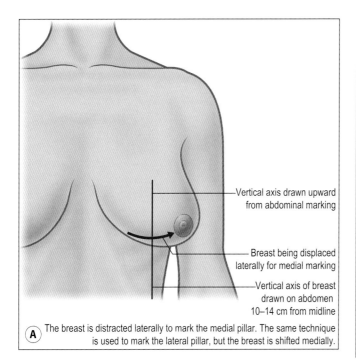

A The breast is distracted laterally to mark the medial pillar. The same technique is used to mark the lateral pillar, but the breast is shifted medially.

- Vertical axis drawn upward from abdominal marking
- Breast being displaced laterally for medial marking
- Vertical axis of breast drawn on abdomen 10–14 cm from midline

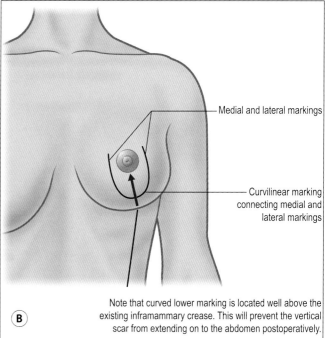

B

- Medial and lateral markings
- Curvilinear marking connecting medial and lateral markings

Note that curved lower marking is located well above the existing inframammary crease. This will prevent the vertical scar from extending on to the abdomen postoperatively.

FIGURE 8.3 Preoperative markings for vertical mastopexy.

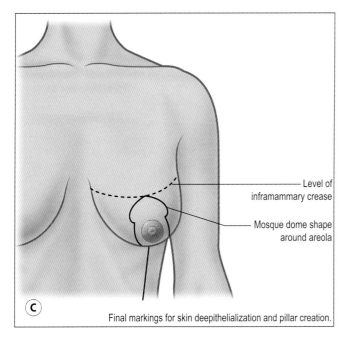

C Final markings for skin deepithelialization and pillar creation.

- Level of inframammary crease
- Mosque dome shape around areola

areola. Failure to suture these two pillars together adequately will allow the superior breast tissue to push down and splay the columns, resulting in recurrent ptosis. At the end of the procedure, the lower pole of the breast should be flat and the upper pole almost excessively full (Fig. 8.10). Although this initial appearance is somewhat exaggerated, it takes into account gravity and natural skin elasticity, which will confer some settling and rounding of the lower-pole tissues in the initial postoperative months. If the lower pole is not flat initially, these same forces will result in bottoming-out as opposed to a natural rounding of the lower pole.

The length of the periareolar marking should range from 14 to 16 cm to prevent a large discrepancy in size between the preserved areola and the newly marked opening. This will minimize periareolar skin redundancy and facilitate closure. Additionally, the new desired point for the superior border of the areola should be marked just at the level of the inframammary crease, or even slightly lower. This will minimize the risk of a high-riding nipple postoperatively.

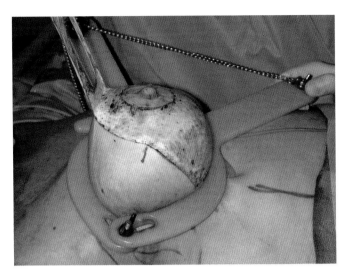

FIGURE 8.4 Use of a mammostat to facilitate de-epithelialization.

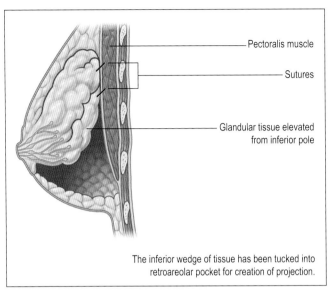

Pectoralis muscle

Sutures

Glandular tissue elevated from inferior pole

The inferior wedge of tissue has been tucked into retroareolar pocket for creation of projection.

FIGURE 8.7 Elevating and securing inferior glandular tissue.

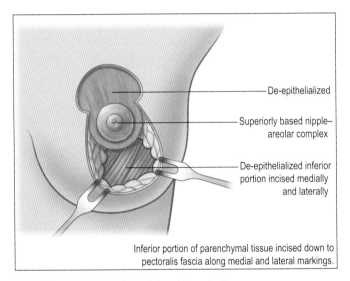

De-epithelialized

Superiorly based nipple–areolar complex

De-epithelialized inferior portion incised medially and laterally

Inferior portion of parenchymal tissue incised down to pectoralis fascia along medial and lateral markings.

FIGURE 8.5 Creation of medial and lateral pillars.

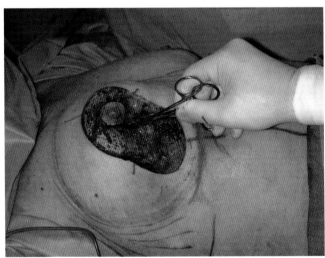

FIGURE 8.8 Invaginating superiorly based flap into retroareolar space.

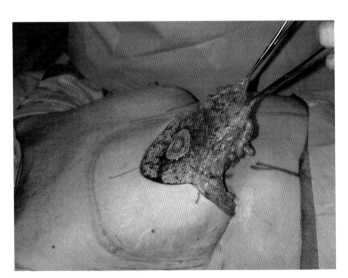

FIGURE 8.6 Elevation of superiorly based flap in vertical scar mastopexy.

Proponents of this technique feel that it yields a superior breast shape with the added benefit of eliminating the more traditional horizontal scar. Unlike many other mastopexy procedures, it does not rely merely on dermal suspension to maintain the breast contour. The sutured pillars of glandular tissue provide a more stable basis for maintenance of form against gravity and natural postoperative settling, which would otherwise contribute to recurrent ptosis. In addition, the ptotic portion of the breast has been repositioned in such a way to recreate projection and superior cleavage. In her 10-year experience with 250 consecutive cases, Lejour[15] reports that at 1-year follow-up only four patients presented with recurrent ptosis. Lassus[16] has demonstrated a maintenance of shape for as long as 20 years following the initial procedure (Fig. 8.11).

The use of a superiorly based dermoglandular pedicle preserves most of the neurovascular supply to the nipple–areolar complex and thus the risk of sensory or vascular compromise is minimized. Lassus[17] reports his 30-year experience using a superiorly based pedicle with no incidence of nipple necrosis in cases where the nipple was elevated 9 cm or less. He emphasizes maintenance of a wide base to the pedicle to ensure adequate venous drainage and preservation of sensory input.[16] Anatomic studies have demonstrated that medial and lateral branches of the second to sixth intercostal nerves contribute to nipple sensation.[18] Because a portion of both medial and lateral parenchyma is preserved with the vertical technique, along with dermoglandular tissue around the nipple–areolar complex, postoperative nipple sensation should be maintained. Clinically, Lejour[15] found in her series that the overwhelming majority of patients had nipple sensitivity that was either unchanged or only temporarily reduced.

Immediate complications are fortunately rare. In Lejour's review of 152 patients who underwent mastopexy, four developed a seroma, six had hematomas, and one developed an infection. No patients had areolar necrosis or delayed skin healing.[19] Lassus' technique, which does not rely on skin undermining or liposuction, seems to have fewer associated problems with seroma. Berthe et al.[20] also found that the incidence of hematoma and seroma was less in those cases where skin undermining and liposuction were not included.

Long-term complications tend to be focused more on scarring and breast shape. An often-cited shortcoming is the poor quality of the scars, particularly at the inferiormost end of the vertical scar and in the periareolar region. Because of the excess skin in these areas, puckering often persists even after the scars have had time to soften and settle. Tension can also lead to widening of the scars, particularly if it is so great as to cause superficial wound breakdown. Placement of purse-string sutures in these areas may offset tension and help improve quality. Lejour feels that her undermining of the pillar skin edges also improves the quality of the resultant scar, although this must be weighed against the potential risk of skin flap devascularization. Lockwood[21] describes suturing a superficial fascial system as a distinct layer from breast tissue or dermis, which minimizes tension and creates finer scars. Most cases of poor scar quality can be corrected by revision under local anesthesia. Whereas the vertical technique has a higher associated rate of secondary minor procedure for scar revision, Lassus[16] states that this is a small price to pay for elimination of the horizontal scar altogether. In cases where the vertical scar is too long, correction can be achieved with a triangular excision of skin, which will leave a small horizontal scar. This can be avoided by ensuring that the lowest extent of the vertical incisions is several centimeters above the original inframammary fold.

Nipple–areolar complex

Medial and lateral pillars

Sutures

Pillars sutured together. This will support the now elevated nipple areolar complex.

FIGURE 8.9 Reapproximating medial and lateral pillars of tissue.

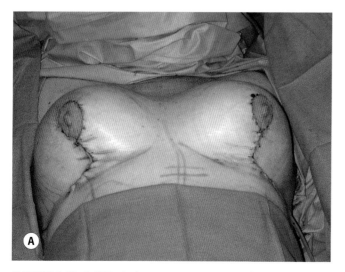

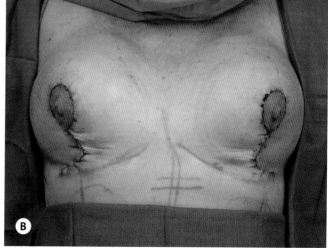

FIGURES 8.10 A, B Vertical scar mastopexy at completion of case. Note the flatness in the inferior poles and the almost exaggerated fullness in the superior poles. In this case, a small lateral extension has been added to the vertical incision to accommodate skin redundancy.

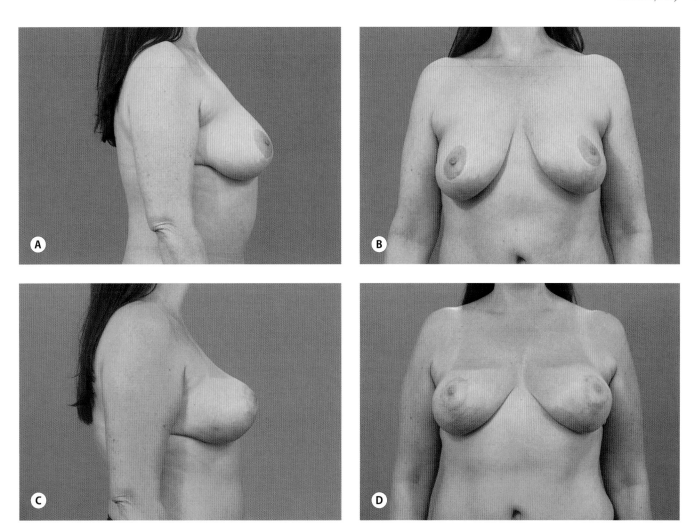

FIGURES 8.11 AP and lateral views of a 44-year-old woman before (**A, B**) and after (**C, D**) vertical scar mastopexy. Results are demonstrated 5 months postoperatively.

Poor postoperative shape or asymmetry in terms of nipple position is usually related to inadequate tightening of the lower-pole pillars. The key to avoid this is to ensure adequate tightening of the lower-pole pillars intraoperatively, and to compare the two sides on the operating table with the patient in a sitting position. Failure to do so initially can then only be corrected by a reoperation to recreate the pillars and tighten them sufficiently to create a flat lower breast. In cases where the nipple–areolar complex is situated too high, a crescent excision in the inframammary fold can remove some skin and bulk and situate the complex in a lower and more natural location. Once again, this complication can be avoided by suturing the pillars together so that they form a solid column of parenchymal tissue that resists gravitational forces leading to bottoming-out. Additionally, placement of the nipple–areolar complex slightly below the anterior projection of the inframammary fold can offset this tendency.

Periareolar mastopexy

The appeal of periareolar mastopexy is that it limits scarring even more than the aforementioned vertical techniques.

Realistically, though, it is applicable to only a small subset of patients who present with mammary ptosis. Potential candidates have minor degrees of ptosis and typically require 3 cm or less of nipple elevation. Additionally, these patients possess a greater degree of glandular tissue than fatty tissue, which confers some firmness and preservation of shape to the breast.

The doughnut mastopexy relies on skin excision to raise the ptotic nipple–areolar complex to its desired position. The new placement of the nipple–areolar complex is marked on the breast along the breast meridian. Comparing sternal notch to nipple distances between the two sides will aid in achieving symmetry. In the operating room, the circle of areola to be preserved is marked. The skin between these two markings is then de-epithelialized. This newly created skin edge can then be elevated off the glandular tissue, particularly in the superior direction to facilitate upward mobility of the nipple–areolar complex. The dermal edge encircling the complex is then tacked to the glandular tissue now freed from the skin edge, in effect elevating the nipple to its new position. A Gore-Tex or Mersilene purse-string suture is placed in the dermis of the skin edge and cinched down to the size of the areola. The areola is then inset with interrupted dermal sutures followed by a subcuticular stitch.

Experience in both breast and facial surgery suggests that reliance on skin only to maintain the new shape and position is typically fraught with failure and early recurrence of ptosis. A natural extension of this procedure, then, would incorporate some degree of glandular reshaping via the periareolar incision to improve durability of results. This was in fact popularized by Benelli.[22] His preoperative markings include points A–D as follows: point A, the future superior border of the areola denoted 2 cm above the anterior projection of the inframammary fold along the breast meridian; point B, the future inferior border of the areola measured 5–12 cm above the fold with the patient supine; points C and D, the medial and lateral limits of the areola, with point C 8–12 cm from the midline and point D equidistant from the nipple. These points are connected in what will be an eccentric oval. Once in the operating room, the amount of areola to be preserved is marked and the area between the two markings de-epithelialized. The dermis is then incised from the 2 o'clock to the 10 o'clock position and continued in the subcutaneous plane down to the inframammary crease (Fig. 8.12B). A semicircular incision is made through the glandular tissue about 3 cm away from the inferior areolar edge, but still parallel to it. This is carried down to the level of the prepectoral space. The glandular tissue is then additionally incised along the breast meridian, leaving the areola on a superiorly based dermoglandular flap with medially and laterally based flaps of parenchyma below. The glandular tissue on the deep side of the superior flap is then tacked higher up on the chest wall to the pectoralis fascia. This maneuver will elevate the nipple–areolar complex and initially produce an unnatural bulge in the superior pole, which will gradually relax as the tissues settle in the first few weeks postoperatively. The lower medial flap is then turned and tacked behind the areola with sutures fixing it to the pectoralis fascia. The lateral flap is then rotated over this and sutured to the medial flap. In so doing, the base of the breast is narrowed and the newly elevated areola now has a column of glandular tissue to support it, rather than a skin brassiere only. The areola is now sutured to the superior skin edge. A purse-string suture is then passed through the dermal edge and tied down to the appropriate diameter of the areola. A vertical and horizontal U-shaped suture is passed in the retroareolar plane to prevent herniation in this region. A subcuticular periareolar stitch is the last to be placed.

The use of the Benelli round block technique is an important addition for optimizing the results of periareolar mastopexy. By cinching the dermal skin edge down to the areolar border, tension across the closure is minimized and the risk of scar widening reduced. Many advocate using a permanent Gore-Tex suture for the cerclage stitch which can maintain the circular shape and prevent widening of the areola.

Patient selection is also a critical determinant in achieving aesthetic results with periareolar mastopexy. Despite the appeal of hiding the scar at the areolar edge, the results in terms of shape and scar quality will be poor in those not well suited for the procedure. Ideal candidates have large areolas to begin with, usually >45 mm, and require less than 3 cm of elevation. In this sense it can be a particularly useful technique in patients who have either congenital or acquired asymmetries that require minor degrees of adjustment. Patients with tuberous breast deformities may also benefit from this technique. On the other hand, patients with significant ptosis and a small areolar diameter are poorly suited for periareolar mastopexy. Accurate preoperative assessment and sound clinical judgment are therefore crucial to ensure that a periareolar technique will appropriately address the problems a patient presents with. In cases where a periareolar technique is not suitable, discussion of the limitations of that particular procedure can lead to acceptance of one with additional scars if it means overall improved outcome in terms of shape and ptosis correction.

Spear et al.[23] also championed the notion that modest skin excision helps to achieve superior results in terms of scar quality and areolar diameter. He recommends that the diameter of the excised circle should be less than three times that of the inner circle and in general less than 10 cm. This, particularly in combination with a purse-string suture, will once again minimize tension around the closure and increase the likelihood of fine scars with minimal areolar spread.

Additionally, those periareolar techniques that rely on more than just skin excision for maintenance of form have greater success and improved aesthetic outcomes. Thin skin with multiple striae will not provide durable breast support, and the weight of retained breast tissue will result in bottoming-out. The concept of glandular reshaping for internal support is therefore important in optimizing the outcome of periareolar techniques. Goes' periareolar tech-

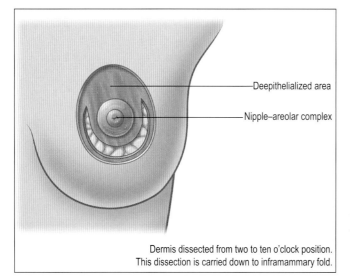

Deepithelialized area

Nipple–areolar complex

Dermis dissected from two to ten o'clock position. This dissection is carried down to inframammary fold.

FIGURE 8.12 Breast de-epithelialization and dissection in Benelli mastopexy.

nique,[7,24] which uses a combination of dermal flaps and a prosthetic mixed mesh to support the gland, is based on this same notion.

Despite the appeal of a limited scar, the complication rate of periareolar mastopexy is not insignificant. Rohrich's[10] survey published in 2006 showed that this technique had the highest rate of revision and the lowest physician satisfaction. An inherent drawback of the periareolar design is that it tends to flatten the areola and can lead to loss of central breast projection. This can result in an unnatural, boxy postoperative appearance to the breast. In this sense, it is a useful technique for patients with a tuberous breast deformity who possess an abundant herniation of breast tissue in the retroareolar region. The problem of areolar distortion is exacerbated if areolar spreading or widened scars develop as well. This situation is difficult to correct and best avoided altogether. Once again, limiting the technique to only patients requiring minimal elevation will offset tension across the closure and the tendency for areolar spreading and flattening. The purse-string suture works in a similar manner and can even help to recreate some of the areolar protrusion. In those instances where this complication does develop, scar revision can be attempted with scar excision, undermining of remaining skin edges, and placement of a cerclage stitch to advance tissue and effect some tissue eversion. Additional measures, such as prolonged use of Steri-strips or silicone sheeting, can be considered. If scar hypertrophy appears to develop early, intralesional triamcinolone injections are an option. These measures, however, are often unsuccessful, and the most effective means of correcting an enlarged or flattened nipple–areolar complex can be conversion to another form of mastopexy, such as the vertical or inverted T.

Inverted T mastopexy

Still the most popular among North American surgeons, the inverted T mastopexy relies on a periareolar, vertical, and inframammary scar pattern. The addition of a horizontal component makes it very useful for severe grades of ptosis requiring significant skin removal.

As with most other techniques, the breast meridian and inframammary crease are marked preoperatively. The position for the areolar apex is marked by transposing the level of the crease anteriorly on to the meridian. Limbs extending from this point down and around the areola are drawn for a distance of about 8 cm. These are then connected to the inframammary crease marking.

In the operating room, the diameter of the desired areola is drawn and the skin between this and the preoperative markings is de-epithelialized. At this point, several techniques for glandular reshaping exist. Superior, inferior, and central mound pedicles are commonly used to preserve the nipple–areolar complex. Once the chosen pedicle is dissected, the remaining flaps of parenchyma are elevated off the pectoralis muscle to free them. In this way, the flaps can be rotated, transposed, and fixed with sutures in their new desired position. The skin is redraped and closed along its horizontal and vertical limbs. At a distance of 5–6 cm up the vertical limb of the T incision a circle of tissue is marked and excised and the nipple–areolar complex brought out in this new location.

Because of the liberal use of incisions, even large amounts of skin can easily be excised with this technique. This may have particular relevance given the increasing popularity of bariatric procedures for massive weight loss. Such patients typically present with significant mammary ptosis and an abundance of overly stretched, striated skin heretofore previously seen only rarely. In these difficult cases, an inverted T mastopexy is often the best option, and in some instances can be combined with implant or autoaugmentation using nearby de-epithelialized excess tissue to achieve reasonable aesthetic results.

Proponents of the inverted T technique like the immediacy of the results. The new shape can be assessed with the patient still on the operating table, allowing for adjustments or correction of asymmetries. Control of the shape remains in the hands of the surgeon rather than being dependent on postoperative settling and gravity, which are to a certain extent unpredictable. This potentially minimizes the need for postoperative surgical revisions. Additionally, patients can appreciate their new shape and correction early on, as there is no reliance on tissue settling to correct overly exaggerated upper-pole fullness.

However, unlike the vertical mastopexy, the inverted T places heavy reliance on a skin brassiere for maintenance of shape. This inherently increases the risk of bottoming-out, with high-riding nipples and the bulk of breast tissue centered below this in the inferior pole. Such is often the case when an implant is placed simultaneously, as this adds to the weight behind the skin envelope and puts greater stretch on it. The use of an inferior pedicle, where tissue is left in the lower pole and not resuspended, would also increase this risk. Internal shaping sutures or tacking glandular tissue to higher points on the pectoralis fascia may help offset this risk. Others have begun to incorporate some form of actual glandular reshaping into the technique to improve long-term results.[25,26] Once again, prevention of the bottoming-out phenomenon is easier than its correction. Options for dealing with this long-term complication include a crescent excision of skin and parenchyma along the inframammary crease to shorten the vertical distance from the inferior edge of the areola. Placement of an implant to add superior fullness and projection can to some extent camouflage bottoming-out when it occurs.

The other limitation of this technique is its scarring. The length of the scar across the crease is an obvious disadvantage, coupled with the fact that this portion of the scar has a tendency for widening and hypertrophy. As with all scars, minimizing tension at the time of incision closure can improve scar quality. Often, in the case of longstanding scars, there will be some relaxation of the tissues surrounding the scar, and revision can have some success as there will be less tension. Attempts should be made to limit scar length, particularly along the medial leg, as permanent scarring near or across the midline can be conspicuous and limit clothing options for the patient.

POSTOPERATIVE CARE

Postoperative recommendations follow those routinely advocated for most breast operations. Most surgeons recommend several days of antibiotics, narcotics for pain control, and limiting strenuous upper-body activity for several weeks after surgery. If drains are used, they are typically removed when output is less than 30 mL/24 h. Because of the usual combination of glandular rearrangement and skin redraping, most surgeons advocate some type of external support to help splint the breast in its new position until some scar tissue can develop and maintain this on a permanent basis. A well-fitting bra can be helpful in achieving this. In addition, some use Tegaderm laid over the upper and lower poles to reinforce positioning and provide support even when the bra is removed. After several weeks, scar massage and the application of scar creams can be started to eliminate pleating and facilitate settling. Scar revisions may ultimately be necessary for persistent wrinkles, puckering, or dog-ears, but are usually delayed till at least 6 months postoperatively.

CONCLUSION

Many factors can contribute to the development of breast ptosis. Although manual elevation of the breast by either pinching or pulling on the skin seems straightforward enough to correct this problem, plastic surgeons can attest to the difficulty of reproducing these results surgically to last over an extended period. The sheer number and variety of techniques attest to the fact that no one procedure is applicable to all patients. Success in mastopexy surgery probably rests in having some facility with more than one surgical method and applying those methods appropriately to meet individual patient needs and anatomy. Future refinements of this procedure will no doubt focus on better preservation of shape over time while simultaneously minimizing scars. Continued research into scarless surgery and improved wound healing may one day positively affect the results of mastopexy surgery. The slow but demonstrated trend towards increasing use of vertical scar techniques highlights the fact that surgeons are critically assessing their results and open to ways to improve them.

REFERENCES

1. Penn J. Breast reduction. Br J Plast Surg 1955; 7: 357.
2. Smith DJ Jr, Palin WE Jr, Katch VL, et al. Breast volume and anthropomorphic measurements: Normal values. Plast Reconstruct Surg 1986; 78: 331.
3. Westreich M. Anthropomorphic breast measurement: protocol and results in 50 women with aesthetically perfect breasts and clinical application. Plast Reconstruct Surg 1997; 100: 468–479.
4. American Society for Aesthetic Plastic Surgery. Percent of change in select procedures: 1997–2006. American Society for Aesthetic Plastic Surgery, 2006.
5. Lejour M. Vertical mammaplasty and liposuction of the breast. Plast Reconstruct Surg 1994; 94: 100.
6. Graf R, Biggs TM, Steely RL. Breast shape: A technique for better upper pole fullness. Aesthetic Plast Surg 2000; 24: 348.
7. Goes, JCS. Periareolar mammaplasty: Double skin technique with application of polyglactin or mixed mesh. Plast Reconstruct Surg 1996; 97: 959.
8. Hauben DJ, Adler N, Silfen R, Regev D. Breast–areola–nipple proportion. Ann Plast Surg 2003; 50: 510–513.
9. Regnault B. Breast ptosis: Definition and treatment. Clin Plast Surg 1976; 3: 193–203.
10. Rohrich RJ, Gosman AA, Brown SA, Reisch J. Mastopexy preferences: a survey of board-certified plastic surgeons. Plast Reconstruct Surg 2006; 118: 1631–1638.
11. Lassus C. A technique for breast reduction. Int Surg 1970; 53: 69.
12. Lassus C. Breast reduction: Evolution of a technique – a single vertical scar. Aesthetic Plast Surg 1987; 11: 107.
13. Lejour M. Vertical mammaplasty and liposuction of the breast. St Louis: Quality Medical Publishing, 1994.
14. Hidalgo DA. Vertical mammaplasty. Plast Reconstruct Surg 2005; 4: 1179–1197.
15. Lejour M. Vertical mammaplasty: update and appraisal of late results. Plast Reconstruct Surg 1999; 104: 771–781.
16. Lassus C. Update on vertical mammaplasty. Plast Reconstruct Surg 1999; 104: 2289–2298.
17. Lassus C. A 30-year experience with vertical mammaplasty. Plast Reconstruct Surg 1996; 97: 373.
18. Schlenz I, Kuzbari R, Gruber H, Holle J. The sensitivity of the nipple areola complex: an anatomic study. Plast Reconstruct Surg 2000; 105: 905–909.
19. Lejour M. Vertical mammaplasty: early complications after 250 consecutive cases. Plast Reconstruct Surg 1999; 104: 764–770.
20. Berthe JV, Massaut J, Greuse M, et al. The vertical mammaplasty: a reappraisal of the technique and its complications. Plast Reconstruct Surg 2003; 111: 2192–2199.
21. Lockwood T. Reduction mammaplasty and mastopexy with superficial fascial system suspension. Plast Reconstruct Surg 1999; 103: 1411–1420.
22. Benelli L. A new peri-areolar mammaplasty: the 'round block' technique. Aesthet Plast Surg 1990; 14: 93–100.
23. Spear SL, Giese SY, Ducic I. Concentric mastopexy revisited. Plast Reconstruct Surg 1999; 107: 1294–1299.
24. Goes J. Peri-areolar mammaplasty: double skin technique. Rev Soc Bras Cir Plast 1989; 4: 55–63.
25. Flowers RS, Smith EM. Flip-flap mastopexy. Aesthet Plast Surg 1998; 22: 425.
26. Nicolle F, Chir M. Improved standards in reduction mammaplasty and mastopexy. Plast Reconstruct Surg 1982; 69: 453.

Breast Augmentation

Bernadette Wang Ashraf and Diane Z. Alexander

INTRODUCTION

Augmentation mammaplasty has always been among the top cosmetic surgical procedures performed in the United States. In 2006, breast augmentation became the most popular cosmetic procedure for the first time since the American Society of Plastic Surgeons (ASPS) began collecting statistics. Over 329 000 women underwent augmentation mammaplasty in 2006, a 55% increase from 2000 and more than triple the number from 1997. With the November 2006 approval of silicone gel breast implants by the Food and Drug Administration (FDA), it is likely that the number of breast augmentations will continue to increase.

Breast implants can be used to enhance the size, shape and symmetry of breasts in cases of developmental hypomastia, mild asymmetry, involutional breast changes, or just a desire for larger breasts. The results of augmentation mammaplasty are influenced by the patient's preoperative anatomy. Implants are capable of modifying the volume and shape of the breasts. Despite these strengths, implants alone cannot change the patient's skin quality nor significantly change the location of the breast or nipple. In situations where this is desired, an augmentation mastopexy may be necessary, especially when there is significant breast ptosis or asymmetry (Figs 9.1–9.3).

Breast implants should not be placed in any patient who has an active infection, is pregnant or breastfeeding, or has untreated breast cancer or mental health issues.

PREOPERATIVE CONSIDERATIONS

Important factors to consider prior to breast augmentation include patient motivation and expectations, as well as anatomy. Women who desire an improvement in their body image are usually appropriate candidates. Studies have shown that incorporation of the implant into body image after augmentation mammaplasty results in positive changes in outlook, personality and behavior with improved self-esteem.[1]

The importance of adequately assessing breast anatomy and patient body habitus cannot be overemphasized. It is important preoperatively to note the patient's skin quality; the configuration of the chest wall; breast shape, including any degree of ptosis or breast base constriction; breast asymmetries, including differences in volume; inframammary fold position; and asymmetry of the size and location of the nipple and areola. An analysis of 100 random patients who presented for breast augmentation[2] demonstrated that nearly 88% of women are naturally asymmetric, and that 72% of these women had more than one area of asymmetry. These findings should be pointed out to the patient before surgery and documented with preoperative photographs. Subtle differences preoperatively will most likely still be

---

BOX 9.1 Indications for breast augmentation

- To enhance the body contour of a woman who, for personal reasons, feels her breast size is too small
- To restore breast volume lost due to weight loss or following pregnancy
- To achieve better symmetry when breasts are slightly disproportionate in size and shape
- To improve the shape of breasts that are sagging or have lost firmness, often used with a breast lift procedure

---

BOX 9.2 Contraindications to breast augmentation

- Active infection anywhere in the body
- Breast cancer or lesions that have not been adequately treated
- Pregnancy or nursing
- Untreated mental health disorder

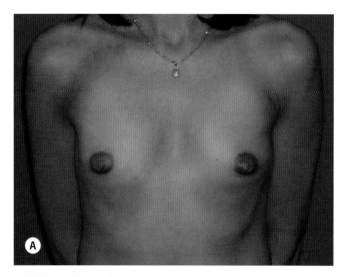
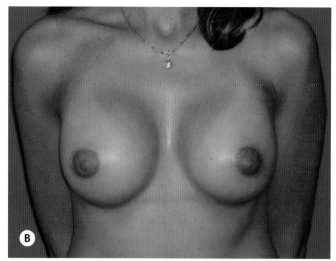

FIGURE 9.1 Pre- and postoperative views of patient with developmental hypomastia.

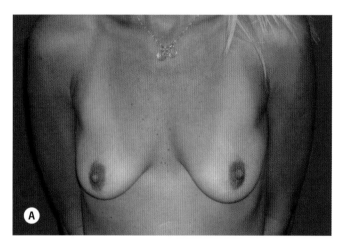
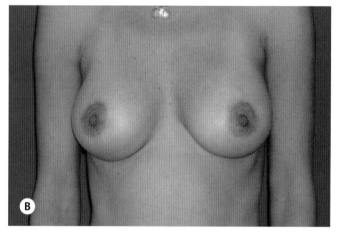

FIGURE 9.2 Pre- and postoperative views of patient with involutional breast changes.

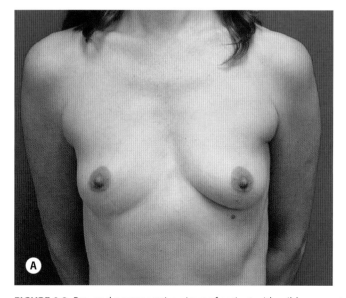
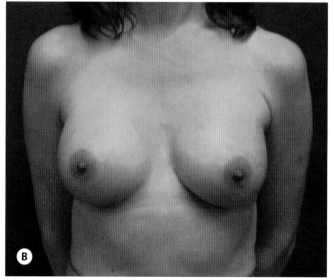

FIGURE 9.3 Pre- and postoperative views of patient with mild asymmetry.

present after breast augmentation, and may even be more pronounced (Figs 9.4–9.6).

Although implants can improve size discrepancies and enhance the breast shape, a mastopexy at the time of augmentation may be indicated in cases of ptosis, low or laterally positioned breasts, tubular breasts, enlarged areolae, or significant asymmetry of the breast shape or nipple position.

During the initial consultation, a thorough history and physical examination should be performed. Emphasis should be placed on existing breast disease, breast changes during pregnancy, and family history of breast cancer. The breast examination should include careful palpation for breast and axillary masses. Any woman who has suspicious findings in the history or on examination should be properly evaluated prior to surgery. A baseline preoperative mammogram is recommended for all women aged 35 and over.

Important surgical decisions include choice of implant, incision location, and implant placement sites in the subglandular, subpectoral or dual-plane locations.

Silicone or saline

The November 2006 FDA decision to approve silicone breast implants has provided women with more choices and

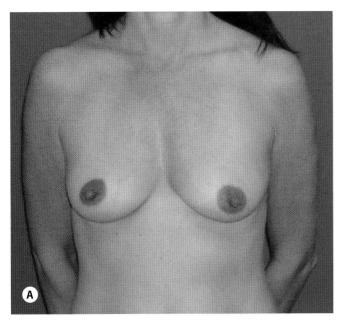 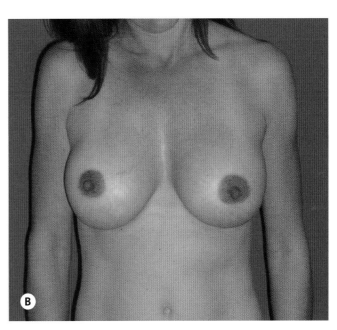

FIGURE 9.4 Patient with asymmetry of her nipple–areolar complex position evident in both pre- and postoperative photos.

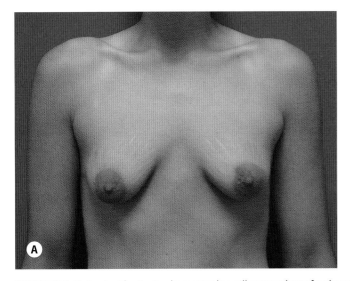 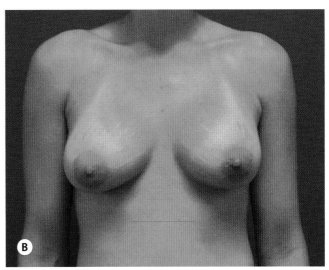

FIGURE 9.5 Patient with ptosis whose nipples still appear low after breast implants.

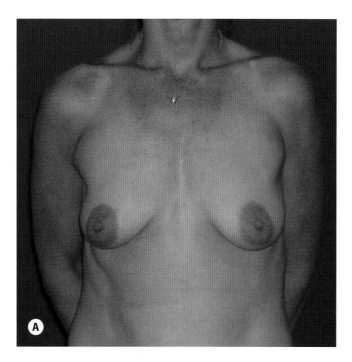

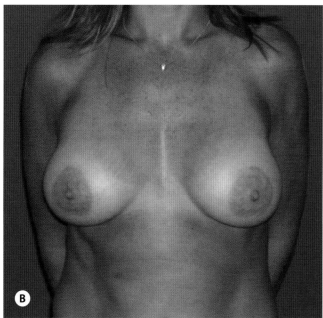

FIGURE 9.6 Patient with ptosis whose implants appear very low and lateral. She would have had better results with mastopexy augmentation.

The obvious advantage of silicone over saline implants is the more natural look and feel of silicone. Silicone devices are less likely to result in implant visibility, rippling, wrinkling, and palpability. During the last decade, significant improvements have been made in silicone implant design, specifically more durable low-bleed silicone elastomer shells and more cohesive silicone gels. Unlike the earlier generation of silicone gel implants, the more recent silicone gel implants that are now available in the USA for cosmetic use have been reported to be equally as good as saline implants in avoiding capsular contracture.[4] A disadvantage of silicone compared to saline implants is that the incision may need to be larger, especially for the larger silicone implants and more cohesive gels. The transaxillary incision, which has become popular for saline implants, may be more difficult when placing a larger silicone implant. The transumbilical incision is not advised for breast augmentation using silicone gel implants. Another consideration is that silicone gel implants are more expensive than saline implants.

Despite the most recent data, there are still women who are anxious and concerned about the use of silicone gel and prefer to have saline implants. An advantage of saline breast implants is that they can be placed in any of the main four incision sites (inframammary, periareolar, transaxillary, and transumbilical). Because they are not prefilled, the final fill volume can be adjusted intraoperatively. Another factor that can influence the decision as to which device to choose is that saline implants are less expensive than silicone.

Implant size

One of the most common reasons for reoperation in an augmentation patient is for a size change. Therefore, it is very important to have good communication with the patient preoperatively about the desired size and to understand that a specific bra cup size may not mean the same thing between the surgeon and patient. During the consultation, patients will often place a breast implant in their bra to better appreciate the size changes that are possible with augmentation. For the plastic surgeon, this technique is used primarily as a communication tool to discuss the size the patient would like to be, rather than to pick the exact implant size to use during surgery. The surgeon can then select an implant within a given range based on volume, base diameter, and desired size and profile.

Some women present with unrealistic expectations and expect to increase their breast size from an 'A' cup to a 'D' cup. It is important to adequately educate patients and convey that their current breast characteristics may not be

options in breast augmentation. After rigorous scientific review, the FDA approved silicone gel-filled implants for breast reconstruction in women of all ages and for breast augmentation in women aged 22 and older. In the past decade, a number of independent studies have examined whether silicone gel-filled implants are associated with connective tissue disease or cancer. The conclusion, including a report by the Institute of Medicine, was that there is no convincing evidence that breast implants are associated with either of these diseases.[3]

able to accommodate an implant that is too large based on base diameter measurements. In addition, their skin may be insufficiently compliant and lack the elasticity to accommodate a large device. This may be the case in women with severe micromastia or developmental deficiency.

Implant shape

There are two basic shapes currently available for breast augmentation: round and contoured. Their availability and usage appear to be geographically diverse. In the USA, round implants are more commonly used than contoured implants. Round implants can be effective for a variety of patient shapes and can appear anatomic when they are placed under the pectoralis muscle, especially when the breast has more existing parenchymal tissue. A disadvantage of round devices is that they can cause excessive upper pole fullness in patients with minimal breast tissue.

Anatomic or teardrop-shaped implants can provide greater volume to the lower pole of the breast and diminish upper pole roundness. These devices can be placed in the subglandular or subpectoral positions. With the availability of silicone gel implants, these contoured devices may provide added benefits for some women. A potential concern, however, is the risk of implant rotation and a visible breast abnormality. To reduce this risk it is important not to overdissect the implant pocket and to stabilize the implants postoperatively with a support bra and binder.

Implant shell: smooth or textured

The ideal shell surface characteristics have long been debated. With older implants, the textured surface devices resulted in a lower incidence of capsular contracture.[5] However, both the Mentor and the Allergan Core Studies were unable to demonstrate a difference in the likelihood of developing capsular contracture with textured versus smooth implants.[6] In addition, any potential difference between textured and smooth seemed to decrease when both were placed submuscularly.[7] One caveat when considering a textured device is that the textured surface may result in more rippling and wrinkling than a smooth surface. In addition, the textured devices may require a slightly larger incision.

INCISIONS

The optimal incisional approach for breast augmentation continues to be debated. The decision is usually based on a combination of factors that include patient desire, the surgeon's recommendation, and the characteristics of the breast. The most commonly used incisions are periareolar, inframammary, and transaxillary (Fig. 9.7). Silicone gel implants can be inserted through the inframammary and periareolar approaches, and in some women may be inserted through the transaxillary approach. Saline breast implants can be inserted through each of these and also through the transumbilical incision.

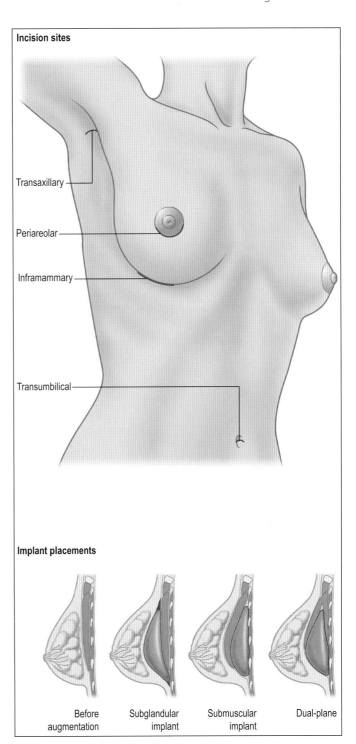

FIGURE 9.7 Four incision sites: periareolar, inframammary, transaxillary and transumbilical.

Periareolar

The periareolar incision is well concealed and very versatile. It gives access to the subglandular and submuscular pockets, and the inframammary fold can easily be lowered if necessary. The breast parenchyma can also be manipulated in cases where the breast is constricted. Candidates for a periareolar incision include women with a relatively large areola in whom an incision can be made that will permit the insertion of an implant. Women with a small areolar diameter may not be suitable for this approach. The dissection can proceed through the breast parenchyma or along the subcutaneous plane from the base of the areola to the inframammary fold. Dissection through the breast gland has not been shown to increase contamination and infection rates.[8] However, there have been preliminary reports of an increased risk to nipple sensation and increased difficulties with future breastfeeding.[9] Perhaps the principal advantage of this approach is that the incision is nicely concealed and barely visible at the junction of the skin and areola.

Inframammary

This incision is a very straightforward approach to breast augmentation and may in fact be the most commonly performed. It allows for direct access to either the subglandular or the submuscular pocket without disrupting the breast parenchyma. This can allow for precise pocket dissection and is ideally suited to augmentation using contoured devices. The length of the incision can be varied based on the size of the implant and whether or not it is silicone gel-filled. This incision is best concealed in patients who have a well-defined inframammary fold that is in already in a good location. In patients who have a high, tight fold or an ill-defined fold, the incision may be visible.

Transaxillary

The transaxillary incision has gained increased acceptance over the past decade, especially as endoscopic techniques have improved. The main advantage of this technique is that no scars are created on the breast skin itself. The breast parenchyma is usually completely unviolated. A disadvantage is that precise pocket creation is compromised because visibility is somewhat limited. Because of this, the chances of asymmetry and implant malpositioning are increased. It is also more difficult to manipulate the breast parenchyma in cases of tight, constricted breasts.

Transumbilical

The transumbilical incision is the most recent approach to breast augmentation and leaves a well-concealed scar. It is used for placing saline implants in either the subglandular or the submuscular pockets. Like the transaxillary incision, the transumbilical incision has the advantage of creating no scars on the breast; however, it has a similar disadvantage related to the distant access with an increased potential for implant malposition. A unique risk of this approach is that the implant may be more frequently damaged. Its application in complex situations such as with a tuberous breast deformity will be limited because of the inability to properly manipulate the breast parenchyma. Furthermore, problems with hemostasis or secondary procedures will most likely require a direct-access approach.

IMPLANT PLACEMENT SITES

There has always been debate as to which implant position is best, subglandular or subpectoral. There are advantages associated with each, and the decision as to which to choose is ultimately related to the characteristics of both the patient and the breast. Current thinking is that the subglandular position is more natural because the implant will directly augment the parenchyma. This is especially true in women with some degree of natural breast volume. However, in women with smaller breasts the subpectoral position may be preferred, to provide an additional layer between the cutaneous surface and the implant.

Subglandular

The subglandular location has been traditionally advocated for very active or muscular women in whom the submuscular location may cause distortion or weakness. However, based on the experience of many of our European colleagues, the subglandular position may be ideal for women interested in using contoured silicone gel devices. Outcomes with these devices in this position appear to be improved. As previously mentioned, this position may be accessed via an inframammary, periareolar, or transaxillary incision. A prerequisite for the subglandular position is that there should be sufficient soft tissue coverage to minimize palpability and visibility issues. One disadvantage of the subglandular position is that it is associated with a higher incidence of capsular contracture.[10] It may also cause more difficult imaging during mammography.[11]

Subpectoral

The subpectoral location usually refers to a partial muscle coverage of the implant, with the pectoralis muscle covering the implant superiorly and medially and sometimes partially inferiorly. This location is generally associated with less capsular contracture and less implant visibility or palpability than with the subglandular location. In addition, when round implants are used the upper pole has a more natural appearance. A disadvantage of this position is that there may be more postoperative discomfort, muscle spasm, distortion of breast shape with pectoralis contraction, and the implants may take more time to descend and for breast shape to settle. Postoperative imaging via mammography may be facilitated because the technician is better able to delineate the junction of the breast parenchyma with the pectoralis muscle, ensuring total visibility.

Dual plane

The difference between the dual plane and a subpectoral location is the deliberate division of the pectoralis muscle inferiorly and the calculated subglandular dissection that extends from above the inframammary fold. The amount of subglandular dissection can range from a few centimeters from the inframammary fold to the level of the areola for the more ptotic or constricted breast. Purposeful dissection in the subglandular planes alters the breast parenchyma–pectoralis interface, which repositions the inferior portion of the pectoralis muscle. This in turn can help create a more desirable breast shape, while minimizing muscle distortion and avoiding a double-bubble deformity.[12]

OPERATIVE APPROACH

Surgical anatomy

The main innervation to the nipple–areolar complex arises from the fourth lateral intercostal nerve. However, anterior and lateral branches of the third and fifth intercostal nerves can contribute to nipple sensation. Regardless of the incisional approach, diminished sensation of the nipple–areolar complex can occur as a result of stretching or injury to the anterior and lateral nerve fibers when the lateral breast pocket is dissected.

Preoperative markings

Markings should be made with the patient in the standing position. Important landmarks include the vertical midline and the inframammary folds. When the inframammary fold is to be lowered, the desired location is delineated. It is also useful to determine the exact dimensions of the breast and appreciate any asymmetries. Relevant distances include the sternal notch to nipple distance, the nipple to inframammary fold distance, and the nipple to mid-sternal distance.

Preoperative medications

Prophylactic antibiotics (first-generation cephalosporin) are routinely administered to all patients undergoing breast augmentation. An anti-nausea protocol of scopolamine patch, Zofran, Decadron and Benadryl has also been demonstrated to be effective. Robaxin is given to patients undergoing submuscular implants.

Exposure

Periareolar

A curved incision is made with the scalpel just slightly inside the inferior border of the areola. Using electrocautery, we dissect directly through the breast tissue to the prepectoral fascia. If a subpectoral or dual-plane location is to be used, the lateral border of the pectoralis muscle is identified.

Inframammary

A 2.5–4 cm incision is made at the level of the inframammary fold. If the fold needs to be lowered, the incision is usually made at the level of the new fold. The incision is easily carried to the prepectoral fascia.

Transaxillary

A 4–5 cm incision should be placed in a line that starts not less than 1 cm posterior to the lateral border of the pecto-

ralis, going through the apex of the axilla and continuing high in the posterior axilla to maximize visibility. The dissection proceeds to the level of the axillary fat but does not continue through it. The lateral pectoral fascia, which is anterior to the axillary fat, is identified perpendicular to the skin incision.

Transumbilical

A superior periumbilical incision is made, and an obturator is used to tunnel under the skin to the inframammary fold. An endoscope is inserted to identify the prepectoral fascia.

Implant pocket

Subglandular

Once the pectoralis muscle has been identified by the periareolar, inframammary, or transaxillary approaches, dissection between the breast and prepectoral fascia is initially performed using electrocautery. This is facilitated using a lighted retractor. This direct vision allows for improved hemostasis. Once the implant pocket is partially formed, a temporary sizer can be obtained and inflated to assist with pocket dissection.

Subpectoral or dual-plane

Once the pectoralis muscle has been identified, the subpectoral plane is initially established by inserting the end of a lighted retractor immediately beneath the muscle. This allows for direct vision and the use of an electrocautery device to dissect the pocket. Inflating a temporary sizer further assists in creation of the pocket. The inferior origins of the pectoralis muscle should be divided. It is important *not* to divide the medial origins of the pectoralis muscle. If a dual-plane pocket is to be used, a subglandular dissection from the inframammary fold is performed. This can be just a few centimeters or, in cases of ptosis, all the way up to the level of the areola.

Meticulous hemostasis is achieved, and the pockets are irrigated with antibiotic solution. We routinely instill Marcaine with epinephrine into the pockets for postoperative analgesia. The use of postoperative drains is not usually necessary.

For the transumbilical approach, both the subglandular and subpectoral pockets can be accessed. The endoscope is used to confirm the correct plane of dissection. An implant sizer is guided up the tunnel into the proper plane. The pocket is dissected by inflating the sizer to a dimension somewhat larger than the final implant to be placed. The sizer is removed and replaced with the saline implant, which is placed and filled in a similar fashion.

Placement of implants

Meticulous sterile technique is advocated throughout the operation, but especially when handling and inserting the implants. This is accomplished by replacing gloves or wiping them with an antibiotic-soaked gauze sponge. The breast is again prepared with an antibiotic solution such as Betadine. The pocket is irrigated with antibiotic solution, as are the implants themselves. Saline implants are rolled up and placed into the pocket. The implant is either partially filled with 50 mL of saline or empty at the time of insertion. Once in place, the implants are filled with sterile injectable saline using a closed system.

The insertion of silicone gel implants is different. It is usually necessary for an assistant to retract the upper edge of the incision with a small Deaver-type retractor. The implants are then placed into the pocket. One hand is used to push the implant into the pocket while the other hand stabilizes and squeezes the implant in. Care and judgment must be exercised to ensure that the incision is of adequate length and that excessive force is not used when pushing the implant into the pocket. Because these devices consist of highly cohesive silicone, gel fracture can occur and has been described.

Once both implants have been inserted, the patient is sat upright and the breasts are examined for size, shape, and symmetry. Occasionally minor finger dissection of the lateral or medial pockets will improve the appearance. Once the appearance is satisfactory, the incisions are closed. A typical closure will consist of glandular, dermal, and finally a subcuticular layer using monofilament sutures. Sterile tape or Steristrips are placed over the closed incisions.

Postoperative care

Patients are placed in a surgical bra. Oral antibiotics are typically continued for 2 postoperative days, but can be used for longer if necessary. Pain is controlled using narcotic medication such as acetaminophen/hydrocodone. A muscle relaxant such as Robaxin is used following subpectoral augmentation.[13] Women are instructed to shower on postoperative day 2 or 3. Implant displacement exercises are routinely initiated in women with smooth round devices.

OPTIMIZING OUTCOMES

Outcomes can be optimized by proper patient selection, proper device selection, attention to surgical details, and good postoperative care. Specific aspects that are most important include the following:
- Identify chest wall abnormalities, ptosis, constricted breasts, and asymmetries preoperatively.
- Communicate with the patient about desired size and realistic expectations.
- Choose the appropriate implant.
- Do not divide the origins of the pectoralis major muscle medially when placing implants in the submuscular or dual-plane locations.
- A lighted retractor aids visualization.
- Prevent known causes of capsular contracture, such as hematoma and infection, with meticulous hemostasis, sterile technique, and pocket irrigation with antibiotic solution.

- Marcaine placed in the pocket and the muscle relaxant Robaxin help with postoperative pain control.
- Use a closed injection system for saline implants.
- Sit the patient up to compare the breasts for size, shape, and symmetry.

COMPLICATIONS

Complications can be divided into two groups. The first consists of those arising from the operation itself and includes complex scarring, hematoma, infection, wound dehiscence, altered sensation of the nipple–areolar complex, implant malposition, and capsular contracture. The second group consists of those that arise from the device and include rupture, rippling, and wrinkling. Other aspects that can lead to patient dissatisfaction include asymmetric breasts as well as inadequate size and abnormal contour.

Perhaps the most valid data regarding complications come from the implant manufacturers themselves. This was compiled in response to the FDA approval process for both saline and silicone gel devices. Prospective studies of the saline-filled breast implants approved by the FDA in May 2000 and prospective studies of the silicone-filled breast implants approved by the FDA in November 2007 provide data on breast augmentation complications. Complications often lead to reoperation, and the rate of reoperation is quite high after breast augmentation (Tables 9.1 and 9.2).

Complex scarring

Hypertrophic scars occur in approximately 3–7% of women following breast augmentation. Placing the incision in a well-concealed location is the best way to minimize the appearance of a scar. A periareolar incision should be placed just slightly within the pigmented border of the areola. An inframammary incision should be placed at the level of the anticipated new inframammary fold. Otherwise there may be a tendency for the incision to be visible and on the lower pole of the breast mound. An axillary incision should be planned and placed such that the posterior aspect of the incision is high in the axilla to minimize scar visibility.

TABLE 9.1 Mentor and Inamed post-approval studies: saline breast augmentation complications[14]

Complication	Mentor 7-year complication rate n = 1264 (%)	Inamed 7-year complication rate n = 901 (%)
Reoperation	25	30
Implant removal	19	15
Capsular contracture III/IV	11	16
Implant deflation	16	10
Breast pain	12	25

TABLE 9.2 Mentor and Allergan pre-approval core studies: silicone breast augmentation complications[6]

Complication	Mentor 3-year complication rate n = 551 (%)	Allergan 4-year complication rate n = 455 (%)
Reoperation	15.4	23.5
Capsular contracture III/IV	8.1	13.2
Breast pain	1.7	8.2
Implant removal with replacement	2.8	7.5
Nipple complications	10.4	4.9
Implant malposition		4.1
Hypertrophic scarring	6.7	3.7
Implant rupture	0.5	2.7
Implant removal without replacement	2.3	2.3
Hematoma	2.6	1.6
Infection	1.5	<1

Hematoma

The incidence of hematoma formation following breast augmentation is low and ranges from 1% to 3%. Meticulous hemostasis during the operation is the best way to avoid the formation of a hematoma. However, hematomas occurring up to 4 weeks later have been observed and are usually the result of sudden bleeding from a vessel that had been controlled intraoperatively.

All significant hematomas should be evacuated in the operating room, as undrained hematomas have been linked to an increased incidence of capsular contracture and infection.[15] After the incision has been opened, the implant and clot are removed and any active bleeding is controlled. Copious irrigation with an antibiotic solution is recommended prior to reinsertion of the implant and closure. The use of a postoperative drain may be considered in these situations.

Infection

Infection is a very uncommon complication after breast augmentation, with an incidence of <2%. Preventative measures include the administration of preoperative intravenous antibiotics, and careful sterile technique both in the operating room and throughout the operation. The breast pocket and the implant are irrigated with an antibiotic solution. When filling saline implants, a closed system is used to inject sterile saline.

When cellulitis occurs early in the postoperative course, a superficial versus a deep space infection must be determined. Patients are usually admitted for intravenous anti-

biotics. Early resolution of the cellulitis with a normal white blood count and afebrile state is suggestive of a superficial infection. Failure to respond to antibiotics usually suggests a deep space infection that is frequently associated with implant removal. Although there have been reports of infected implants salvaged by operative drainage and intravenous antibiotics, the standard and safe treatment is implant removal, allowing the infection to clear and the breasts to soften before replacing the implant. It is generally recommended to wait at least 6 months before reinserting breast implants.

Nipple sensation changes

The incidence of diminished sensation in the nipple–areolar complex has been reported to be as high as 15% following breast augmentation.[16] Aggressive pocket creation, especially with sharp dissection of the lateral pocket, is the most common cause of stretching or injury to the fourth lateral intercostal nerve. Sensory changes in the nipple–areolar complex can occur with any incision and any pocket location. Return of sensation may continue for months or even years.

Unsatisfactory size

The Mentor Core Study found that the second most common reason for reoperation in an augmentation patient was for a change of size.[6] Thus, it is very important to have good communication with the patient preoperatively about the desired size. Patients should be informed that their preoperative breast dimensions and characteristics may not be able to accommodate the desired volume. This may be because the breast diameter is too small for the implant base diameter, or that the skin may be too tight if they have a severe developmental deficiency.

Unsatisfactory shape: implant malposition, double bubble, synmastia

Malposition

Implant malposition may be defined as too high, too low, or too lateral. The malposition often is not apparent until the implant has settled into its permanent position. This may take several months as the pocket matures.

A high-riding implant (Fig. 9.8) can result when the inframammary fold is not lowered adequately, especially in the case of a large submuscular implant placed in a small breast. A compression strap worn postoperatively may assist with implant descent. If the implant does not descend enough over the next several months, surgical release of the inferior capsule may be required to lower the implant.

A low-riding implant is usually associated with a device that descends below the desired inframammary fold. This usually results in a breast with a bottomed-out appearance and nipples that are sitting too high. The implant can also drift too far laterally. A compression support bra worn several weeks postoperatively may minimize the occurrence of this problem. Correction of a malpositioned implant

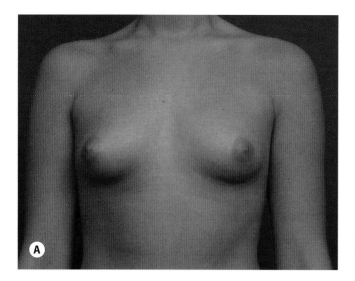

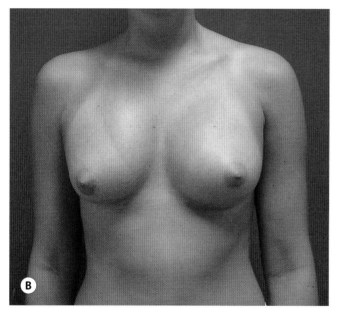

usually requires reoperation. For a bottomed-out implant (Fig. 9.9), a crescent of inferior capsule can be excised and the subcutaneous tissue of the inferior flap can be sutured to either the underlying fascia or the chest wall, depending on whether the implant was placed subglandularly or submuscularly, to create the new inframammary fold. Careful suturing is required to prevent fold irregularities. Similarly, if an implant has drifted too laterally, then lateral capsulorrhaphy sutures can be placed to reduce the width of the pocket and to redefine the lateral border (Fig. 9.10). This technique can fail if the sutures do not hold during the early healing phase. An alternative surgical correction of the

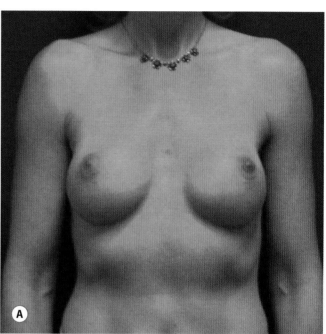

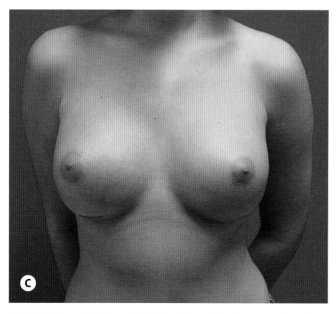

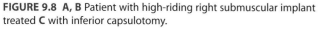

FIGURE 9.8 **A, B** Patient with high-riding right submuscular implant treated **C** with inferior capsulotomy.

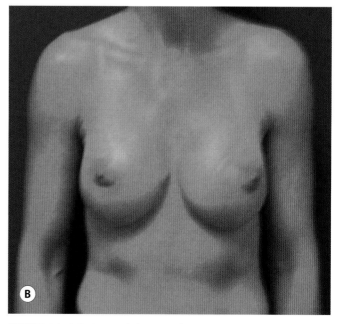

FIGURE 9.9 **A** Patient with bottomed-out implants. **B** Correction was by recreating the inframammary fold.

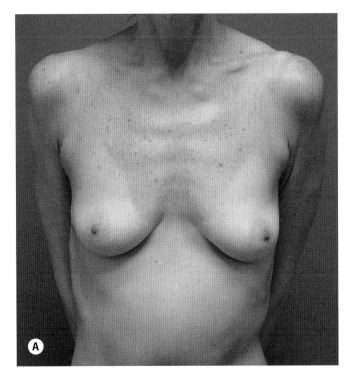

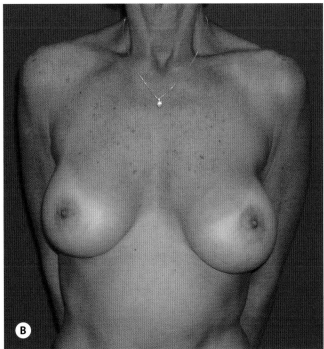

FIGURE 9.10 A Patient with left breast submuscular implant that has fallen too low and laterally **B. C** Correction was with capsulorrhaphy sutures.

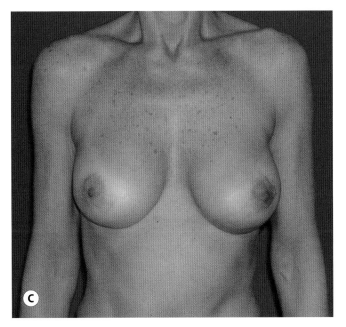

malpositioned implant is to change the implant site from subglandular to submuscular.

Double bubble

A 'double-bubble' appearance can occur when the inframammary fold has been lowered and there is persistent constriction at the old fold (Fig. 9.11). This typically occurs when a submuscular implant is placed in a breast with a tight, constricted high fold and the breast parenchyma does not redrape well. Releasing and stretching the old fold with radial scoring may help. Converting to a dual-plane location may avoid the double-bubble deformity. This is done by an inferior subglandular dissection to allow the pectoralis

muscle to ascend a little and the soft tissue to redrape better. In some cases a mastopexy may be needed to lift the breast tissue up from the old fold.

Synmastia

Synmastia after breast augmentation is rare, but is difficult to fix. It is usually the result of overaggressive medial dissection, resulting in an implant that can cross the midline and distorts the cleavage. It can result after either submuscular or subglandular implant placement. Prevention is preferable to successful repair. The repair usually consists of placing a row of sutures along the medial border of the breast pocket. Techniques that use the medial capsule as a

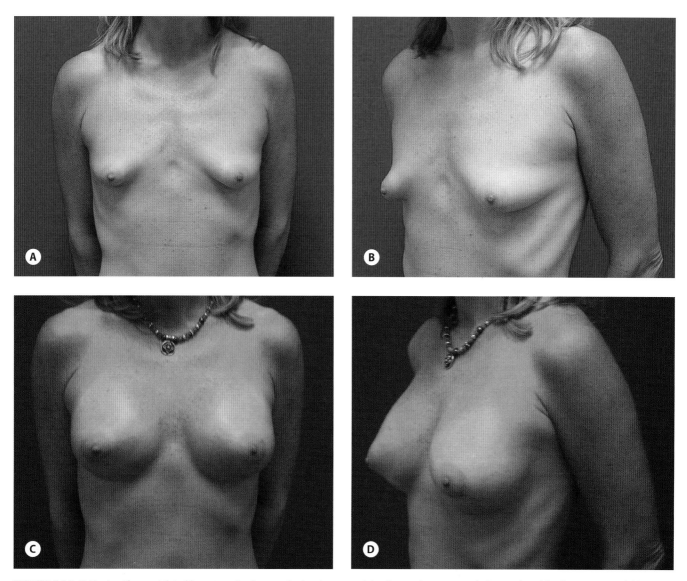

FIGURE 9.11 Patient with constricted breast and submuscular implants resulting in persistent constriction at the old inframammary fold despite radial scoring.

turnover flap may also be useful to eliminate the communication between the two pockets. Another method of correction is to stage the repair by removing the implants and then reinserting them in a different pocket at a later date.

Asymmetry

Shape asymmetry usually occurs because the breasts have different shapes before surgery; this cannot usually be corrected with implants alone. Other reasons for asymmetry may be related to chest wall irregularities that were not appreciated preoperatively. When preoperative asymmetry is noted, it should be explained to the patient before breast augmentation. When the asymmetry is due solely to a volume discrepancy, then intraoperative sizers can be helpful. If, following the augmentation, there is new or persistent volume discrepancy (not just differential swelling or implants settling at different rates), the implants can be easily exchanged for another size.

Capsular contracture

Capsular contracture remains a significant complication after breast augmentation. Both the Mentor and Allergan pre- and post-approval studies have demonstrated that capsular contracture is the main reason for reoperation in both saline and silicone breast augmentations.[6,14] The incidence has been reported to be 36–81% for silicone-gel filled implants and 8–41% for saline-filled implants.[3] Prospective studies of the saline-filled implants approved by the FDA in May 2000 showed grade III or IV capsular contracture rates of 9% at 3 years and 11–16% at 7 years for breast augmentation patients[14] (Table 9.1). Similarly, prospective studies of silicone breast implants approved by the FDA in November 2006 showed grade III or IV capsular contracture rates of 8–13% at 3 years[6] (Table 9.2).

The etiology of capsular contracture is multifactorial. Although undrained hematomas are known to increase the rate of contracture, the overall low incidence of hematomas in breast augmentation cannot account for the much higher observed incidence of capsular contracture. There is also a well-established correlation between infection and capsular contracture.[17] Reducing the incidence of infection with antibiotic breast irrigation has been shown to reduce the rate of contracture.[18] **M**odern silicone implants have more durable low-bleed shells and more cohesive gel, and have been reported to be equally as good as saline implants in avoiding capsular contracture.[4] Possible explanations why the subglandular position is associated with a higher incidence of capsular contracture compared to the submuscular location include the continuous muscle contraction over the implant, and that the submuscular space may be less vulnerable to bacterial contamination.

Earlier treatments of capsular contracture included closed or open capsulotomy and open capsulectomy with replacement of subglandular implants. These techniques

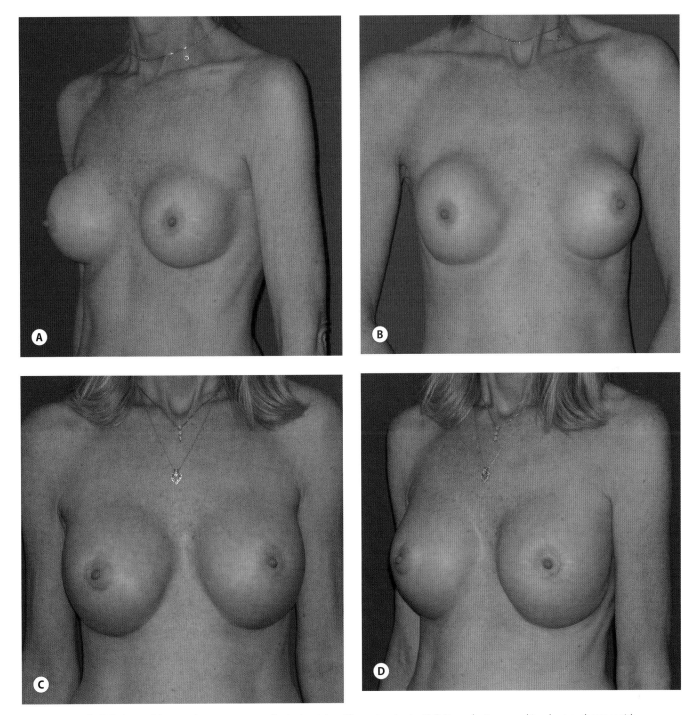

FIGURE 9.12 A, B Patient with capsular contracture of subglandular silicone implants. **C, D** Capsulectomy and implant exchange with submuscular conversion.

had varying degrees of success initially, and were associated with high recurrence rates. To give the patient the best chance to avoid redeveloping capsular contracture, the replacement implant should be placed in the best environment with the least amount of scar tissue. This means total or subtotal capsulcctomy and moving the pocket to a new location. After the capsulectomy has been performed, relocation to the dual-plane position has been shown to be an effective means of correcting capsular contracture (Fig. 9.12).[4]

Rupture

A ruptured saline breast implant is obvious as the implant deflates through a damaged valve or a break in the implant shell. Deflation usually happens immediately, but can occur over a period of days, becoming obvious by a loss of size or shape. Replacement of a saline implant is relatively simple and can be performed at any time. Recovery is usually uncomplicated, and women are able to resume normal activities within a month (Fig. 9.13).

The earlier saline implant models had more frequent deflations than modern models. It is estimated that 1–3% of modern saline-filled breast implants will rupture by the first year, and that this rate will increase over time. The Mentor and Inamed post-approval studies for saline implants showed a deflation rate of 3–5% at 3 years and 7–10% at 5 years for augmentation patients[14] (Table 9.1).

A ruptured silicone implant is usually undetected initially because the shape and feel of the breast are often unchanged. With the widespread use of cohesive gel devices, the issue of 'silent ruptures' has been debated. Detection of

silicone implant rupture can be difficult because physical examination may not provide clues. Mammography is the least sensitive imaging method for examining silicone gel breast implant rupture, with a sensitivity of 11–69%. Magnetic resonance imaging (MRI) has been reported to have a sensitivity of 39–76% when radiologists used a body coil, and 52–95% when they used a breast coil.[19]

The Mentor and Allergan Core Studies for silicone implants show a rupture rate of 0.5% at 3 years and 2.7% at 4 years, respectively[6] (Table 9.2). Further data on Allergan silicone implants come from the International MRI Study, which showed that silent rupture occurred in approximately 15% of patients, whose average age of implant was 11 years.[20] Studies in Danish women showed that about 75% of silicone implant ruptures found on MRI were intracapsular and 25% extracapsular, and that over a 2-year period about 10% of intracapsular ruptures progressed to extracapsular rupture as detected by MRI.[21,22] Thus, it would appear that removal of any ruptured silicone implant is indicated before intracapsular rupture progresses to extracapsular. It may be easier to remove the ruptured silicone implant in conjunction with a capsulectomy. Extracapsular silicone and siliconomas should be cleaned out.

CONCLUSION

Breast augmentation is a very popular cosmetic operation, and based on current trends it can be assumed that the use of this procedure will continue to increase. It is estimated that more than 34% of American women are dissatisfied with their breast size or shape and are interested in augmentation.[3] The periareolar, inframammary, transaxillary, and transumbilical incisions are all commonly used today, as are the subglandular, subpectoral, and dual-plane pocket locations. With the November 2006 FDA approval for silicone gel implants, it is expected that silicone gel breast implants will gain in popularity, especially in the United States, where their use has been most restricted. More choices will be available for breast augmentation when the cohesive shaped silicone gel implants are permitted for unrestricted use.

REFERENCES

1. Killmann P, Sattler J, Taylor J. The impact of augmentation mammaplasty: a follow-up study. Plast Reconstruct Surg 1987; 80: 374.
2. Rohrich RJ, Hartley W, Brown S. Incidence of breast and chest wall asymmetry in breast augmentation: A retrospective analysis of 100 patients. Plast Reconstruct Surg 2003; 111: 1513.
3. Committee on the Safety of Silicone Breast Implants. Safety of silicone breast implants. In: Bondurant S, Ernster V, Herdman R, eds. Washington, DC: Division of Health Promotion and Disease Prevention, National Academy Press, 1999.
4. Spear SL, Carter ME, Ganz JC. The correction of capsular contracture by conversion to 'dual-plane' positioning: Techniques and outcomes. Plast Reconstruct Surg 2003; 112: 456.
5. Pollack H. Breast capsular contracture: A retrospective study of textured versus smooth silicone implants. Plast Reconstruct Surg 1993; 91: 404.
6. Augmentation Patient Labeling for Mentor, November 2006 and Augmentation Patient Labeling for Allergan, November 2006 at FDA's website: http://www.fda.gov/cdrh/breastimplants/.

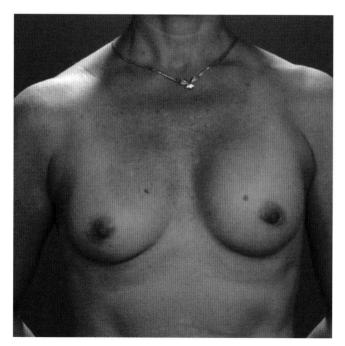

FIGURE 9.13 Patient with ruptured right breast implant is shown 4 years after undergoing subpectoral breast augmentation with saline implants.

7. Spear SL, Bulan EJ, Venturi ML. Breast augmentation. Plast Reconstruct Surg 2004; 114: 73e.

8. Courtiss EH, Webster RC, White MF. Selection of alternatives in augmentation mammaplasty. Plast Reconstruct Surg 1974; 54: 522.

9. Hurst NM. Lactation after augmentation mammoplasty. Obstet Gynecol 1996; 87: 30–34.

10. Henriksen TF et al. Surgical intervention and capsular contracture after breast augmentation: a prospective study of risk factors. Ann Plast Surg 2005; 54: 343–351.

11. Silverstein MJ, Handel N, Gamagami P. The effect of silicone gel-filled implants on mammography. Cancer 1991; 68: 1159.

12. Tebbetts JB. Dual plane breast augmentation: Optimizing implants–soft-tissue relationships in a wide range of breast types. Plast Reconstruct Surg 2006; 118: 81S.

13. Schneider MS. Pain reduction in breast augmentation using methocarbamol. Aesthet Plast Surg 2004; 21: 23.

14. Patient Labeling for Mentor saline breast implants, January 2004 and Patient Labeling for Inamed saline breast implants, November 2004 at FDA's website: http://www.fda.gov/cdrh/breastimplants/.

15. Hipps CJ, Raju DR, Straith RE. Influence of some operative and postoperative factors on capsular contracture around breast prostheses. Plast Reconstruct Surg 1978; 61: 384.

16. Courtiss EH. Goldwyn RM. Breast sensation before and after plastic surgery. Plast Reconstruct Surg 1976; 58: 1.

17. Cortiss EH, Goldwyn RM, Anastasi GW. The fate of breast implants with infections around them. Plast Reconstruct Surg 1979; 63: 812.

18. Adams WP Jr, Rios JL, Smith SJ. Enhancing patient outcomes in aesthetic and reconstructive breast surgery using triple antibiotic breast irrigation: Six-year prospective clinical study. Plast Reconstruct Surg 2006; 118: 46S.

19. Brown SL, Middleton MS, Berg WA, et al. Prevalence of rupture of silicone gel breast implants revealed on MR imaging in a population of women in Birmingham, Alabama. Am J Roentgenol 2000; 175: 1057.

20. Heden P, Nava MD, van Tetering JPB, et al. Prevalence of rupture in Inamed silicone breast implants. Plast Reconstruct Surg 2006; 118: 303.

21. Holmich LR, Friis SF, Fryzek JP, et al. Untreated silicone breast implant rupture. Plast Reconstruct Surg 2004; 114: 204.

22. Holmich LR, Friis SF, Fryzek JP, et al. Prevalence of silicone breast implant rupture among Danish women. Plast Reconstruct Surg 2001; 108: 848.

10

Augmentation/Mastopexy

Scott L. Spear and Joseph H. Dayan

INTRODUCTION

Augmentation/mastopexy is an operation that can present significant challenges. The added risk and conceptual difficulty of a one-stage procedure are reflected in its well-known common association with malpractice litigation. When performed individually, breast augmentation or mastopexy carries minimal risk. However, the combined maneuvers of expanding breast volume and reducing the skin envelope alter the blood supply and place greater stress on the closure. These factors increase the risk of skin and nipple necrosis, distortion of the nipple–areola complex (NAC), poor scarring, and even implant extrusion. Quantified in one study by Spear, complication rates comparing breast augmentation, primary augmentation/mastopexy[28], and secondary augmentation mastopexy were 1.7%, 17%, and 23%, respectively.[28] Because of the obvious convenience, as well as patient preference for a single-stage procedure, careful preoperative planning and thoughtful execution of this operation are essential to reduce both the severity and frequency of complications.

INDICATIONS AND CONTRAINDICATIONS

A systematic preoperative evaluation of the nature of the patient's ptosis is critical in achieving a favorable result. Breast ptosis is most commonly described using the Regnault classification.[20] Grade I ptosis is a nipple lying at the fold, grade II is a nipple below the fold but still on the anterior portion of the breast, and grade III is when the nipple is at the most inferior portion of the breast. However, deciding whether to perform a mastopexy and what type of excision pattern to use requires more information. The size of the breast and the surface area of the skin envelope, as well as the relationships between nipple position, breast parenchyma, and inframammary fold, are all important.

The assessment begins with two key elements: nipple position related to the inframammary fold, as classified by Regnault, and the amount of breast tissue that overhangs the fold. The more the skin and glandular tissue overhang the inframammary fold, the less likely an implant will be able to successfully fill out the breast in a cosmetically acceptable fashion unless skin is excised. Similarly, the lower the nipple, the less likely a prosthesis will raise the nipple adequately onto the surface of the breast (Fig. 10.1).

Identifying the primary motivation of the patient is also important. If the patient is focused on augmentation, a mastopexy may not even be necessary. Because the implant increases the breast size and the amount of skin necessary to cover it, skin excision patterns should not be finalized until after the implant is placed. In our experience, mastopexy may not be required if the nipple lies on the anterior surface of the breast with non-pigmented skin visible below it in the upright position, and where there is less than 2 or 3 cm of breast overhanging the inframammary fold. In these patients, placement of an implant alone may be sufficient to fill out the breast and achieve an acceptable aesthetic result.

In the vast majority of cases a circumareolar or circumvertical technique is sufficient, leaving a formal 'Wise' pattern only for the most severe cases. A periareolar mastopexy works well for a patient in whom the nipple lies near or just below the fold, with the inferior border of the areola no lower than the inferior curve of the breast on frontal view, and where there is less than 4 cm of breast overhanging the fold, leaving an initial nipple-to-fold distance of 6–8 cm. When planning a circumareolar mastopexy, as a guideline the ratio of the outer to the inner diameter of the circumareolar markings should ideally be no greater than 2:1, or at most 3:1. Overzealous use of the circumareolar pattern is one of the more common errors, especially when the patient insists on a minimal scar pattern. If used too aggressively, the resulting excess tension will probably lead to poor circumareolar scars, distortion of the NAC, and flattening of the breast.

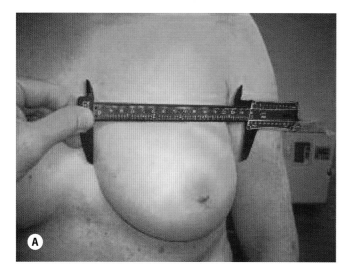

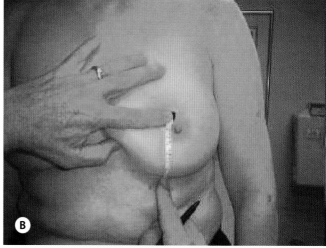

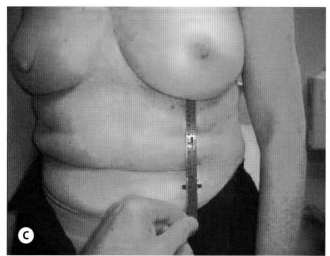

FIGURE 10.1 Thorough evaluation includes measuring the base width **A**, glandular ptosis **B**, and nipple-to-fold distance **C**.

The circumvertical or vertical technique offers greater versatility, and is most helpful when there is a greater degree of ptosis. This technique is most appropriate when the nipple is more than 2 cm below the inframammary fold, a portion of the areola lies on the inferior curve of the breast, the nipple-to-fold distance is greater than 8 cm, or the breast overhangs the fold by 4 cm or more.

For patients in whom the mastopexy is the primary goal, the implant should be just large enough to fill the skin envelope. If the plan includes attempting to correct significant asymmetries, particularly with substantial removal of parenchyma, then staging the procedure by performing a mastopexy initially may be better in the long run than trying to accomplish everything in one operation. Although inconvenient for the patient, trying to account for too many variables in one stage will probably increase the risks of the procedure and may lead to a poor outcome.

As a general principle, the final extent and pattern of the excision should not be committed to until the implants are placed. The skin envelope and nipple position are then tailor-tacked with the patient sitting upright, and finally adjusted to the dimensions of the newly augmented breast.

PREOPERATIVE HISTORY AND CONSIDERATIONS

There are a number of variables that may increase the risks of performing a single-stage augmentation mastopexy, including smoking, or a previous breast augmentation or reduction. Smokers are counseled about the increased risk and are cautioned to stop smoking. As the blood supply to the NAC is impaired to some extent in all of these patients, the procedure is performed very carefully with minimal undermining. Previously augmented patients have some degree of thinning of the tissues from the implant, so for the same reasons a cautious and conservative approach is necessary.

CHOOSING THE IMPLANT

The choice of implant size is an integral part of mastopexy planning, even when the two procedures are to be staged. The larger the implant, the less aggressive the skin excision should be. The decision-making process in augmentation mastopexy patients is complex, certainly more complex than for simple augmentation alone. Much depends on the fundamental indication for the mastopexy: is it a loose, pendulous, typically postpartum deflated breast that has an excess of capacity? or is it the opposite, such as a youthful tuberous breast with a deficiency of skin and an abnormally high, tight fold?

For the deflated pendulous breast it is important to measure the base diameter, both in the natural state and while simulating the mastopexy by pinching the breast to narrow it from side to side. In most cases the more important base width is the one simulated by pinching. If the breast is naturally 14 cm wide, 2 cm thick and pinches to 13 cm wide when the mastopexy is simulated, then an 11 cm wide implant is probably preferable to a 12 cm wide one. Because of the excess of space available in the involuted breast, higher-profile devices are often preferable to help fill the space. Discussion with the patient regarding the anticipated results helps finalize implant selection.

Conversely, for the constricted or tuberous breast the implant diameter chosen must often exceed the original breast base width. For this reason, mastopexy in these patients must be very conservative – often just enough to move the nipple superiorly or to reduce the areolar diameter. In these cases the implant diameter is chosen to help create a breast of more normal proportions and dimensions.

OPERATIVE APPROACH

Markings

With the patient standing upright, markings begin with the midline, breast meridians and inframammary fold (Fig. 10.2). A line is drawn tangential to the inframammary folds across the front of the chest for use as a reference. The midline is marked from the sternal notch to the xiphoid process. Careful attention is paid to marking the breast meridians, as there are often lateral asymmetries of the NAC that should be corrected as much as possible by adjusting the planned excision.

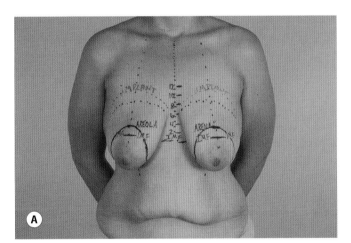
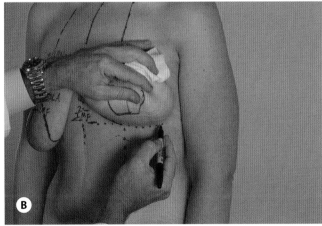
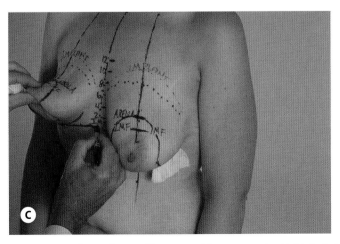
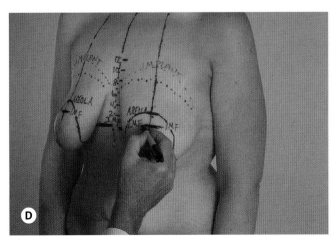

FIGURE 10.2 The midline and breast meridians are marked initially **A**. Inframammary folds (IMF) are then marked and a line tangential to the folds is drawn across the anterior chest **B, C**. This IMF level is then transposed over each breast **D**.

The degree of ptosis is then evaluated, noting the relationship of the nipple to the inframammary fold, as well as the nipple-to-fold distance and the amount or volume of breast that overhangs the fold. Sternal notch-to-nipple distance is variable among patients with different heights, and so the absolute numerical measurement is not as helpful as the previously mentioned measurements. However, it is used as a guide to assess the symmetry of the NAC. Based on these measurements, an appropriate excision pattern is planned as described. If there is significant asymmetry between the breasts, logically the planned skin excisions may be different, and it is made clear to the patient that although the intention is to achieve a more symmetric result, perfect symmetry virtually never happens (Fig. 10.3).

After evaluating the degree of breast and nipple ptosis and forming an operative plan, measurements for the implant are made. The base width of the breast is measured, as well as the superior pole pinch thickness. The difference between these values is a guide to the upper limit for the diameter of the implant. Using the implant diameter measurement, the anticipated height of the breast is marked from the inframammary fold. Markings are made to visualize the implant position on the chest wall and predict appropriate nipple placement.

As part of the initial skin marking in the examination room, the NAC is manually pinched and tailor-tacked so that the upper border of the planned new areola can be marked on the chest with the nipple at or slightly below the center of the projected dimensions of the breast mound. Gentle downward traction is placed on the superior pole breast skin to simulate the tension that will be created by the mastopexy. Unlike breast reduction procedures, in augmentation mastopexy the NAC is invariably marked to lie somewhere above the inframammary fold. Whereas the most serious error is to place the nipple too high, the most common error is inadequate elevation. It is important to note the presence of tan lines, as the nipple should never violate these borders, which may change once the breast is enlarged. It is also useful to have the patient wear a bra and mark its upper boundaries. These maneuvers can serve as important guides to prevent too-high placement of the nipple. The final position is decided intraoperatively after placement of the implant, tailor-tacking the planned excision, and sitting the patient upright (Figs 10.4 and 10.6).

Circumareolar technique

An ellipse is drawn from the previously marked upper areolar border, skirting the edges of the NAC and around the lower half of the areola, leaving 5–7 cm of skin between this mark and the fold. Measurements are taken from the midline to the medial edge of the markings on both sides to help provide reasonably symmetric placement of the NAC on the vertical axis. If there is significant asymmetry, the side with the relatively malpositioned NAC is addressed by adjusting the medial or lateral extent of the ellipse. Finally, the nipple-to-fold distance is measured again to ensure symmetry of the NAC in the transverse plane.

The procedure itself begins with the patient in the supine position with the arms tucked or abducted 90° or less. A 42 mm cookie cutter is centered over each nipple

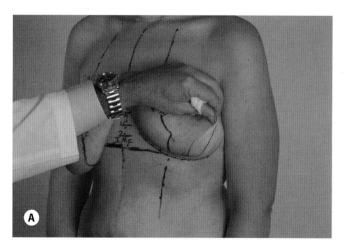

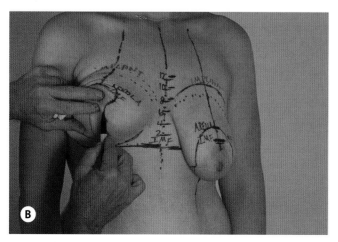

FIGURE 10.3 The medial and lateral pillars are marked in alignment with each breast meridian as superolateral and superomedial traction is applied to each breast.

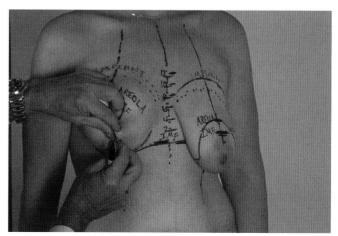

FIGURE 10.4 Manual tailor-tacking is used to evaluate the projected breast shape after placement of the pillars and ensure closure without undue tension.

without undue tension on the skin. In patients where it is unclear whether any mastopexy procedure will be necessary, the procedure begins with a periareolar incision for placement of the implant without de-epithelialization. The incision is usually made along the inferior border of the areola and dissection is carried down to the pectoralis major muscle.

Dissection and implant placement then proceed, with our preference being the dual-plane or partly retropectoral technique. The inferior third of the pocket is dissected in the subglandular plane, whereas the upper two-thirds or so of the pocket lie in the subpectoral plane. Meticulous hemostasis and irrigation with a triple-antibiotic solution are routinely performed to minimize the risk of capsular contracture or infection. After completing the dissection, the implant is soaked in antibiotic solution, the field is reprepared with a Betadine paint stick, and gloves are changed prior to implant placement. After insertion, the incision is stapled closed and the patient is positioned sitting fully upright. If there is still significant ptosis, the

previously planned circumareolar pattern is tailor-tacked using a skin stapler. The nipple position is then reassessed and remeasured, and may be fine-tuned as required. Circumareolar de-epithelialization may then be performed as necessary. This strategy may avoid unnecessary placement of scars on the breast in borderline cases (Fig. 10.5).

Following de-epithelialization, the outer circumference of the dermis is incised with the Bovie on cutting mode, ensuring that the incision is about 5–7 mm away from the skin edge, leaving a dermal cuff. Minimal undermining in the subcutaneous plane is performed to redrape the skin. Care is taken not to dissect deep and violate the breast parenchyma in order to preserve blood supply to the nipple. Usually only 1–2 cm of undermining is required. Classically, a 'blocking' purse-string suture is used by purse-stringing the dermal cuff with a permanent 3/0 suture. More recently we have adopted the interlocking Gore-Tex suture technique described by Hammond. Using a CV-3 Gore-Tex suture, eight equally spaced bites are placed between the dermal cuff and the dermis of the NAC. Finally, the skin is closed with interrupted and running buried Monocryl sutures.

Circumvertical technique

In this technique, the excision pattern extends vertically down to or just above the inframammary fold. If required, a small transverse skin excision can be placed in the inframammary fold to eliminate any dog-ear. This allows for coning of the breast in cases where greater skin excision is necessary.

The preliminary markings are essentially the same as in the circumareolar technique. The nipple position is determined as described. Superomedial and superolateral traction is applied to the breast and vertical marks are drawn on the surface of the skin over the projected breast meridian. These markings extend from the circumareolar

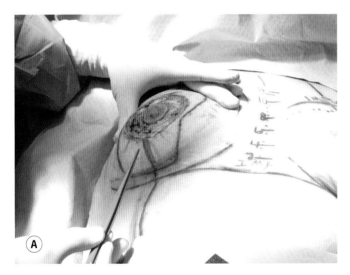

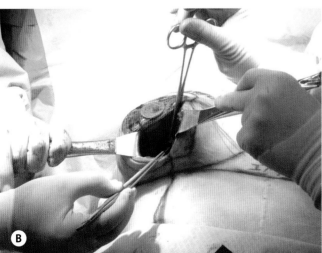

FIGURE 10.5 Conservative circumareolar de-epithelialization is performed **A**. The breast parenchyma is transected vertically and a subpectoral pocket is created **B**.

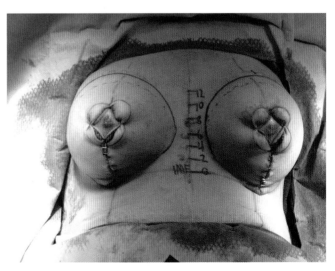

FIGURE 10.6 Implants are placed in the subpectoral position and intraoperative tailor-tacking with a skin stapler is performed prior to committing to preoperative markings.

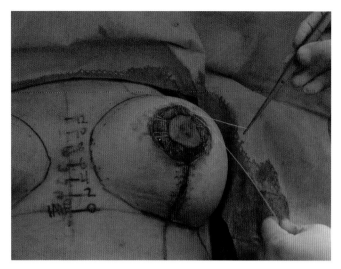

FIGURE 10.7 The interlocking Gore-Tex suture technique may be used for added stability when closing the circumareolar incision.

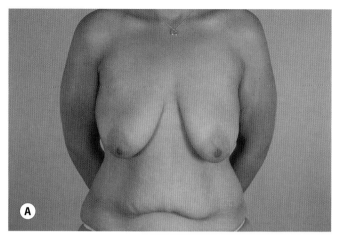

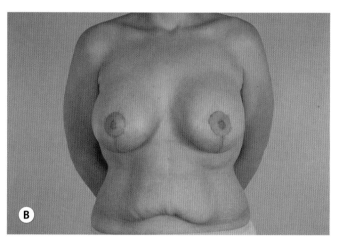

FIGURE 10.8 Pre- and early postoperative views showing improved contour and nipple viability.

marks and join in a 'V' or 'U' shape down to or just above the fold. These lines are then pinched together to check whether skin closure is possible while anticipating the effect of the implant. The length of the vertical limb is directly related to the amount of ptosis, but never extends beyond the inframammary fold. If necessary, after tailor-tacking, any residual dog-ear can be excised, leaving a small transverse scar in the inframammary fold (Figs 10.2, 10.3 and 10.4).

As previously described, the planned skin excision is not committed to until intraoperative tailor-tacking is performed with the implant in place. If the ptosis is severe and the surgeon is confident that a vertical technique is required, then the safest way to enter the breast is in a vertical manner within the planned area of de-epithelialization. Theoretically this dissection would be parallel to the neurovascular supply to the nipple. However, if there is any question about the need for a vertical excision, a periareolar approach is used (Fig. 10.5).

Once the implant is in place, the design is tailor-tacked with the patient sitting upright (Fig. 10.6). The amount of excess skin that can safely be removed is now more accurately determined. These areas are de-epithelialized and then minimal subcutaneous undermining is performed around the areola after incising the dermis, leaving a 5–7 mm dermal cuff. The vertical closure is usually 6–8 cm in length, depending on the implant and final total breast size. Greater vertical lengths are addressed with small transverse triangular excisions based at the inframammary fold. Sometimes, a small amount of excision of breast tissue is required both in the vertical and transverse components of the design. However, these maneuvers should be conservative, as they increase the risk of implant exposure and vascular compromise. All incisions are then closed using buried interrupted and running Monocryl sutures. If the circumareolar area of excision is significant, the interlocking Gore-Tex suture technique may be used for added stability, even with the vertical technique (Fig. 10.7).

Optimizing outcomes

- Setting the nipple at the right height
- Not expecting too much out of the circumareolar technique
- Purse-string or interlocking purse-string suture
- Excising the dog-ear at the inframammary fold as needed

Pearls and Pitfalls

- When in doubt, stage the procedure, performing the mastopexy first
- Devascularizing the nipple
- Setting the nipple too high or too low

COMPLICATIONS AND SIDE EFFECTS

As previously mentioned, the most common complications in augmentation/mastopexy arise from inappropriate use of the circumareolar excision pattern. When used too aggressively, poor scarring, areolar distortion, and flattening of

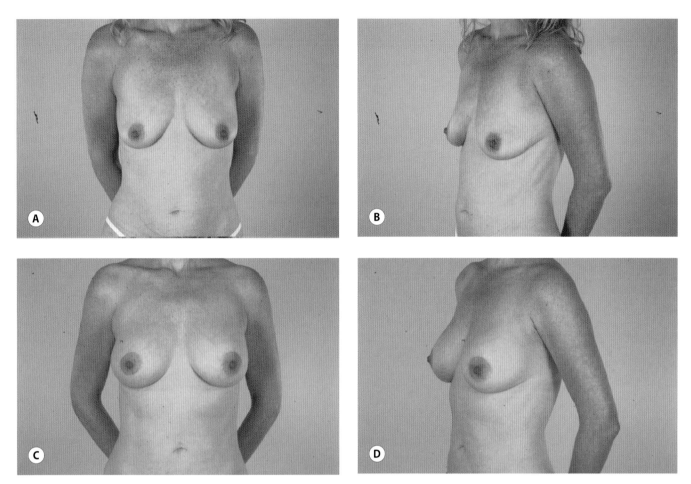

FIGURE 10.9 A, B This 44-year-old woman presented with mild ptosis and 1 cm of gland overhanging the fold. **C, D** Circumareolar augmentation/mastopexy was performed using McGhan style 40 silicone 200 mL implants.

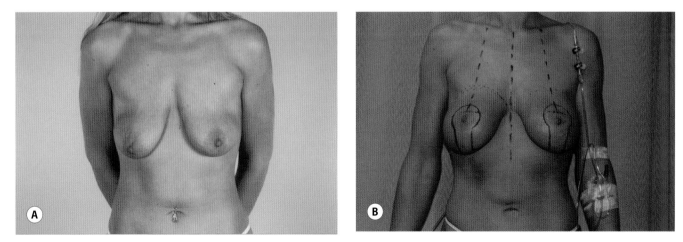

FIGURE 10.10 A This 33-year-old woman previously lost 100 lb and presented with 5 cm of gland overhanging the fold and a nipple-to-fold distance of 12 cm, necessitating a circumvertical approach. **B** Her initial augmentation mastopexy was performed using McGhan style 40 silicone 280 mL implants.

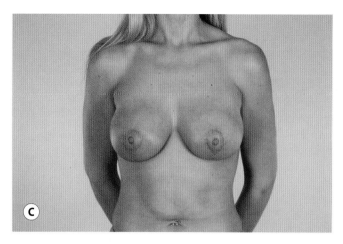
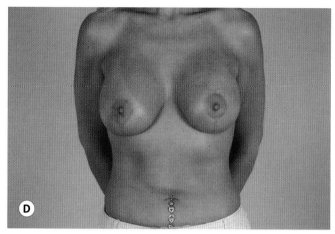

FIGURE 10.10, cont'd C The patient presented 10 months later with some residual gladular ptosis, and requested larger implants. **D** A revision mastopexy was performed by de-epithelializing the skin and simple closure without any undermining. Implants were replaced with Allergan style 20 silicone 500 mL implants (**D**).

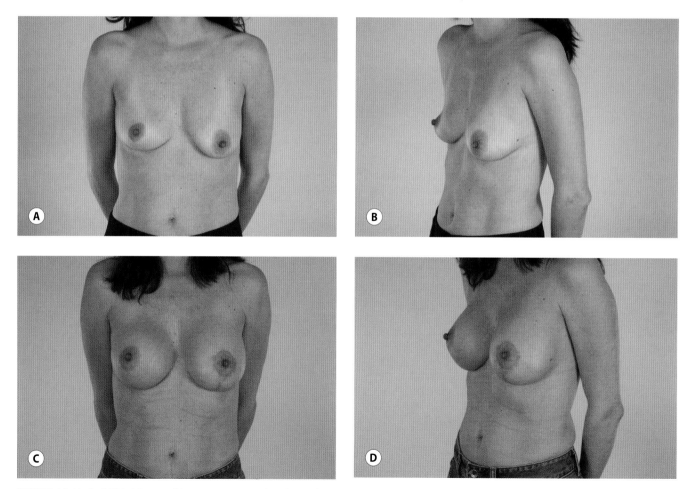

FIGURE 10.11 A, B This 38-year-old woman presented with significant breast asymmetry and desired fuller and larger breasts. The nipple lies below the fold on the left and there is 3 cm of gland overhanging the fold on the left, as opposed to 1 cm of overhang on the right. Additionally, the base width on the right is 12.5 cm and 11 cm on the left. **C, D** An augmentation was performed on the right using an inframammary incision and a 300 mL medium-profile saline implant filled to 305 mL with a base width of 11.9 cm. A circumvertical augmentation mastopexy was performed on the left with a 250 mL low-profile saline implant filled to 245 mL with a base width of 11.7 cm.

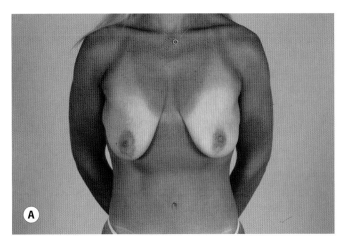

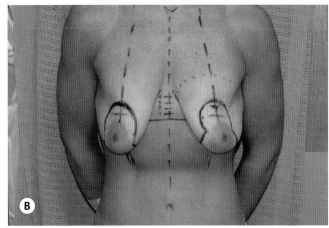

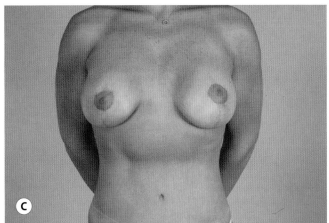

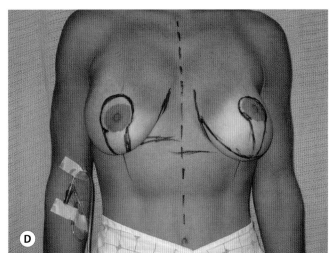

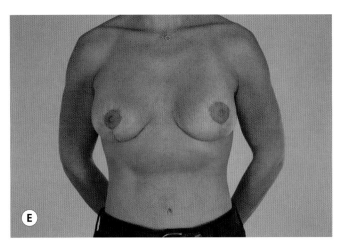

FIGURE 10.12 A This 35-year-old woman previously lost 120 lb and presented with severely deflated breasts. **B, C** Augmentation mastopexy was performed with a circumvertical technique using 268 mL Inamed style 15 silicone implants. She returned with some bottoming-out and nipple asymmetry that were addressed with revision mastopexy. **D, E** Simple de-epithelialization and closure were performed and implants were exchanged for 240 mL silicone implants.

the breast may occur. To avoid these potential problems, when in doubt use a circumvertical pattern, especially when the ratio of the outer to inner circumareolar diameters is greater than 3 : 1.

A malpositioned NAC is usually the result of poor preoperative planning and/or committing to the planned excision without intraoperative tailor-tacking. These maneuvers are critical because it is not always possible to accurately predict the new dimensions of the breast once the implant is placed. Most commonly the nipple is inadequately raised, which can be addressed with a simple revision. However, an NAC that is too high is a more difficult problem, as surgical correction is difficult and may leave the patient with a visible scar in the superior pole of the breast – a scar that may be visible in a swimsuit or low-cut dress.

Finally, perhaps the most dreaded complication is nipple necrosis. In patients who have previously undergone breast reduction the risks may be significant. In secondary cases, when in doubt the mastopexy may be performed using de-epithelialization only, without undermining the skin. If redraping is necessary, undermining should always be performed conservatively (1–2 cm) in a superficial subcutaneous plane.

POSTOPERATIVE CARE

Patients are placed in a soft bra and followed closely for the first few days to monitor the nipple and flaps.

CONCLUSION

Although augmentation/mastopexy may be a common elective procedure, it carries increased risks that require particularly thoughtful planning and caution. In patients with asymmetric breasts it should be stressed that these asymmetries can be improved upon but that achieving true symmetry is rare. For mild asymmetries, a symmetric approach is preferred. For significant asymmetries, different excision patterns may be more appropriate. Undermining around the areola should avoid violating the parenchyma and be limited to the minimal amount required to redrape the skin. Finally, the implant dictates the final nipple position, and so intraoperative tailor-tacking is critical in avoiding NAC malposition (Figs 10.8–10.12).

FURTHER READING

1. Adams WPJr, Rios JL, Smith SJ. Enhancing patient outcomes in aesthetic and reconstructive breast surgery using triple antibiotic breast irrigation: six-year prospective clinical study. Plast Reconstruct Surg 2006; 118: 46S–52S.
2. Baran CN, Peker F, Ortak T, et al. Unsatisfactory results of periareolar mastopexy with or without augmentation and reduction mammoplasty: enlarged areola with flattened nipple. Aesthet Plast Surg 2001; 25: 286–289.
3. Benelli L. A new periareolar mammaplasty: the 'round block' technique. Aesthet Plast Surg 1990; 14: 93–100.
4. Brink RR. Evaluating breast parenchymal maldistribution with regard to mastopexy and augmentation mammaplasty. Plast Reconstruct Surg 2000; 106: 491–496.
5. Cardenas-Camarena L, Ramirez-Macias R. Augmentation/mastopexy: how to select and perform the proper technique. Aesthet Plast Surg 2006; 30: 21–33.
6. Ceydeli A, Freund RM. 'Tear-drop augmentation mastopexy': a technique to augment superior pole hollow. Aesthet Plast Surg 2003; 27: 425–432; discussion 433.
7. de la Fuente A, Martin del Yerro JL. Periareolar mastopexy with mammary implants. Aesthet Plast Surg 1992; 16: 337–341.
8. Don Parsa F, Brickman M, Parsa AA. Augmentation/mastopexy. Plast Reconstruct Surg 2005; 115: 1428–1429.
9. Elliott LF. Circumareolar mastopexy with augmentation. Clin Plast Surg 2002; 29: 337–347.
10. Friedman RM. Augmentation/mastopexy: 'Surgeon beware.' [Letter] Plast Reconstruct Surg 2004; 113: 2230–2231.
11. Gasperoni C, Salgarello M, Gargani G. Experience and technical refinements in the 'donut' mastopexy with augmentation mammaplasty. Aesthet Plast Surg 1988; 12: 111–114.
12. Gonzales-Ulloa M. Correction of hypotrophy of the breast by exogenous material. Plast Reconstruct Surg 1960; 25: 15–26.
13. Gruber R, Denkler K, Hvistendahl Y. Extended crescent mastopexy with augmentation. Aesthet Plast Surg 2006; 30: 269–274; discussion 275–266.
14. Hoffman S. Some thoughts on augmentation/mastopexy and medical malpractice. Plast Reconstruct Surg 2004; 113: 1892–1893.
15. Karnes J, Morrison W, Salisbury M, et al. Simultaneous breast augmentation and lift. Aesthet Plast Surg 2000; 24: 148–154.
16. Nigro DM. Crescent mastopexy and augmentation. Plast Reconstruct Surg 1985; 76: 802–803.
17. Owsley JQ Jr. Simultaneous mastopexy and augmentation for correction of the small, ptotic breast. Ann Plast Surg 1979; 2: 195–200.
18. Persoff MM. Vertical mastopexy with expansion augmentation. Aesthet Plast Surg 2003; 27: 13–19.
19. Puckett CL, Meyer VH, Reinisch JF. Crescent mastopexy and augmentation. Plast Reconstruct Surg 1985; 75: 533–543.
20. Regnault P. The hypoplastic and ptotic breast: a combined operation with prosthetic augmentation. Plast Reconstruct Surg 1966; 37: 31–37.
21. Snow JW. Crescent mastopexy and augmentation. Plast Reconstruct Surg 1986; 77: 161–162.
22. Spear S, Davison SP. Breast augmentation with periareolar mastopexy. Op Tech Plast Reconstruct Surg 2000; 7: 131–136.
23. Spear S, Giese SY. Simultaneous breast augmentation and mastopexy. Aesthet Surg J 2000; 20: 155–165.
24. Spear S, Giese SY, Ducic I. Concentric mastopexy revisited. Plast Reconstruct Surg 2001; 107: 1294–1299.
25. Spear S. Augmentation/mastopexy: 'Surgeon, beware.' Plast Reconstruct Surg 2003; 112: 905–906.
26. Spear S, Venturi M. Augmentation with periareolar mastopexy. In: Spear SL, ed. Surgery of the breast: principles and art, 2nd edn. Vol. 2. Philadelphia: Lippincott Williams & Wilkins, 2006.
27. Spear SL. Augmentation/mastopexy: 'surgeon, beware.' Plast Reconstruct Surg 2006; 118: 133S–134S; discussion 135S.
28. Spear SL, Boehmler JH, Clemens MW. Augmentation/mastopexy: a 3-year review of a single surgeon's practice. Plast Reconstruct Surg 2006; 118: 136S–147S; discussion 148S–149S, 150S–151S.
29. Spear SL, Kassan M, Little JW. Guidelines in concentric mastopexy. Plast Reconstruct Surg 1990; 85: 961–966,.
30. Spear SL, Low M, Ducic I. Revision augmentation mastopexy: indications, operations, and outcomes. Ann Plast Surg 2003; 51: 540–546.
31. Spear SL, Pelletiere CV, Menon N. One-stage augmentation combined with mastopexy: aesthetic results and patient satisfaction. Aesthet Plast Surg 2004; 28: 259–267.
32. Tebbets JB. Dual plane breast augmentation: Optimizing implant-soft-tissue relationships in a wide range of breast types. Plast Reconstruct Surg 2001; 107: 1255–1272.

Breast Reduction: Wise Pattern Techniques

11

Steven P. Davison and Mark W. Clemens

INTRODUCTION

Reduction mammaplasty is a challenging combination of aesthetic and functional reconstructive plastic surgery. In breast reduction, a technique that provides a safe and predictable result with nipple–areolar preservation is paramount. The preferred technique is ideally versatile and predictable. The end result should be judged on volume, scar pattern, shape, symmetry, and nipple position with projection. The American Society of Plastic Surgeons reports a 25% increase in reduction mammaplasty over the last 4 years. Over 105 000 breast reductions were performed in 2004.[1] This trend is likely to continue as the incidence of obesity in the general population rises. Rohrich et al.[2] have previously reported that the inferior pedicle and Wise pattern techniques were the most popular, based on a survey of Board-certified plastic surgeons. We believe the most common technique for breast reduction surgery remains the inferior pedicle with an inverted-T or Wise skin pattern. This chapter addresses the versatility of the Wise inverted-T technique skin pattern by giving particular attention to its variety of applications.

Historical background

There are two components to breast reduction: the pedicle, and the skin excision. Although related, they are independent of each other.[3–5] The Wise pattern skin excision has been described with a variety of pedicles.

At the turn of the century, most incisions and breast reductions were oriented as vertical-only or horizontal-only. The first breast reductions using a vertical incision with a short horizontal component were described by Lexer in 1925.[6] The Wise keyhole pattern was introduced in 1956, to answer unpredictability concerns raised by limited incision techniques.[7] The Wise pattern or inverted-T gained

much support in the United States, where surgeons were more likely to functionally address moderate to severe mammary hypertrophy. Limited vertical incision techniques tended to predominate in South America and Western Europe, where surgeons were more likely to cosmetically address smaller-volume breast reductions. Surveys among reduction mammaplasty patients indicate that in the United States today, the major concerns revolve around the burden of heavy breasts, and less on aesthetic scars.[8] At our institution, we used the Wise pattern with 133 superomedial-based pedicles and nine free nipples.[9] Average excisions were 1188 g and 1929 g, respectively.

Wise produced a predictable pattern for breast reduction by creating a technique that allowed for three-dimensional control of the breast. Today, there are various pedicles that use the inverted-T pattern skin incision, among them the inferior pedicle, the McKissock vertical bipedicle, and the superomedial, superolateral, and medial pedicles. The idea of a dermoglandular pedicle was introduced when Strombeck in 1960 first used a horizontal bipedicle of dermis and subcutaneous tissue to transpose the nipple–areolar complex superiorly with consistent safety.[10] In 1973, Weiner et al.[11] described a single superior dermal pedicle. Orlando and Guthrie[12] followed in 1975 with a description of the superomedial dermoglandular pedicle. This technique was further popularized by Hauben, who described the associated safety and speed of this particular design.[13,14] Nevertheless, the inferior pedicle technique had been the predominant method used for reduction mammaplasty at our institution.[15] Described in 1972, the McKissock technique involves a central breast reduced around a vertical bipedicle. The vertical limbs are established by breast meridians with the medial and lateral dermoglandular wedges plus portions of the upper flap removed down to fascia, creating a 'bucket handle' as part of the reduction. The inferior pedicle breast **145** reduction relies on a mostly dominant inferior blood supply based on parenchyma and chest wall musculature.

Breast reductions have been classically described by their pedicles (e.g., McKissock, inferior pedicle, etc.) yet this has been interchanged with the terminology Wise pattern.[2] **These are two separate entities.**

Pedicle type

The underlying goal of the pedicle is to provide blood supply to the nipple. The secondary rule is to provide the volume of breast tissue in the correct position so the reduction achieves a pleasing shape, i.e., a round, projecting breast with a superior fullness. Bottoming-out of the pedicle or a flat mound are compromised results. **Getting the pedicle correct is what dictates the volume of breast size.**

Skin pattern

The type of skin pattern is a separate entity from the pedicle. The Wise pattern, discussed here, has been used with a number of pedicles, including the McKissock,[15] the inferior pedicle, and the superomedial dermatoglandular pedicle.

Calvin Johnson, when he described open rhinoplasty, discussed the bony framework of the nose and the soft tissue envelope.[16] He described the soft tissue forming to the framework, often shrinking to it. The breast reduction skin envelope is analogous, but the inverse. We believe that the soft tissue envelope or skin molds the pedicle shape. It is similar in that manner to a bra: too small or tight an envelope and the breast flattens; too large and it becomes ptotic. **Getting the envelope correct is critical to shape.**

INDICATIONS AND CONTRAINDICATIONS

The indications for Wise pattern breast reductions are the same as for most breast reductions that include complaints of macromastia, brassiere shoulder grooving, upper back pain, neck pain, and inframammary intertrigo. Contraindications include any previous chest scars which interfere with skin flaps or the chosen pedicle, which may compromise the blood supply. For mammaplasty reoperations it is critical for the surgeon to be aware of the previously used pedicle orientation. Our current preference is for a superomedial pedicle with Wise pattern.

Anatomy and advantages of superomedial pedicle technique

The blood supply is as reliable as the inferior or central pedicle as it originates from the internal mammary perforators. In larger reductions, feathering of the pedicle can extend the perforators from the lateral thoracic artery and associated lateral intercostal and thoracoacromial vessels.[9] Flaring away from the pedicle also allows for the acquisition of the lateral rami of the fourth intercostal nerve. Additional sensory contributions may be made by the third and fifth intercostal nerves.[17] Objectively, the medial or supero-

medial pedicle techniques compare favorably in postoperative breast sensitivity with the inferior pedicle.

The superomedial pedicle has a better superior blood supply owing to its shorter length compared to an inferiorly based pedicle in an equivalently sized breast. Despite very large reductions, Finger and associates showed that the mean length of the superomedial pedicle was 11.6 cm, and Hall-Findlay utilized the superomedial glandular technique extensively in a wide range of mammaplasties.[5,18] With an inferior pedicle technique, the distance from the nipple to inframammary fold could be closer to 16–19 cm for a similar-sized reduction and potentially necessitate a free nipple graft. The arc of rotation is favorable and the pedicle needs to be rotated no more than 110°.

The skin excision pattern is not dictated by the amount of breast tissue to be removed. In our experience, varying amounts of breast parenchyma can be excised for the same skin patterns. This highlights the principle that it is the amount of excess skin that influences the pattern of excision and not the size of the breast reduction. It is the final size that dictates the amount of skin to be left and, conversely, the amount removed. Using the superomedial technique, the progressive skin excision from circumvertical to a short transverse scar or Wise pattern allows the surgeon to achieve a more ideal breast in one operation.

The superomedial pedicle inherently provides a substantial amount of superomedial fullness by preserving the upper-inner quadrant of the breast. Although this was not measured objectively, we believe it accentuates this area and resists the glandular bottoming-out phenomenon associated with the inferior pedicle. The inferior pedicle technique attempts to raise the inferior breast tissue superiorly while basing it inferiorly, thereby involving two inherently opposing vectors. Attempts to support the pedicle with suturing have had moderate success. Results of a study by Hsia and Thomson[19] comparing breast shape preferences between plastic surgeons, lay people, and patients seeking breast augmentation showed that the latter two groups preferred a convex breast shape, or a fuller superior pole. In patients seeking breast reduction, we find a similar preference for superior fullness and also elimination of inferolateral excess.

Free nipple reduction

When does a surgeon decide to perform a free nipple reduction with the Wise pattern skin excision? Historically, with the inferior pedicle it was the length of the pedicle. A greater than 19 cm pedicle length dictated a free nipple. With the superomedial technique, we use the sternal to nipple distance as a guide. At 39–41 cm, it is difficult to reduce the pedicle size sufficiently while preserving blood flow to create a significant reduction. Interestingly, the more ptotic and atrophic the breast, the more likely it is that the superomedial glandular pedicle will rotate and add to the reduction.

Free nipple transfers are accomplished using the same Wise pattern excision. The nipple is transferred in the

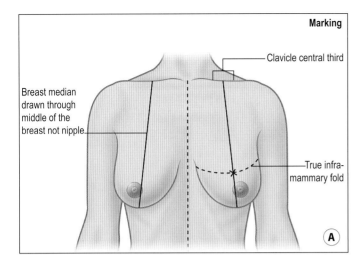

Marking

- Clavicle central third
- Breast median drawn through middle of the breast not nipple
- True infra-mammary fold

A

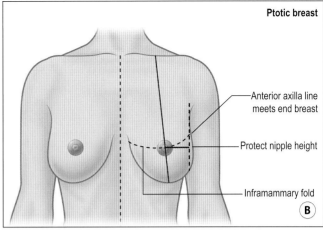

Ptotic breast

- Anterior axilla line meets end breast
- Protect nipple height
- Inframammary fold

B

FIGURE 11.1 Markings for the Wise pattern breast reduction. Note that the Wise pattern can be adjusted to be wider or narrower.

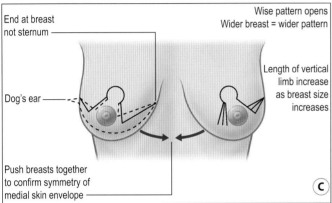

- End at breast not sternum
- Wise pattern opens Wider breast = wider pattern
- Dog's ear
- Length of vertical limb increase as breast size increases
- Push breasts together to confirm symmetry of medial skin envelope

C

standard fashion onto a modified superomedial pedicle that maintains the normal width but does not extend in length to the original nipple–areolar complex. Enough length is maintained to rotate the pedicle toward the new location of the nipple–areolar complex. Free nipple grafts are placed directly on the de-epithelialized pedicle.

OPERATIVE APPROACH

Marking – the Wise wire pattern

The Wise wire pattern is an invaluable tool (Fig. 11.1). However, it is only a tool if it can be modified and applied to a variety of breast types. There is a tendency among residents to use it as it comes, without widening or closing it. This should be performed to accommodate the pattern to breast size. The size of the nipple–areolar keyhole is dictated by the size of the nipple cutter ring – 38, 42, or 45 mm – the surgeon might use. The circle can be drawn inside or outside the wire. The limbs of the wire are graduated, allowing the vertical to be modified to final breast size: 6–6.5 cm for an approximate C cup to 7.5 cm for a D cup, to 8 cm for DD. The wire pattern can be expanded for a broad breast and narrowed for the thin-based breast. To

check and compare the length of the medial limbs for symmetry, the breasts can be approximated together.

Reductions larger than 1000 g with excess skin are performed using the superomedial pedicle with a Wise pattern excision. The preoperative markings are drawn with the patient in the standing position. Breast meridians are determined using the suprasternal notch and acromion to measure the meridian of each breast. A vertical line is drawn through the center of the breast, usually but not necessarily through the nipple–areolar complex. The inframammary fold is marked. Nipple placement is then marked along the breast meridians at the level of the fold.

The nipple to sternal notch distance on larger reductions is in the range of 22–26 cm. Another guide to nipple height is either midhumeral, or estimated by folding the breast skin and looking for the maximum height of the mound. The length of skin from the areola to the bottom of the Wise pattern is marked at 6–8 cm. If the breast is large, a longer vertical limb of 7–8 cm is selected in order to avoid pulling the abdominal skin and the final scar superiorly onto the breast. Often the medial skin contracts less than the lateral, so any length discrepancy should favor a longer lateral limb. On average for our reductions, a C cup breast corresponds to 6.5–7 cm, D cup to 7.5 cm, and D+

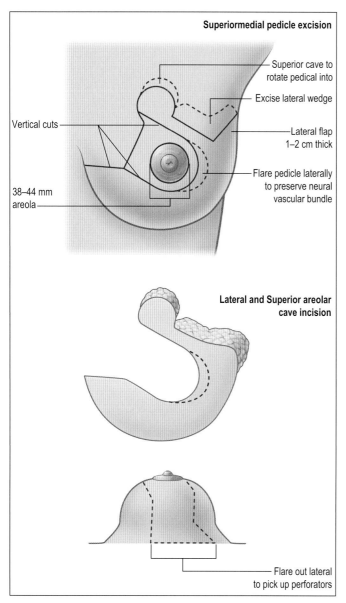

FIGURE 11.2 Diagram outlining the resection in the superomedial glandular pedicle – note that the majority of the removal is lateral.

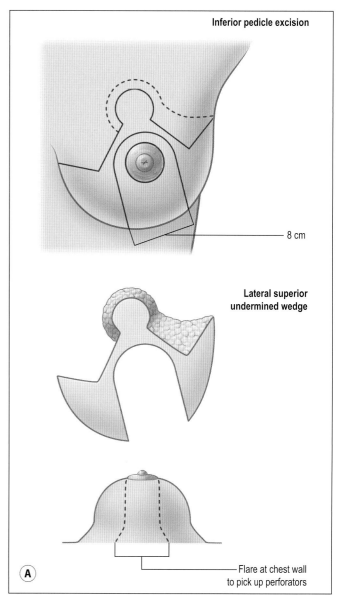

cup to 7.5–8 cm. The superomedial pedicle is then marked 6–8 cm wide (Fig. 11.2). The longer the pedicle and the wider the base, the larger will be the reduced breast.

The majority of the reduction comes from the inferolateral portion of the breast, and care is taken to avoid parenchymal excision from beneath the superomedial flap. A wedge of tissue is excised as an arc above the areola to provide space to rotate the pedicle, and is removed en bloc with the main specimen (Fig. 11.3). The superomedial pedicle is flared at the chest wall to maximize the intercostal perforators. The pedicle is then fixed by the skin envelope, not sutures. A set-up suture is placed at the T junction of the skin flaps with the inframammary fold. This suture is classically placed at the meridian of the breast. However, if it is moved 1–2 cm medially, greater coning of the breast is achieved.

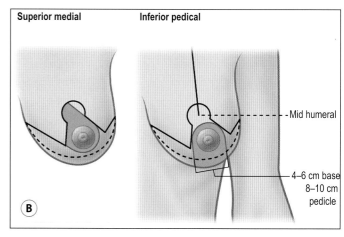

FIGURE 11.3 Diagram outlining the resection in the inferior pedicle. The bulk of the tissue is removed from under the skin flaps.

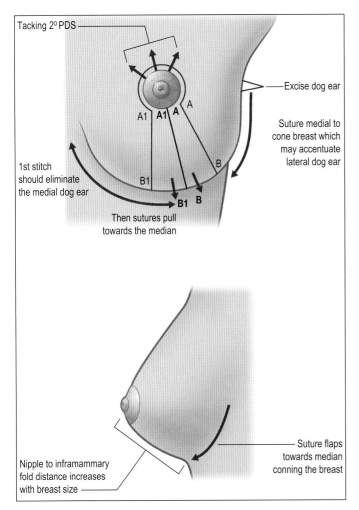

FIGURE 11.4 Diagram of the closure of the Wise pattern. Coning of the breast helps the shape.

Irrelevant of pedicle type, closure of the Wise skin pattern sets up the shape; a T-junction suture positions the flaps. The medial junction where the sternal skin meets the inframammary fold (IMF) is carefully sewn to eliminate a dog-ear. However, laterally we force the dog-ear to the axilla and extend the incision to eliminate it. Patients are uniformly unhappy with a dog-ear medially and better accept a larger scar, especially when combined with anterior axillary line liposuction. The shape of the breast should not be compromised to shorten the length of the axillary scar.

The medial and lateral skin flaps are sewn towards the meridian with some tension. The oblique suture bites with 2/0 PDS are greater at the edges and become progressively more neutral toward the T junction. This cones the breast, creating a pleasing round profile. Laterally, it defines the breast from the axilla.

The nipple–areolar complex is inset to give it support. One potential disadvantage of the superomedial glandular pedicle is that it is a short pedicle with a medially placed nipple which can be difficult to rotate. To facilitate this and avoid inverting the nipple, the dermal bridge of the de-epithelialized pedicle is incised (Fig. 11.4). This is possible in the superomedial glandular technique, as the pedicle is

shorter, which should augment the amount of blood coming in from the base. To cut the dermal pedicle in the inferior or McKissock pattern would be closer to heresy.

The nipple–areolar complex is supported by three to four 2/0 PDS deep dermal sutures, or breast capsule sutures placed at the 3, 9, and 12 o'clock positions. This restricts tension on the scar as the reduction heals, ultimately minimizing hypertrophic scar formation.

If an inferior pedicle is chosen for some reason, such as previous inferior reduction, or the need to include a superior cyst or mass. An inferior pedicle is created 3 or 4 cm in either direction from the breast meridian. The de-epithelialization is extended 2 cm above the nipple–areolar complex. Therefore, the total pedicle is 8–10 cm long.

OPTIMIZING OUTCOMES

One of the most time-consuming parts of a reduction is de-epithelialization. The other is sitting the patient up to confirm volume, symmetry, and nipple position. The predictability of the Wise pattern, with the on-table reproducibility of the superomedial glandular pedicle, allows a minimum of up/down positioning. We recommend closing the first breast, then tailor-tacking the second breast and sitting the patient up at this point. This allows volume and symmetry adjustments. Liposuction can be used to reduce the size of the lateral first breast if needed. The second side is then reopened and changes made, before proceeding to final closure.

Sutures and scars

Although absorbable sutures, both braided and monofilament, have made an enormous contribution to plastic closures, they come with a price. They are absorbed by an inflammatory process and cause localized skin reactions. We find that Vicryl sutures spit excessively. PDS 2/0 is used for deep tension sutures. Limited 3/0 Monocryl sutures are used for deep dermis closure. Note that excessive suture use leads to spitting later, but without the skin reaction of the braided sutures. In patients prone to poor scarring, we now use a 4/0 Prolene running subcuticular suture which is left in place beyond the 8 weeks needed for maximal wound strength.[20] The nipple–areolar complex is inset with a circumareolar Monocryl or simple interrupted Prolene sutures. A loop of Prolene is left out to facilitate easy removal.

COMPLICATIONS AND SIDE EFFECTS

Commonly described reduction mammaplasty complications include reduced sensation in the nipple–areolar complex, complete or partial loss of the nipple–areolar complex, delayed healing, fat necrosis, nipple retraction, hypertrophic scars, dog-ears, infection, and hematoma. Some or all of these occurrences may require a secondary operation. For all women considering reduction mammaplasty, a detailed informed consent should include a discussion of these possible complications as well as a questionnaire to ascertain the importance of future breastfeeding, nipple sensation, hypopigmentation of the nipple, hypertrophic and keloid scars. Incidences differ in the literature with respect to which pedicle was utilized. Revision rate is a very important marker of a reduction technique. At our institution, for 133 Wise pattern superomedial-based pedicles and nine free nipples, results were an overall 4.6% revision rate, for hematomas (1.4%), contour improvements (1.4%), and revision of the surgical scar (1.8%).[9] No nipple losses were observed. We have found immediate treatment with hyperbaric oxygen to be beneficial in selected patients when nipple ischemia is suspected early; however, large prospective studies are still required to completely elucidate its role. At our institution we have observed a link between sickle cell trait and flap necrosis in a breast reduction patient.[21] Risk factors associated with flap survival, such as smoking, obesity, radiation, and diabetes, should be well addressed preoperatively.

POSTOPERATIVE CARE

The postoperative care following reduction mammaplasty is generally routine. Steri-strips are usually placed along the incisions and women are instructed to wear a compressive breast garment. The compressive garment or bra is worn 23 hours a day for 4–6 weeks. Drains are usually inserted and removed after 24 hours. Sometimes the drains will remain in place for 2–3 days if the output is elevated. Women are instructed to shower on postoperative day 2 or 3. Activity restrictions are necessary for the first 6 weeks following the operation. Women are encouraged to refrain from any strenuous or bouncing activities, such as aerobic exercise, jogging, or running. After 6 weeks they can resume all normal activities.

CONCLUSIONS: WISE PATTERN

The key advantages of a Wise pattern, and specifically when combined with a superomedial pedicle, are:

CASE 11.2 Surgical procedure. Photo of the superomedial pedicle. Width of the superomedial pedicle prior to excision of breast parenchyma.

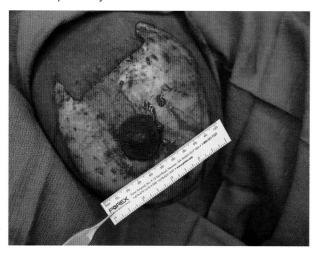

- Adaptability. The Wise pattern as a skin excision scar can be applied to a variety of pedicle or free nipple reductions.
- Shape. The skin pattern can be used to cone and shape the breast.
- Reproducibility and predictability. This pattern features an advantage in the learning curve and ability to teach.
- Progressive. The Wise pattern can be used with increasing degrees of ptosis, skin excess, and breast volume.

CASE 11.1 Surgical procedure. Photo of surgical excision of skin flaps with a superomedial pedicle pattern. Excision of an arc of tissue above the areola to create space for the new position of the nipple–areolar complex. Note that the bulk of the tissue is removed laterally.

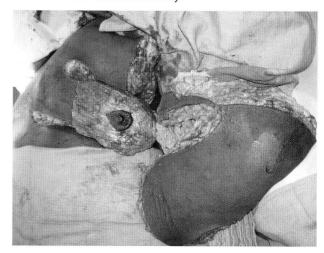

CASE 11.3 Preoperative markings on a 34-year-old woman with macromastia.

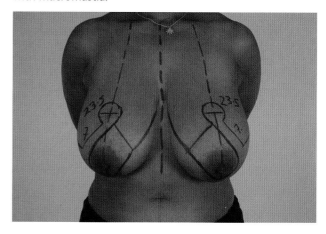

CASE 11.4 A, B The 34-year-old woman with macromastia from Case 11.3. **C, D** 7 months post superomedial pedicle Wise pattern breast reduction. Right and left breasts were reduced 950 g and 1100 g, respectively. Patient demonstrates no settling period or tissue adaptation.

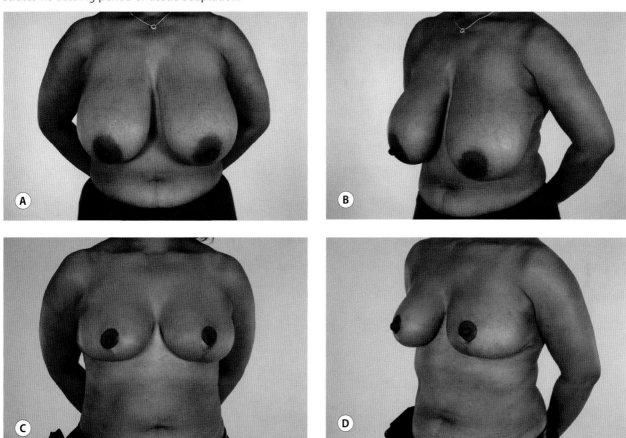

CASE 11.5 A, B A 24-year-old woman with macromastia. **C, D** 6 months post 800 g breast reduction, and **E, F** 14 months post-reduction.

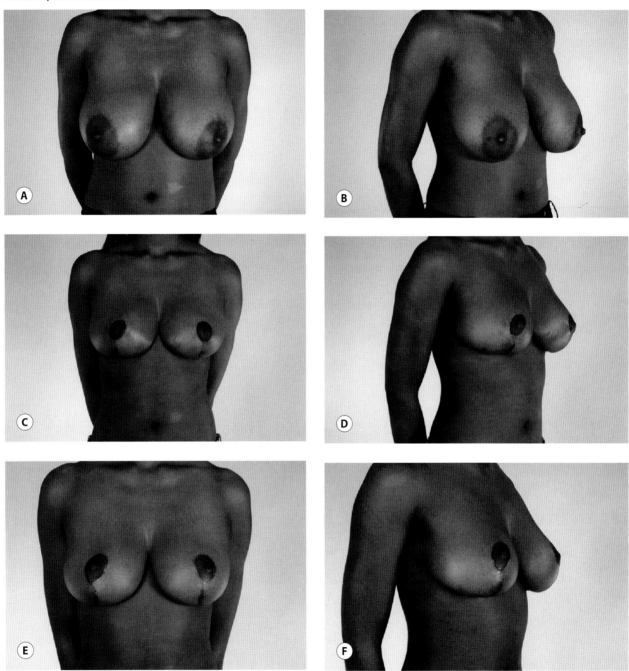

CASE 11.6 A, B A 19-year-old woman with macromastia, and **C, D** 1 year after 740 g reduction right breast and 680 g reduction left breast.

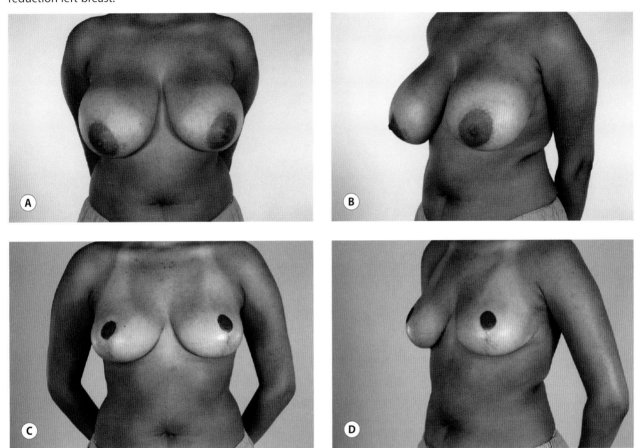

CASE 11.7 A 47-year-old woman with macromastia. **A, B** Preoperative views, and **C, D** 10 months after 1770 g reduction right breast and 1840 g left breast.

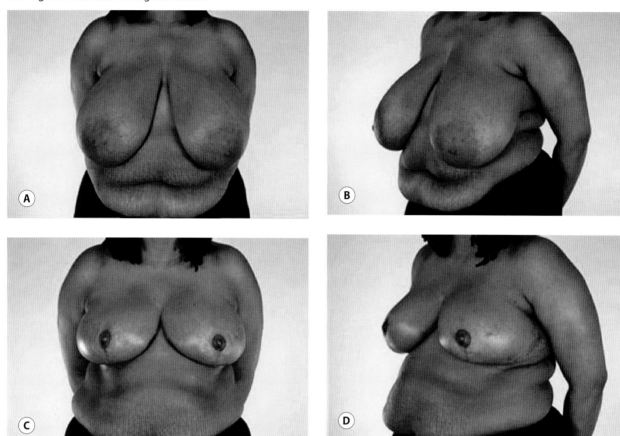

CASE 11.8 A 44-year-old woman with macromastia. **A, B** Preoperative views, and **C, D** 10 months after 565 g reduction right breast and 725 g reduction left breast.

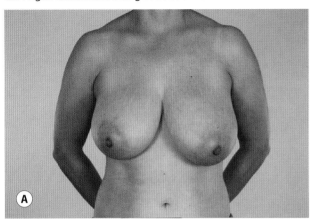
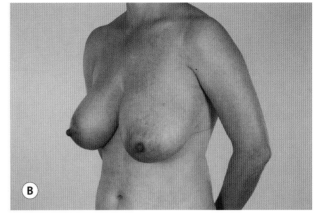
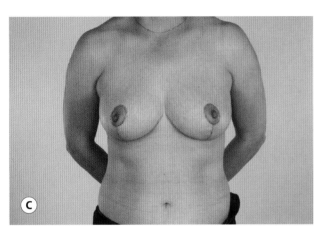
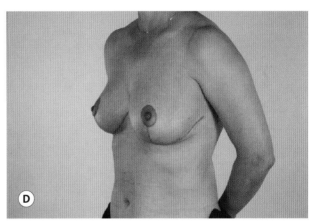

REFERENCES

1. American Society of Plastic Surgeons. www.plasticsurgery.org
2. Rohrich RJ, Gosman AA, Brown SA, et al. Current preferences for breast reduction techniques: a survey of board certified plastic surgeons. Plast Reconstruct Surg 2004; 114: 1724–1733.
3. Hammond DC. Short scar periareolar-inferior pedicle reduction (SPAIR) mammaplasty. Op Tech Plast Reconstruct Surg 1999; 6: 106.
4. Hammond DC. Short scar periareolar–inferior pedicle reduction (SPAIR) mammaplasty. Plast Reconstruct Surg 1999; 103: 890–901.
5. Hall-Findlay EJ. Discussion. Plast Reconstruct Surg 2005; 115: 1278.
6. Lexer E. Zur Operation der mammahypertrophie und der Hangebrust. Dtsh Med Wochenschr 1925; 51: 26.
7. Wise RJ. A preliminary report on a method of planning the mammaplasty. Plast Reconstruct Surg 1956; 17: 367.
8. Cruz-Korchin N, Korchin L. Vertical versus Wise pattern breast reduction: patient satisfaction, revision rates, and complications. Plast Reconstruct Surg 2003; 112: 1573–1578.
9. Davison SP, Mesbahi AN, Ducic I, et al. The versatility of the superomedial pedicle with various skin reduction patterns. Plast Reconstruct Surg In press.
10. Strombeck JO. Report of a new technique based on the two pedicle procedure. Br J Plast Surg 1960; 13: 79.
11. Weiner DL, Aiache AI, Silver L, Tittiranonda T. A single dermal pedicle for nipple transposition in subcutaneous mastectomy,
reduction mammaplasty, or mastopexy. Plast Reconstruct Surg 1973; 51: 115–120.
12. Orlando JC, Guthrie RH Jr. The superomedial dermal pedicle for nipple transposition. Br J Plast Surg 1975; 28: 42–45.
13. Hauben DJ. Experience and refinements with the superomedial dermal pedicle for nipple–areola transposition in reduction mammaplasty. Aesthet Plast Surg 1984; 8: 189–194.
14. Hauben DJ. Superomedial pedicle technique of reduction mammaplasty. Discussion. Plast Reconstruct Surg 1989; 83: 479.
15. McKissock PK. Reduction mammoplasty with a vertical dermal flap. Plast Reconstruct Surg 1972; 49: 245.
16. Johnson CM Jr, To WC. A case approach to open structure rhinoplasty. Philadelphia: WB Saunders, 2004.
17. Farina MA, Newby BG, Alani HM. Innervation of the nipple–areola complex. Plast Reconstruct Surg 1980; 66: 497–501.
18. Finger RE, Vasquez B, Drew GS, Given KS. Superomedial pedicle technique of reduction mammaplasty. Plast Reconstruct Surg 1989; 83: 471–478.
19. Hsia H, Thomson JG. Differences in breast shape preferences between plastic surgeons and patients seeking breast augmentation. Plast Reconstruct Surg 2003; 112: 312–320.
20. Mustoe TA, Cooter R, Gold M, et al. International clinical guidelines for scar management. Plast Reconstruct Surg 2002; 110: 560–572.
21. Spear SL, Carter ME, Low M, et al. Sickle cell trait: a risk factor for flap necrosis. Plast Reconstruct Surg 2003; 112: 697–698.

Breast Reduction: Short Scar (Vertical) Techniques

12

Elizabeth J. Hall-Findlay

INTRODUCTION

Breast reduction techniques have tried to balance the removal of excess tissue with preservation of circulation to the nipple–areolar complex. In the 1970s the introduction of the vertical bipedicle technique as described by McKissock[1] made breast reduction safe, reproducible, and reliable. Once surgeons realized that the nipple could survive on either pedicle the procedure was further simplified. The inferior pedicle[2-4] became the standard in North America, whereas in South America and Europe both superior and inferior pedicles were used.

The vertical bipedicle technique relied on a horizontal excision of skin and breast tissue with removal of the skin in the Wise[5] pattern. These techniques were applicable to every breast size, with free nipple grafts[6] being usually reserved for the extremely large breast.

There was, however, some dissatisfaction with the often unsightly scar along the inframammary fold. South American[7-10] and European[11-15] surgeons tried various shorter scar techniques which often relied instead on a vertical resection of breast tissue. Not only were the scars shortened, but often the breast had a better shape because of the coning effect, which resulted in narrowing of the breast and better projection. Unfortunately, the learning curve was somewhat difficult and surgeons the world over felt more comfortable with the inverted-T techniques.

Surgeons need to realize that these procedures are not limiting. They can apply the vertical wedge resection principles in the breast tissue while still using an inverted T skin resection pattern when needed. The choice of pedicle is not limited. Different pedicles can be used with different parenchymal resection patterns, and both can be used with different skin resection patterns.[16-20]

INDICATIONS AND CONTRAINDICATIONS

Short scar breast reduction techniques which rely on a vertical skin scar rather than incorporating a full inverted T pattern are usually best reserved for small to moderate-sized breasts.[21-23] Extremely large breasts, or those with lots of poor-quality skin, will still need an inverted T to take care of the skin excess. But the same principles discussed below can be used for the parenchyma even in the larger breast.

The very short circumareolar techniques are best confined to reductions or mastopexies where there is only a very small amount of excess skin.[24,25]

The vertical wedge resection of skin and parenchyma results in two dog-ears: one superior, which disappears into the nipple, and one inferiorly, which usually disappears but which may need revision either at the time of the surgery with a small T or J or L, or a later revision in the office.

The inverted-T techniques also have two dog-ears. Because the resection of breast tissue and skin is performed mainly in a horizontal direction in inverted-T cases, there is a dog-ear both medially and laterally. These are often more difficult to correct than the vertical dog-ears. This then results in an artificially low revision rate than with the vertical techniques. Each surgeon needs to take these different factors into consideration.

Breast size

- Very small – short circumareolar techniques
- Small to medium – vertical techniques as described in this chapter
- Large – various pedicles and parenchymal resection patterns with inverted T skin incision
- Extremely large – amputation techniques with consideration of free nipple grafts.

Liposuction-only breast reduction techniques[26,27] can also be considered for fatty breasts. Liposuction will not work in very young patients who are close to their ideal body weight. It is best reserved for older women with fatty breasts and relatively high nipples. The nipples can rise to some degree, but often at the expense of losing some upper pole fullness. Some patients are less concerned about shape, and liposuction-only may be a good choice. The same reasoning could be applied to patients who are more concerned about nipple sensation, or those who are not willing to accept some risk of nipple necrosis.

PREOPERATIVE HISTORY AND CONSIDERATIONS

Breast size and surgeon experience will be the main determinants in the choice of breast reduction procedure. Other factors to be taken into consideration are the nature of the skin excess and elasticity, previous biopsies (which might limit pedicle choices), and concerns about nipple sensation and blood supply. This chapter concentrates on a medial pedicle vertical approach, but many of the principles can apply from small to large reductions by using the same type of pedicle with a mainly vertical skin resection pattern, and then deciding on the final skin resection pattern.

There is no one 'vertical' or 'short scar' technique, just as there is no one 'inverted-T' technique. Each surgeon will have his or her own preferences, depending on the results they can achieve in their hands. The vertical approaches that have come into more common acceptance are as follows:

Vertical skin resection pattern using a superior pedicle[7–15]

In the technique as described by Lassus[11,12] a superior pedicle is used for the smaller breast reductions and a medial pedicle is used when the nipple has a greater distance to travel. He performs a vertical wedge resection of breast tissue with no horizontal resection of parenchyma. The inframammary fold stays at the original level.

In the technique as described by Marchac and de Olarte[13] a superior pedicle is used. For larger reductions a small T skin resection was added.

In the technique as described by Lejour and colleagues[14,15] a superior pedicle is used. For larger reductions liposuction was performed initially to reduce breast size and make the pedicle more pliable and easier to inset. Lejour directly excised both a vertical wedge of breast tissue and a horizontal wedge just above the inframammary fold, where she undermined the skin. This resulted in an elevation of the inframammary fold.

Vertical skin resection pattern using a medial or lateral pedicle[16,17,19,23]

This chapter describes a vertical skin resection pattern using a medial pedicle.[21,22] The lateral pedicle was used initially by the author because it was thought that it would result in better sensation. Studies have shown that final sensation was the same with the superior, medial, and lateral pedicles. The lateral pedicle unfortunately restricted the ability to excise the excess lateral breast tissue because that excess formed the base of the pedicle. The medial pedicle, on the other hand, has excellent sensation and allows resection of all the excess breast tissue both laterally

and inferiorly. The parenchymal resection pattern relies on a vertical wedge excision, with the horizontal excess along the inframammary fold being removed both directly and with liposuction. The Wise pattern is used to determine what breast tissue should remain rather than what should be excised. The inframammary fold rises.

Vertical skin resection pattern using an inferior pedicle[20]

In the technique described by Hammond[20] an inferior pedicle is used along with a circumvertical skin resection pattern. To reduce the length of the vertical scar many surgeons use a circumvertical skin resection pattern,[28,29] where much of the excess vertical distance is taken up around the areola instead. The surgeon must be comfortable with the techniques used to prevent areolar widening, flattening, and wrinkling when there is a significant discrepancy between the skin circumference and the areolar circumference. The inframammary fold does not rise, and it is important not to violate the fold in order to prevent descent. Descent and bottoming-out is less of a problem with the procedures that use a more superiorly based pedicle and which rely on removal of all the excess inferior breast tissue.

OPERATIVE APPROACH USING A MEDIAL PEDICLE VERTICAL SKIN RESECTION PATTERN

Surgical anatomy

Blood supply
The arterial input for the breast comes mainly from the medial branches of the internal mammary system.[30–33] These vessels are the main source of blood supply for the superior, medial, and inferior pedicles. The lateral pedicle is supplied by the superficial branch of the lateral thoracic artery. The superior and medial pedicles are supplied directly by branches of the internal mammary system, and these vessels are superficial when they reach the areola. The inferior pedicle is supplied by a perforator through the pectoralis muscle, which also originates from the internal mammary system.

The veins do not accompany the arteries (except for the venae comitantes, which accompany the perforator that supplies an inferior or central pedicle). The veins are just beneath the dermis and are often easily visible through the skin. It is a good idea to try to incorporate a visible vein in the base of the pedicle.

Innervation
Although the main innervation to the nipple is described as coming from the lateral branch of the fourth intercostal nerve, there are also significant medial branches[34] as well as superior branches. When the pectoralis fascia is not violated, and when a medial pedicle is kept full thickness, there is a good chance that the deep branch of the lateral fourth intercostal nerve will be preserved.[34]

Ductal anatomy

Breast reduction removes many of the ducts needed for breastfeeding, but because the breast usually comprises 20–25 separate lobules, many of these will be preserved with a full-thickness pedicle.[35] Inferior, lateral, and medial pedicles can easily be kept full thickness, but often a superior pedicle needs to be thinned to allow it to be inset. Full-thickness pedicles are therefore not needed for either arterial or venous input (except for the inferior and central pedicles), but they are more likely to contain both nerves and ducts when they are kept full thickness. If a pedicle is thinned it does need to be thicker as it approaches the source of its blood supply. Thinning a medial pedicle right to the sternal border could be a problem. A medial pedicle may have had its blood supply damaged during the pocket dissection for a prior augmentation. A superior pedicle might be more reliable in such cases.

Markings

New nipple position (Figs 12.1, 12.2)

Determining the new nipple level is often confusing and a source of concern. Although the inframammary fold is a good guideline, the best indication is to actually 'see' where the breast mound starts and to keep the nipple position somewhere between the lower third and the middle of the imagined final breast. Once the surgeon realizes that it is almost impossible to raise the breast on the chest wall, the upper border of the breast is a very important landmark. Suturing the breast to the pectoralis fascia to raise the breast or increase upper pole fullness does not work.

Upper border of the breast

This will not change with a breast reduction and is best marked by starting with the indentation just below the pre-axillary fullness. A dotted line (see Figs 12.1B, 12.2A) is then drawn from this area up and across the breast, where it is usually fairly clear where the demarcation between the breast and the upper chest wall occurs. Placing the new nipple position anywhere close to this demarcation line will cause problems with nipples that are too high.

Inframammary fold

It is important to mark the level of the inframammary fold, as this is a good guideline to help determine the level of the new nipple. When a patient has a lot of upper pole fullness then the new nipple can be positioned higher than the level of the fold (see Figs 12.2B, 12.4A). When the patient has very little upper pole fullness the new nipple position may actually need to be lower than the inframammary fold (see Figs 12.1B, 12.10B, 12.11A). The best guideline is to visualize the final breast, realizing that the demarcation between the upper level of the breast mound and the chest wall will not change. The level of the inframammary fold provides a second checkpoint.

Breast meridian

A line is drawn down the breast meridian – not through the nipple, but where the surgeon wants the final meridian to be (Fig. 12.2B). In an inverted-T reduction the meridian

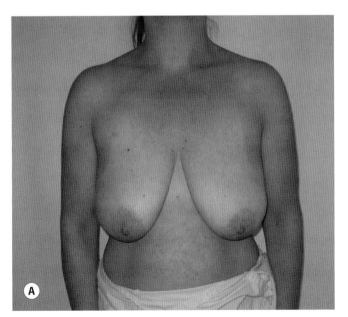 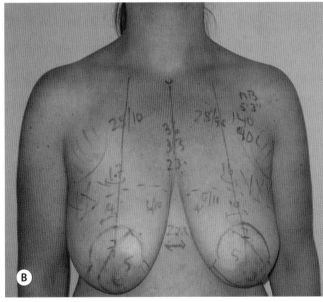

FIGURE 12.1 This patient has breasts which are low on the chest wall. The best way to determine the new nipple position is to mark the upper border of the breast mound where it meets the chest wall. Suturing the breast tissue to the chest wall will only temporarily increase upper pole fullness, and eventually the breast will settle down to its original position. On the other hand, the inframammary fold can be raised slightly by using the vertical techniques, which remove the heavy inferior breast tissue. **A** The breasts are low on the chest wall. **B** The junction of the upper border of the breast where it meets the chest wall is marked with a dotted line. It is important not to mark the new nipple position too close to this border. The nipple is ideally about one-third to halfway up from the lower border of the breast mound. In this case the new nipple position is marked at the level of the inframammary fold, which is shown by a horizontal mark between the breasts.

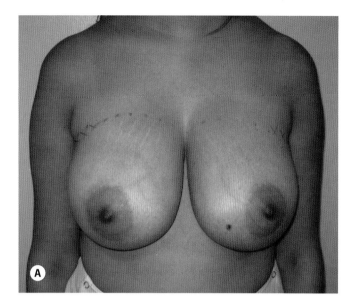

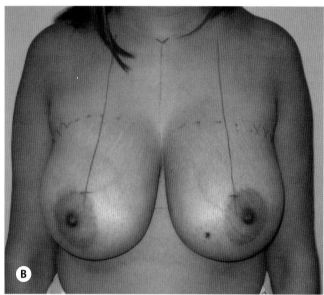

FIGURE 12.2 This patient has breasts which are high on the chest wall. Note the high position of the junction between the upper border of the breast and the chest wall. **A** The dotted line marks the border by starting laterally with x's at the depression just below the pre-axillary fullness and then following the depression medially. **B** In this case the new nipple position is marked higher than the inframammary fold because the patient has so much upper pole fullness. It is best to use the upper border of the breast as the definitive guideline and to use the inframammary fold as a supplementary guide.

will be somewhat more lateral than in a vertical reduction, because the inverted-T techniques do not usually result in as much breast narrowing. At the level of the inframammary fold medially the measurement to the desired breast meridian is usually around 9–11 cm.

The new nipple position is then marked at the intersection of the vertical position (as determined by the top of the breast mound and the inframammary fold; Fig. 12.2B) and the breast meridian. The top of the new areola is

then marked about 2 cm above the nipple position (Fig. 12.3A).

It is important in a vertical reduction to mark the new nipple position slightly lower on the larger breast (Fig. 12.10B), because the weight of the larger breast stretches the skin and a larger vertical wedge resection will push the nipple up higher.

Areolar opening (Fig. 12.3B)

A pattern can be used to determine the areolar opening, or it can be drawn freehand. It will need to be wider if the areola is large and placed laterally, because it is important to remove all the pigmented skin from the flaps that will remain. A large paperclip has a distance of 16 cm – a 5 cm diameter areola has a 16 cm circumference. The original Wise pattern had a 14 cm circumference, which matches a 4.5 cm diameter areola.

An areolar opening that is much larger than 18–20 cm will require knowledge of the circumareolar skin closure techniques to prevent widening of the areola. A large discrepancy between the skin and areolar circumferences will not only cause the areola to stretch, but will also lead to some flattening and loss of projection and could result in permanent wrinkling.

Lejour and colleagues[14,15] would carry the areolar opening out in a mosque dome shape, but it is probably better to try to take out any excess vertically. As long as the final skin shape is circular once it is closed, the original shape is somewhat irrelevant.

Skin resection pattern

The vertical lines that are drawn in a Wise pattern are much the same as those used in a vertical resection pattern. Instead of drawing the vertical limbs for 5 cm and then carrying the lines medially and laterally, the vertical limbs are joined together about 2–4 cm above the level of the inframammary fold (Fig. 12.3E). It is important not to take too much skin. The final closure should be loose and under no tension. It is important to realize that the inverted-T patterns often rely on the skin closure to act as a brassiere, whereas the vertical approaches rely on the parenchymal resection and just allow the skin to redrape.

It is important not to carry the skin resection pattern down to the inframammary fold or the vertical scar will end up below the fold. There are two reasons for this: one is that closure of the skin ellipse will end up longer vertically; the second is that the inframammary fold often rises, and it is important to take this into account. It is also better to keep the skin resection pattern as a 'U' rather than as a 'V,' so that enough skin and subcutaneous tissue is removed. A persistent skin pucker is often more of a problem of residual subcutaneous tissue than of excess skin.

Medial pedicle design

The best way to allow for easy inset of the pedicle is to put half of the base in the areolar opening and half into the vertical skin resection pattern (see Figs 12.3D, 12.4B, 12.7B, 12.10B, 12.11A). If the pedicle is left too low, not enough tissue will be removed inferiorly and there will be

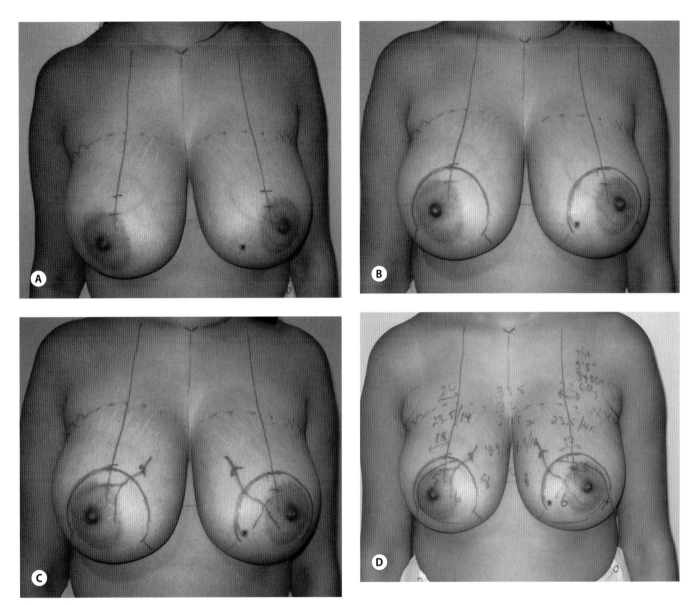

FIGURE 12.3 This series of photos shows the markings for a medial pedicle vertical breast reduction. **A** The initial markings are shown in Fig. 12.2B. Note that the breast meridian is drawn where it should be, not where it currently is. The actual position of the nipple is ignored because drawing the meridian through the current nipple can be misleading and may result in a new nipple that is too medial or too lateral. The new nipple position has been marked in relation to the upper border of the breast rather than directly at the level of the inframammary fold. The top of the areola is marked 2 cm above the new nipple position. **B** The areolar opening is drawn freehand. A large paperclip can be used as a marker because it measures 16 cm, which is the circumference of a 5 cm diameter areola. Care must be taken (as in this case) to draw out the areolar opening to be sure to remove any pigmented skin. The final shape should end up as a circle. **C** Any visible veins should be marked and included in the base of the pedicle if at all possible. **D** A superior pedicle could easily be used in this case, but the medial pedicle still allows easy access to remove the excess breast tissue laterally. The base of the pedicle is usually 6–10 cm. When the pedicle is rotated into position, the inferior border of the medial pedicle becomes the medial pillar.

pseudoptosis and bottoming-out due to inadequate inferior tissue resection.

The base of the pedicle is usually designed from 6 to 10 cm. It is important to try to visualize any veins (see Figs 12.3C, 12.7B, 12.10B) directly under the skin. They are just under the dermis and can often be included in the base of the pedicle. Some surgeons term this a 'superomedial' pedicle,[23] but the blood supply is medial. When the patient

is lying down the medial orientation of the pedicle is more obvious. The superomedial direction is somewhat artificial because it results from ptosis as the patient stands, but the vessels stretch with the skin and breast as they descend and the origin of the vascular supply is medial.

A centimeter of dermis and tissue is left around the new areola, as described by Schwartzmann[36] (Fig. 12.4C) in order to provide some safety margin for the blood supply.

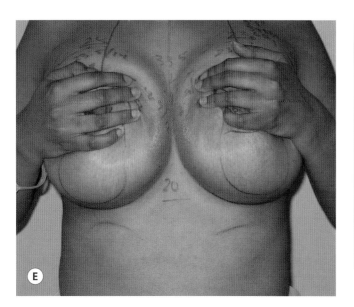

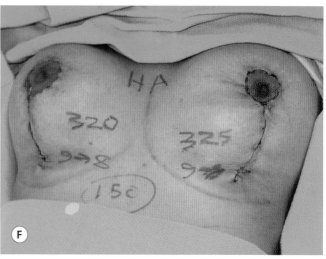

FIGURE 12.3, cont'd E With the breasts pulled up the skin resection pattern is shown. It lies usually 2–4 cm above the level of the inframammary fold and is drawn in the shape of a 'U' rather than a 'V' in order to remove all the redundant skin and subcutaneous tissue. **F** Intraoperative view. The pucker will eventually tuck in without help.

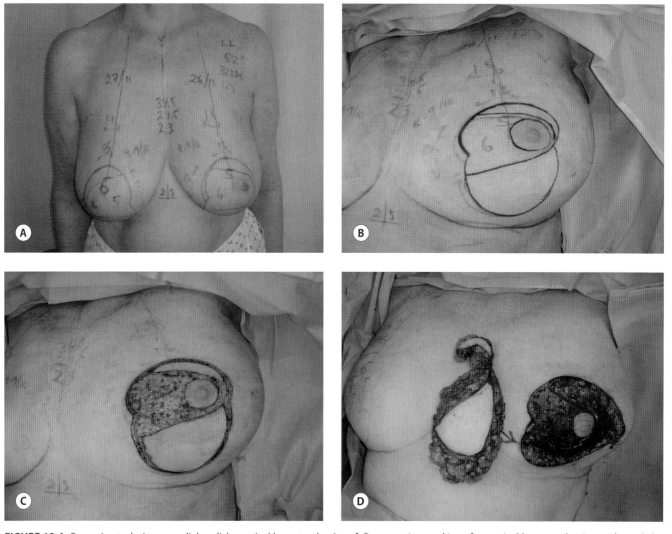

FIGURE 12.4 Operative technique: medial pedicle vertical breast reduction. **A** Preoperative markings for vertical breast reduction with medial pedicle. **B** Intraoperative markings showing base of medial pedicle halfway into the areolar opening and halfway into vertical skin resection pattern. **C** De-epithelialization with skin resection pattern incision made. **D** Resection specimen showing very little skin removal with resection beveled out laterally, medially, and inferiorly.

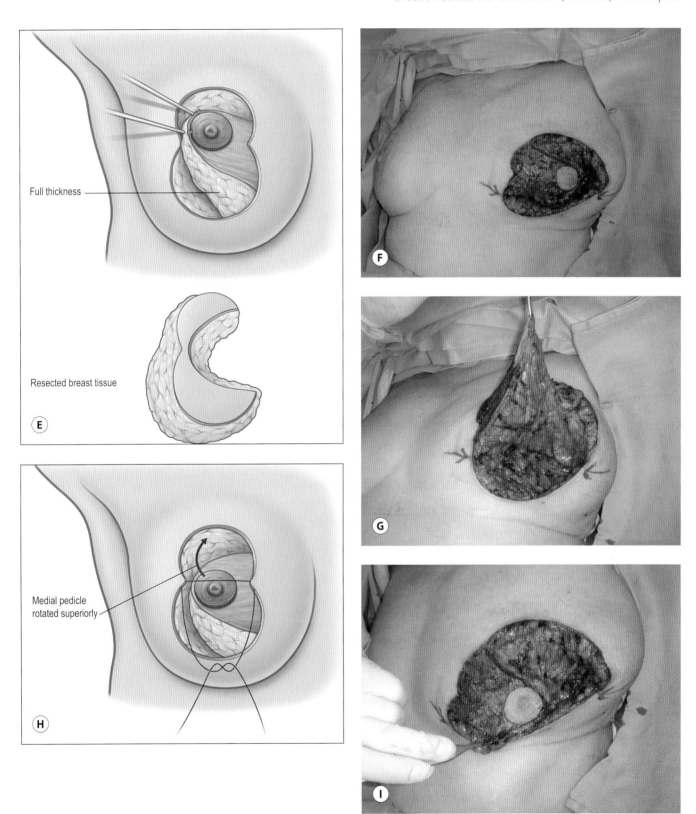

FIGURE 12.4, cont'd E Drawing shows the full-thickness medially based pedicle and the shape of the skin and parenchyma excised. **F** The inferior border of the pillars is marked by the arrows. The pillars are only about 5–7 cm long and do not extend down to the inframammary fold. The inferior border of the medial pedicle becomes the medial pillar. **G** The medial pedicle is full thickness – this is not needed for blood supply but for improved sensation and breastfeeding potential. **H** The base of the areola is closed and the medial pedicle rotates easily into parition. **I** A superior platform is left for the areola to sit on. The medial pedicle will appear to be undermined, much like an inferior pedicle. This superior platform cannot be used to increase upper pole fullness but can be used to help prevent nipple retraction.

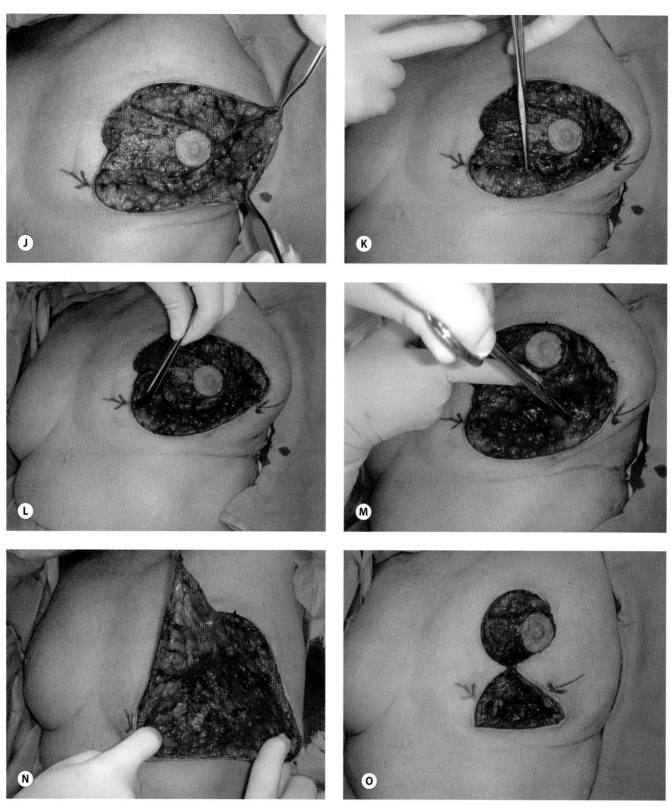

FIGURE 12.4, cont'd **J** The parenchymal excision is beveled out laterally. **K** The Kocher clamp is useful to help undermine the tissue down to the inframammary fold. It is important to leave some fat on the skin to prevent scar contracture. **L** The forceps point to the area where more tissue can be removed directly. Further tapering will be performed with liposuction. **M** Area for further resection laterally. It is important to leave tissue to form a lateral pillar, which should be a couple of centimeters thick. Further tissue should be removed inferior to the lateral pillar and under the pillar parallel to the chest wall. It is difficult to remove enough tissue with the vertical approach, and the tissue under the lateral flap can be excised. Any thick fibrous tissue will need to be directly excised because liposuction is ineffective. **N** Resection is completed. It is important to leave tissue on the pectoralis major muscle to preserve nerves and to help prevent bleeding. **O** The first pillar suture is placed at the inferior border of the pillars. This suture is only a centimeter or so below the surface. It is both unnecessary and unwise to try to pull tissue from deep and lateral. Putting tension on the tissue will not hold in the long term.

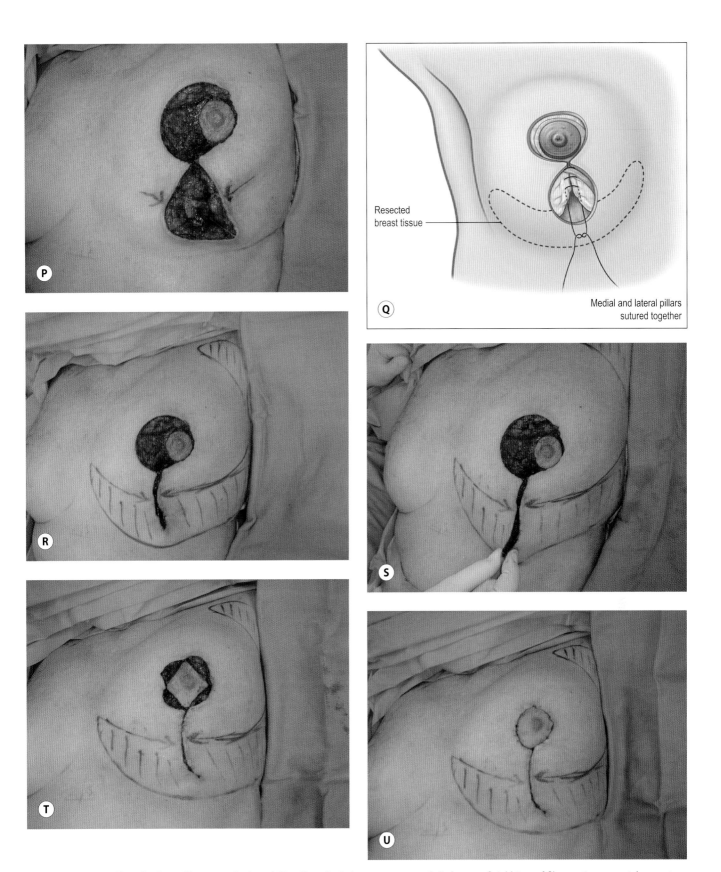

FIGURE 12.4, cont'd P The first pillar suture is closed. Usually only 3–4 sutures are used. Only superficial bites of fibrous tissue are taken, not deep bites of fat. **Q** The red dotted lines show where breast tissue needs to be removed below the pillars by direct excision and tailored out by liposuction. **R** Deep dermal sutures are used just to approximate the skin edges. It is important not to use too many sutures. The dermis is not sutured to the breast tissue. The areas for liposuction are marked. Liposuction is designed to leave a Wise pattern of tissue behind to give the breast a good shape. The lateral chest wall and pre-axillary areas are also suctioned. **S** Care must be taken to remove subcutaneous tissue below the pucker, both laterally and medially, without removing all the fat under the skin. The pucker will then tuck in without being sutured down. **T** Liposuction is completed and the areolar stay sutures placed in the dermis. **U** The areolar and vertical incisions are closed with a subcuticular absorbable suture. Note that the closure is loose so that the circulation to the skin edges is not constricted and the vertical incision is left at its full length and not gathered. The gathering interferes with wound healing and either lengthens over time or stays and leaves permanent pleats in the skin that require revision.

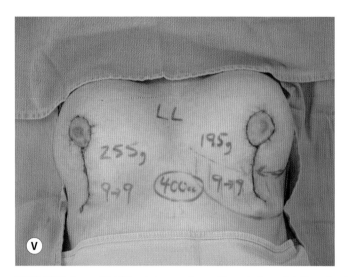
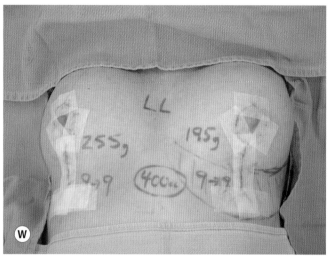

FIGURE 12.4, cont'd V Final closure. A good breast shape is left on the table at the end of the procedure. **W** Paper tape is applied to the incisions and left on for 3 weeks. Patients are allowed to shower the next day and a brassiere is only used to hold the bandages in place.

Operative technique (Fig. 12.4)

Infiltration

It is important not to infiltrate along the incision lines so that the veins are not damaged. Infiltration can be used in the breast tissue itself, but is usually reserved for those areas where liposuction will be performed. Either direct infiltration or a tumescent-type solution can be used. Liposuction is usually performed in the pre-axillary areas as well as the lateral chest wall and along the inframammary fold.

Creation of the pedicle (Fig. 12.4C)

The pedicle is created full thickness after de-epithelialization (Fig. 12.4G). Either a scalpel or cutting cautery is used to cut the pedicle directly down towards the pectoralis fascia. It is important at this stage to make sure the assistant does not pull on the pedicle so that it is not inadvertently undermined. Undermining is not likely to damage the blood supply, but could interfere with sensation and breastfeeding potential. Most of the bleeding that is encountered is superficial.

Parenchymal resection (Fig. 12.4D)

The breast parenchyma is resected en bloc using either a scalpel or cutting cautery. The resection can be beveled out laterally, medially, and inferiorly. It is often difficult to reduce the breasts adequately using the vertical technique, and more tissue can be removed parallel to the chest wall laterally in order to remove more tissue.

It is a good idea to leave a superior platform (Fig. 12.4I) of tissue so that the areola can sit with some support from below. The pedicle will tend to look undermined and be thinned (much as happens with creation of an inferior pedicle), and this platform can help prevent nipple retraction.

It is important to leave about 1–2 cm of tissue attached to the skin laterally to create a lateral pillar (Fig. 12.4M). This tissue should be about 7 cm long and the resection can be more aggressive inferiorly (below the Wise pattern). Further tissue can be removed laterally under the lateral pillar and parallel to the chest wall in order to achieve an adequate parenchymal resection.

It is important to avoid resecting tissue superiorly unless the patient has a great deal of upper pole fullness. The breast tissue below a Wise pattern (Fig. 12.5) is removed either by direct excision under the skin flaps or by liposuction. A combination of beveled resection (rather than undermining) and liposuction for the more distal (and usually fatty) areas works best (Fig. 12.4R). This type of resection is much like that used for gynecomastia, where the glandular tissue is excised directly and the resection tailored distally with liposuction. Partial closure is often completed before the final liposuction is performed (Fig. 12.4R).

It is important to look at what is being removed and what is being left behind. The Wise pattern[5] was developed from a brassiere design and is a good design to guide the surgeon on what to leave behind (Fig. 12.4R). The medial pedicle vertical breast reduction leaves the breast parenchyma attached to the upper skin flaps, and the excess breast tissue inferiorly is removed. The breast will descend to its original position on the chest wall. The inframammary fold may rise slightly, but the upper border of the breast will remain the same unless tissue has been removed there. Suturing breast tissue up to the pectoralis fascia will not raise the breast on the chest wall or increase upper pole fullness. Breast tissue which has been pushed up will just drop with gravity and end up bottoming-out.

Skin resection

The skin that is removed mirrors the vertical wedge parenchymal resection. If the patient has good-quality skin and

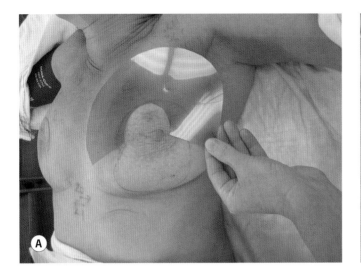

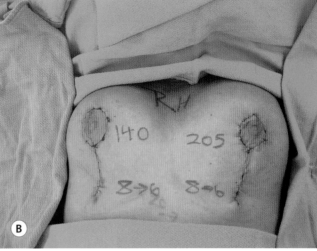

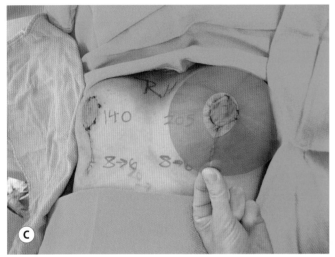

FIGURE 12.5 The Wise pattern was developed from a brassiere design. It is often used now for designing the keyhole opening, but in fact the whole pattern is good for deciding what breast tissue to leave behind. **A** The Wise pattern superimposed on the supine patient preoperatively. **B** The patient at the end of surgery. **C** The Wise pattern superimposed on the breast at the end of surgery. The pattern can be used to help determine what tissue to remove, either by direct excision or by liposuction. The remaining breast is left attached to the skin flaps superiorly, medially, and laterally. The breast tissue is removed inferiorly and laterally and liposuction is used to tailor the breast peripherally.

there is not too much excess, the skin will redrape. Surgeons are often surprised by how much of the extra skin will redrape. Puckers are deliberately left behind (Figs 12.6, 12.8, and 12.9) and they tuck in toward the inframammary fold quite well (Fig. 12.8C). It is often quite difficult to design a further 'T,' 'J' or 'L' resection properly (Fig. 12.10). The surgeon does not know exactly where the new inframammary fold will lie, and any horizontal scar may end up below the fold.

Closure

The closure is started by placing a suture at the base of the areolar opening (Fig. 12.4O). This allows the surgeon to see what has been removed and what is left behind.

The inferior border of the medial pedicle now becomes the medial pillar. The pedicle is rotated up into position and the pillar suturing starts inferiorly with the base of the pedicle inferiorly being sutured to a matching position on the lateral side. This is usually about 7 cm below the areola, where the de-epithelialized pedicle base meets the skin and about 1 or 2 cm below the skin surface (Fig. 12.4O,P). Deep sutures pulling tissue from laterally are not only unneces-

sary but can delay healing. Any tension placed on the parenchymal closure will just stretch out to some degree. Any tension on the skin closure will not only cause wound healing problems but will also stretch out.

Only about two to four sutures are usually needed to close the pillars, and it is important to keep the medial pedicle rotated up into position during closure. Absorbable sutures such as 3/0 Monocryl are used. The dermis is then closed with deep interrupted absorbable sutures (Fig. 12.4R). Here it becomes obvious that too much skin resection will lead to too tight a closure. Wound-healing problems can result. The dermis is usually closed vertically, but a slight hockey stick going out laterally may be indicated (see Figs 12.8C, 12.10D). It is important to do this after the parenchymal resection. A hockey stick-type resection should be confined to skin only, because a similar resection or closure of the parenchyma itself will end up with a medialized breast (much like the Dufourmentel[37] lateral resection).

The skin is then closed with a running subcuticular suture (Fig. 12.4T). Originally surgeons (including the author) thought that this skin needed to be gathered to keep the vertical length as short as possible, but with it

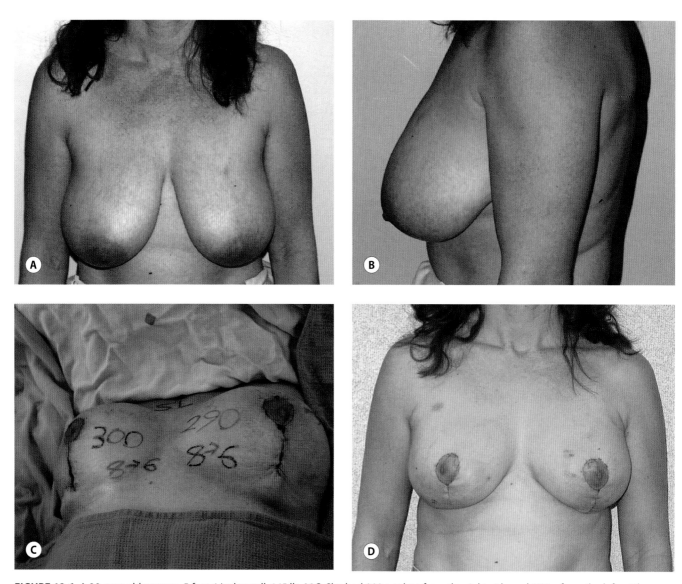

FIGURE 12.6 A 38-year-old woman, 5 feet 4 inches tall, 145 lb, 38C. She had 300 g taken from the right side and 290 g from the left, with 150 mL liposuction peripherally. She had almost complete return of sensation in 3 months. **A** Preoperative frontal. **B** Preoperative lateral. **C** intraoperative view showing initial puckers. **D** 10 days postoperative frontal.

has been realized that gathering is not only unnecessary but is actually contraindicated.[38,39] Measurements have shown that the vertical length stretches out with time, and gathering not only leads to a temporary teardrop-shaped areola but also results in delayed healing, because the gathering constricts the blood supply to the skin margins. The pucker at the inferior end of the vertical incision may look better on the table when it is gathered, but in fact it can cause delayed resolution of the inferior aspect of the breast.[39]

The areola is closed with four interrupted deep dermal sutures and a subcuticular suture (Fig. 12.4T,U). The pedicle is not rotated into position any set number of degrees, but usually sits at about 90° compared to its original position. It is allowed to settle into its own position at the areolar level, but is definitely rotated up in order to close the pillars properly.

It is not necessary to suture dermis to breast tissue or to suture the pucker down to the chest wall. The shape will actually resolve better and faster if the skin is allowed to find its own position.

There are surgeons who believe that they can increase upper pole fullness by undermining superiorly and suturing breast tissue up to the pectoralis fascia. The author has tried this using 3/0 PDS in 30 patients and 3/0 Ticron in another 30 patients, and it has not lasted. Initially it looks as if some increase in upper pole fullness is achieved, but this drops out with time. For this reason, determining the upper border of the breast is a key component in determining the new nipple position.

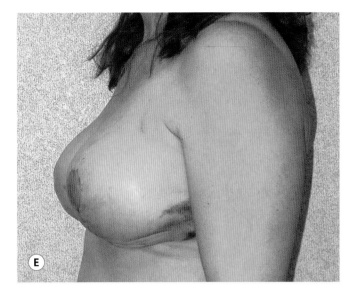

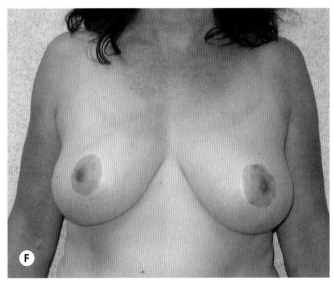

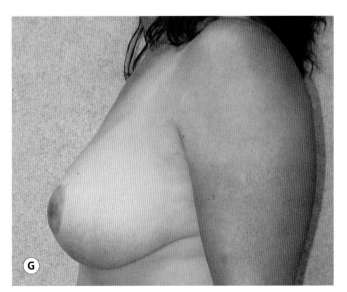

FIGURE 12.6, cont'd E 10 days postoperative lateral. **F** 4 years postoperative frontal. **G** 4 years postoperative lateral. The vertical scars are 11 cm on the right and 10 cm on the left.

Drains and antibiotics

Drains are rarely used. They do not prevent hematomas, and seromas in the breast will disappear fairly quickly without treatment. The author has performed over 1600 breast reductions and has only had two cases of hematoma. The key is to search for known vessels (especially the perforator that supplies an inferior or central pedicle) and make sure that hemostasis is secured (especially when tumescent-type infiltration has been used).

Antibiotics are used routinely at induction and then for several days postoperatively. Not only did they improve the author's infection rate in larger breast reductions, but wound-healing problems in the vertical incision almost disappeared. This was observed before the author stopped gathering the vertical incision, and nothing other than the routine use of antibiotics was changed. Absorbable suture spitting (PDS and Monocryl) cleared up dramatically.

Dressings

The incisions are all covered with paper tape (Fig. 12.4W), which stays in place for 3 weeks and provides an excellent bandage. Patients are encouraged to shower the day after surgery. A surgical brassiere is used mainly to hold the bandages in place, and is usually used for a couple of weeks day and night. Patients are restricted in their activities only as discomfort dictates.

OPTIMIZING OUTCOMES

- Patient selection: small to medium-sized breast reductions
- Markings: nipple position is key
- Base of pedicle halfway into areolar opening, half vertical; incorporate a vein into pedicle
- Do not take too much skin: tension causes healing problems
- Leave 2–4 cm of skin above inframammary fold
- Technical: full-thickness, medially based pedicle
- Excise tissue to leave behind a Wise pattern
- Liposuction for tailoring peripherally
- Leave tissue over pectoralis fascia
- Do not suture breast to pectoralis fascia
- Do not suture dermis to breast
- Do not gather the skin
- Do not put tension on the pillar closure
- Do not put tension on the skin
- Do not suture the pucker down
- Drains are usually unnecessary
- Antibiotic coverage helps wound healing
- Postoperatively: puckers can take months to settle in larger breasts
- A preoperatively informed patient is the surgeon's best ally.

The key to a good result is first to educate the patient. It is not simple to convert a vertical scar with a small T, and seemingly large puckers will disappear with time, leaving a more acceptable result in the long term. Correcting a pucker 1 year postoperatively is usually easy through

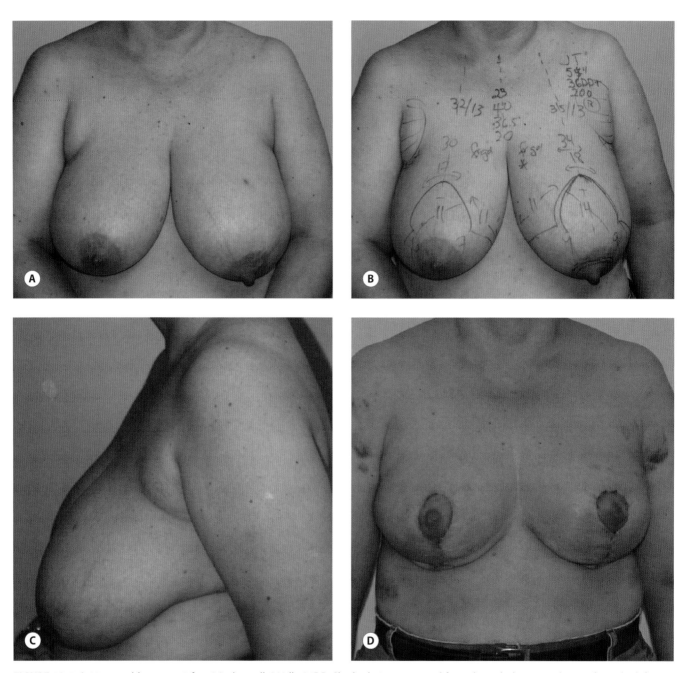

FIGURE 12.7 A 45-year-old woman, 5 feet 3 inches tall, 200 lb, 36DD. She had 625 g removed from the right breast and 740 g from the left breast. Liposuction peripherally totaled 850 mL. The patient had complete return of sensation. **A** Preoperative frontal. **B** Preoperative frontal with markings. Many of the numbers are there only for follow-up statistics. **C** Preoperative lateral. **D** One month postoperative frontal.

a vertical incision in the office under local anesthesia, and is often more a question of excising excess subcutaneous tissue than excess skin. Revision rates depend on the surgeon's threshold for revision as well as getting past the learning curve. Plastic surgeons accept a small revision rate in most other procedures, and a small revision rate should be accepted for breast reduction as well. It is fortunate that in a vertical reduction the puckers can be revised – it is much more difficult to revise the puckers at either end of a horizontal inframammary fold incision.

It is important not to excise too much skin in order to allow the closure to be slightly loose. Tension created on the breast tissue itself by taking deep bites to close the pillars will just stretch out with time and leave a less satisfactory shape. Excision, not tension, is the key to a good shape. Tension on the skin will just lead to wound healing problems. Skin under tension (the principle behind tissue expansion) will eventually stretch and should not be relied upon to hold shape.

It is important not to gather the skin during closure. Excessive gathering just constricts blood supply to the

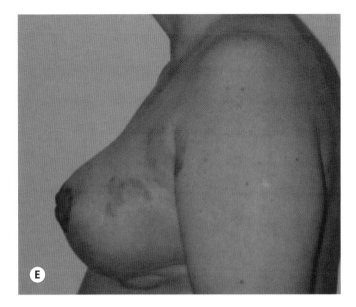

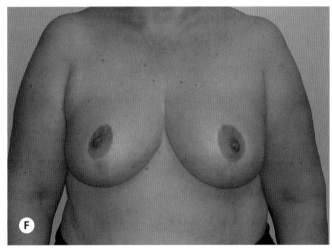

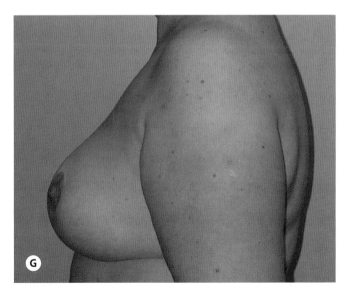

FIGURE 12.7, cont'd E One month postoperative lateral. **F** 4 years postoperative frontal. **G** 4 years postoperative lateral.

wound edges and the vertical length eventually stretches. A long vertical length is not a problem. Most surgeons have trouble switching their thinking from keeping a 5 cm vertical length – which is needed in an inverted-T inferior pedicle breast reduction – to allowing a vertical length of 7–11 cm. An elegant curve to the breast is quite acceptable, a B cup being about 7 cm from areola to inframammary fold, a C cup being about 9 cm, and a D cup being about 11 cm.

Surgeons need to alter their concept of trying to push the breast above the inframammary fold to allowing a nice curve to fall slightly below the fold (see Figs 12.6G, 12.7G, 12.8H, 12.9H). Not only do larger breasts look good with this curve, but the vertical length also allows for better projection because the breast is not compressed by a tight skin brassiere. With an inverted-T inferior pedicle reduction the skin eventually stretches anyway, and the result is some bottoming-out below the scar (which makes the nipples look as if they were placed too high).

Bottoming-out can be avoided by removing enough breast tissue inferiorly. Trying to push breast tissue up into the upper pole will only result in that same tissue settling back inferiorly and bottoming-out. The key to a good final breast shape is to remove all tissue, with the residual parenchyma falling into a Wise pattern. The remaining tissue is left attached to the overlying skin, and all tissue external to a Wise pattern is either directly excised or tailored with liposuction.

COMPLICATIONS (Figs 12.11–12.14)

All complications will occur eventually, especially in a large-volume practice.[40] They cannot be completely avoided. For example, nipple necrosis is probably more likely to occur because of a variation in vascular anatomy that cannot be predicted, and less likely to be a problem of surgical error.

- Hematoma: good hemostasis, especially with tumescent-type infiltration
- Seroma: drains do not help – seromas disappear with time
- Infection: no tension on skin, antibiotic coverage
- Nipple necrosis: care in design and execution of pedicle
- Fat necrosis: avoid large sutures in fat
- Wound healing: no tension on repairs
- Asymmetry: design nipple lower on larger breast
- Under-resection: patient education, remove tissue laterally
- Scarring: avoid tension on skin closure, no gathering
- Indentations: avoid tension on pillar closure
- Bottoming-out: adequate inferior resection is essential
- Shape: leave behind a Wise pattern

POSTOPERATIVE CARE

Paper tape is placed on the incisions and patients may shower daily and pat the tape dry. This forms an excellent bandage and is applied directly from the roll. The first piece is thrown away and the remaining tape is as sterile as needed. 3M Micropore paper tape appears to

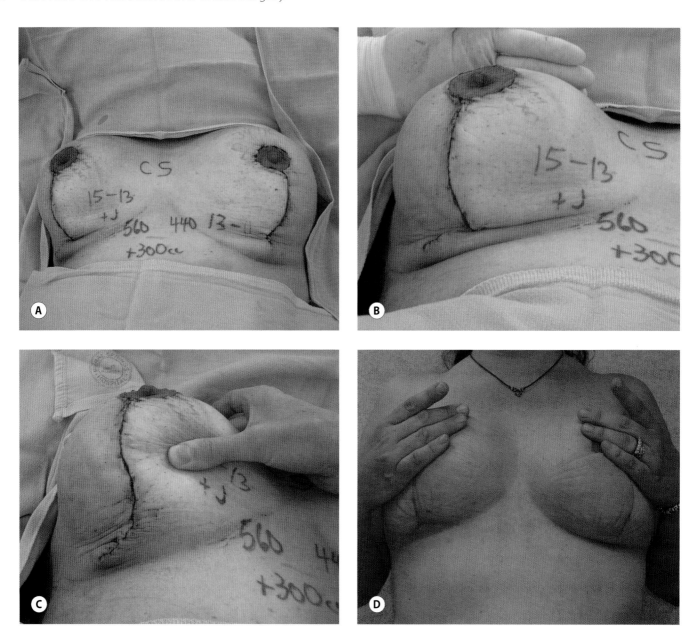

FIGURE 12.8 A 37-year-old woman, 5 feet 8 inches tall, 175 lb, 38F. 560 g removed from right breast and 440 g from left breast; 300 mL liposuction peripherally. She had complete return of sensation at 6 weeks postoperatively. **A** Intraoperative view shows puckers, which are hard for many surgeons to accept. The temptation is strong to convert to a short 'T'. The problem with the T is that it is often not clear where to put it. The inframammary fold rises with the medial pedicle vertical breast reduction. Instead, a small 'J' curve was allowed to settle on the right breast without further skin excision. **B** The new inframammary fold is not at the level when the breast is just pushed down as shown. **C** The actual level of the new fold is better demonstrated when the breast is elevated and pushed down in the manner shown. **D** 6 weeks postoperatively showing the area pulled up. There is a small 'J' curve on the right.

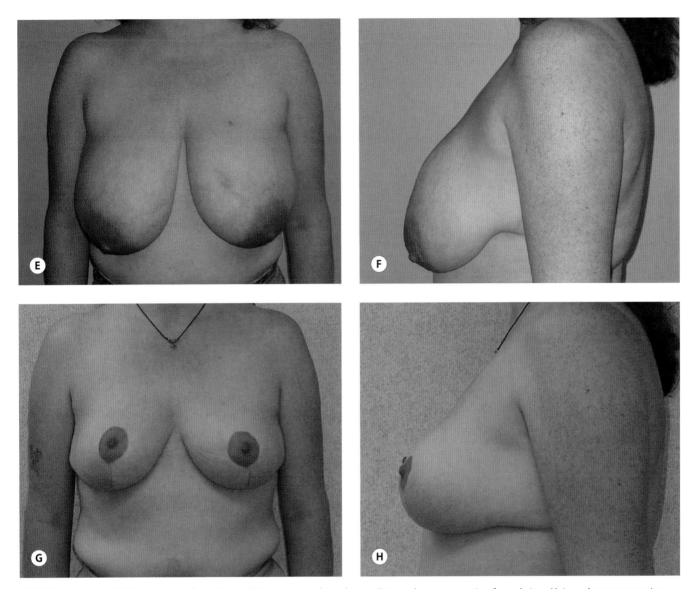

FIGURE 12.8, cont'd **E** Preoperative frontal view. **F** Preoperative lateral view. **G** 6 weeks postoperative frontal view. **H** 6 weeks postoperative lateral view. The vertical scar length on the left breast is 10 cm and on the right is 13 cm.

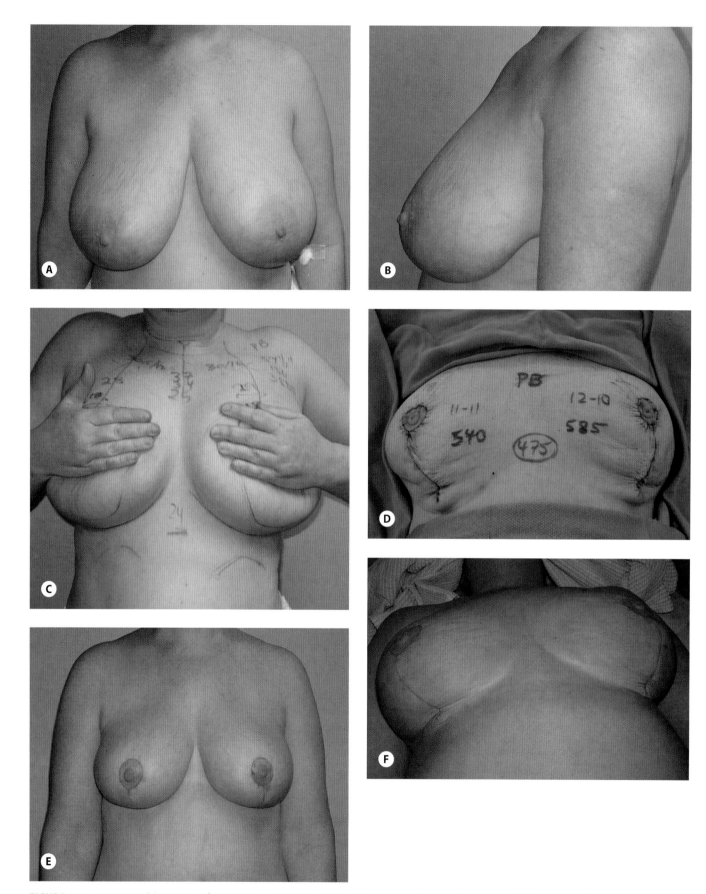

FIGURE 12.9 A 42-year-old woman, 5 feet 5 inches tall, 185 lb, 38DD. 540g removed from right breast and 585 g removed from left breast. 475 mL liposuction peripherally. This series of photos shows how the pucker at the end of the procedure looks as if it should be converted to a 'T' but how it does settle. She had almost complete return of sensation by 2.5 months. **A** Preoperative frontal view. **B** Preoperative lateral view. **C** Preoperative marked with breasts pulled up. **D** Intraoperative view at end of procedure, showing puckers. **E** 3 weeks postoperative frontal view. **F** 3 weeks postoperative view lying down, showing how much the puckers have already tucked in and settled.

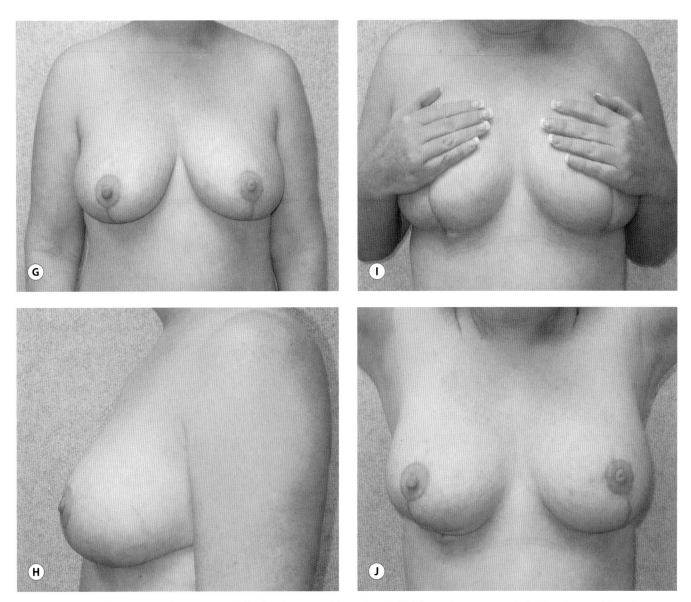

FIGURE 12.9, cont'd G 2.5 months postoperatively, showing a good frontal result. **H** 2.5 months postoperatively, showing good lateral projection and shape. The vertical scar now measures 10 cm. **I** 2.5 months postoperatively with the breasts pulled up. **J** 2.5 months postoperatively with the arms up, showing resolution of left pucker but persistent right pucker. The right will still take some time to settle.

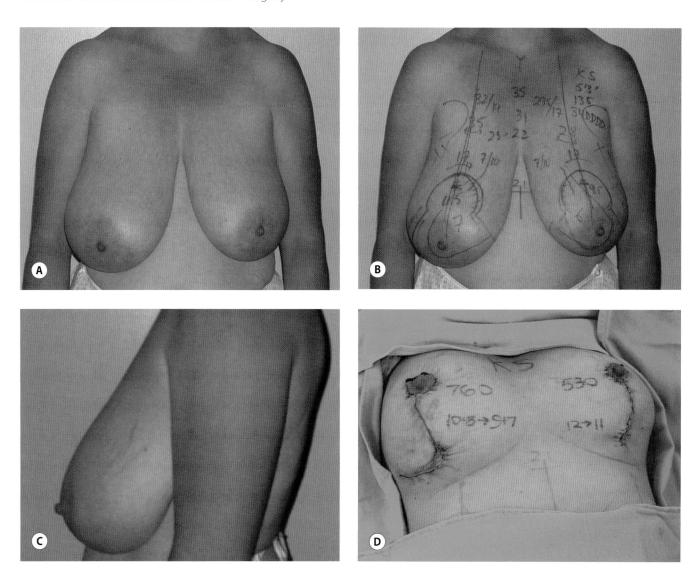

FIGURE 12.10 A 36-year-old patient, 5 feet 3 inches tall, 135 lb, 34DD. 760 g removed from right breast and 530 g from left breast. 300 mL liposuction peripherally. She had partial return of sensation at 2 months but no documentation at 8 months. **A** Preoperative frontal view. **B** Preoperative frontal view with markings. Note that new nipple position on the right (larger) breast is marked lower. Note that veins are marked and preserved in the pedicles. The pedicle may look 'superomedial' with the patient standing, but the blood supply is medial and the orientation of the pedicle is more obviously medial when the patient is lying down. **C** Preoperative lateral view. **D** Intraoperative view showing the vertical scar on the left breast but the scar on the right breast angled out laterally as a 'J'. Note that the 'J' is kept above the original inframammary fold and curved upwards.

stay in place better and last longer than generic tape (Fig. 12.4T).

A surgical brassiere is applied mainly to hold the initial bandages in place and then to give the patient a sense of support. Although it would be ideal to apply pressure to the areas where liposuction has been performed, it would not be appropriate to apply too much pressure to the nipple–areolar complex. Patients are warned that the liposuction areas will be bruised and will remain swollen and firm for several weeks. Patients are allowed to change brassieres or go without completely. Most prefer some support.

Although seromas do occur, they usually do not need to be aspirated. They tend to disappear fairly quickly.

Patients are informed preoperatively that they will not achieve as small a size as they often would like, and the final size will depend on the size of the pedicle needed. The pedicle will be larger in a larger breast and these patients cannot expect a 'B' cup.

Patients are also informed preoperatively that puckers are to be expected. They realize that it may take a full year for the puckers to disappear. They are also informed that if a pucker remains it can usually be corrected in the office under local anesthesia, but they must realize that this will not be performed for a full year. Sometimes it takes that long for a pucker to settle down, but most puckers – especially in the smaller breasts – will take only a few weeks to months to settle.

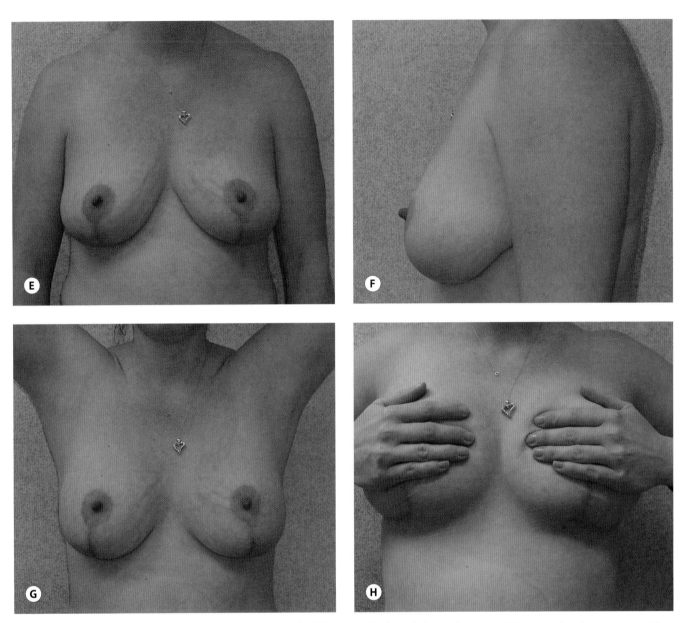

FIGURE 12.10, cont'd E Postoperative frontal view at 8 months. **F** Postoperative lateral view at 8 months. **G** Postoperative view, arms up, at 8 months. **H** Postoperative pulled-up view at 8 months to show how the scar could end up too low – the inframammary fold rises with this procedure.

CONCLUSIONS

Shorter scar reduction techniques are best used for the smaller and medium-sized breast reductions. The circum-areolar techniques can be used for very small reductions, but small to moderate-sized breasts can easily be reduced with some of the many vertical approaches. Several pedicles can be used with different skin resection patterns, but the medial pedicle combined with a vertical skin pattern has proved to be a reliable easy-to-learn technique which gives good results. The medial pedicle principles can also be applied to larger reductions or patients with poor-quality skin where a horizontal excision (T, J, or L) is added.

The principles involved are to use as short a scar as possible but at the same time give the patient an excellent shape with a narrowed breast base and good projection. Removing the heavy inferior breast tissue and leaving the skin attached superiorly, medially, and laterally helps prevent bottoming-out with time. Leaving behind a Wise pattern of tissue and excising or suctioning all excess peripherally will give a good, long-lasting shape. It is important to realize that the skin is not used as a brassiere and needs to be looser to accommodate the increased projection that results with the medial pedicle vertical breast reduction.

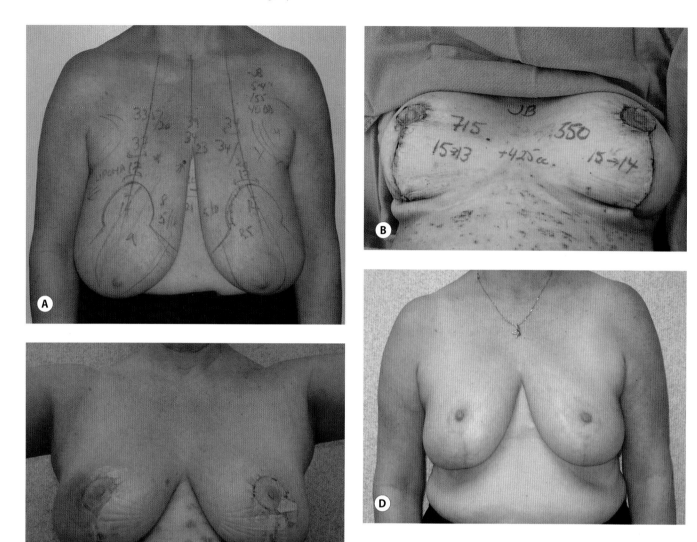

FIGURE 12.11 A–D A 56-year-old woman who had a vertical breast reduction using a medial pedicle. She was 5 feet 4 inches tall, wore a 40DD brassiere and weighed 155 lb. She had 715 g removed from the right breast and 550 g from the left. She also had multiple seborrheic keratoses on the chest wall removed at the same time. She was placed on perioperative cephalosporin but developed an infection in the right breast at 3 weeks. This was successfully treated with ciprofloxacin and healed well without any further treatment. She had full recovery of sensation in her nipples and areolas.

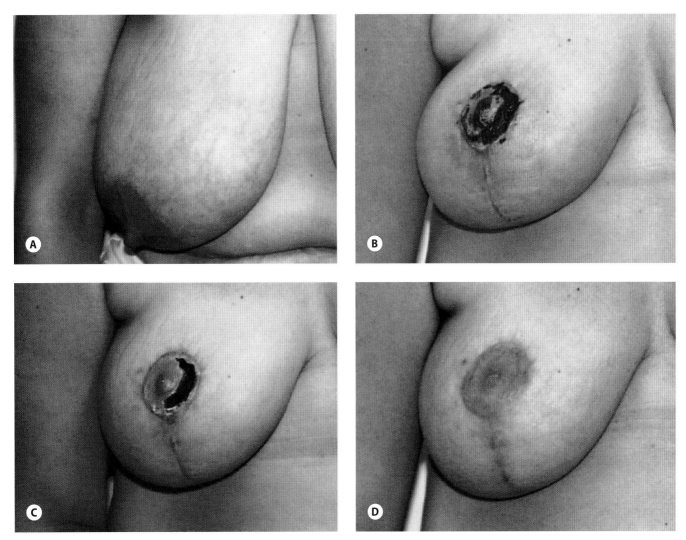

FIGURE 12.12 Nipple necrosis can occur from a lack of arterial input or venous congestion. It is often unpredictable and difficult to assess and treat. This case, shown at 2 weeks, 6 weeks, and 3 months, shows that it can be best to leave the areola to declare itself and heal by secondary intention.

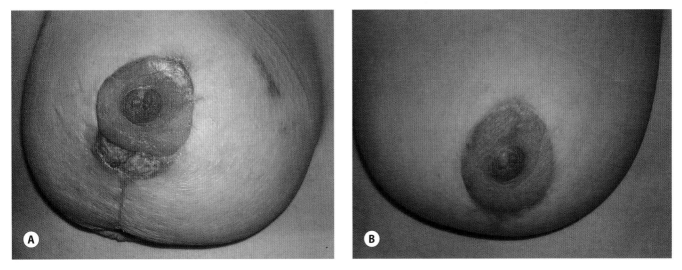

FIGURE 12.13 A, B Dehiscence of the areola at 3 weeks which healed in a few months by secondary intention. The final result is shown at 18 months.

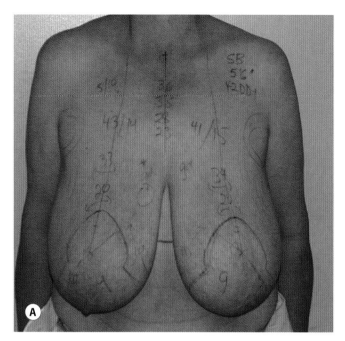
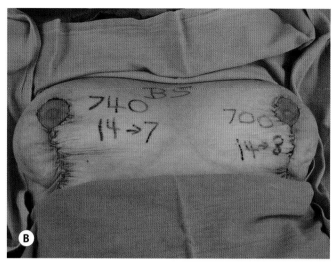
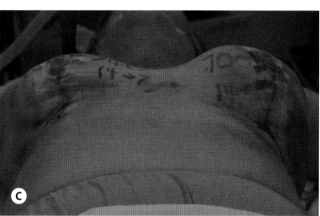
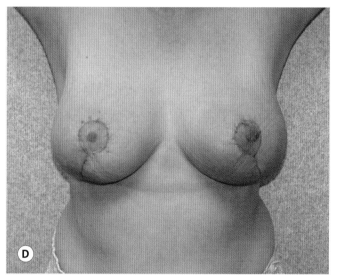

FIGURE 12.14 A Preoperative markings for vertical breast reduction using a medial pedicle. **B** Intraoperative photo with 740 g removed from the right breast and 700 g removed from the left. **C** Hematoma developed postoperative. Tumescent infiltration had been used and the perforator that would normally supply an inferior pedicle was bleeding. It had probably been in a constricted state because of the tumescent infiltration and had not been properly cauterized. **D** Patient seen 2 months postoperatively.

REFERENCES

1. McKissock PK. Reduction mammaplasty with a vertical dermal flap. Plast Reconstruct Surg 1972; 49: 245–252.
2. Robbins TH. A reduction mammaplasty with the areola-nipple based on an inferior pedicle. Plast Reconstr Surg 1977; 59: 64–67.
3. Courtiss EH, Goldwyn RM. Reduction mammaplasty by the inferior pedicle technique. An alternative to free nipple and areola grafting for severe macromastia or extreme ptosis. Plast Reconstruct Surg 1977; 59: 500.
4. Georgiade NG et al. Reduction mammaplasty utilizing an inferior pedicle nipple–areolar flap. Ann Plast Surg 1979; 3: 211.
5. Wise RJ. A preliminary report on a method of planning the mammaplasty. Plast Reconstruct Surg 1956; 17: 367.
6. Gradinger GP. Reduction mammaplasty utilizing nipple–areola transplantation. Clin Plast Surg 1988; 15: 641–654.
7. Arie G. Una nueva técnica de mastoplastia. Rev Iber Latino Am Cir Plast 1957; 3: 28.
8. Pitanguay I. Surgical correction of breast hypertrophy. Br J Plast Surg 1967; 20: 78.
9. Ribeiro L. A new technique for reduction mammaplasty. Plast Reconstruct Surg 1975; 55: 330.
10. Peixoto G, Reduction mammaplasty: a personal technique. Plast Reconstruct Surg 1980; 65: 217.
11. Lassus C. A technique for breast reduction. Int Surg 1970; 53: 69.
12. Lassus C. A 30-year experience with vertical mammaplasty. Plast Reconstruct Surg 1996; 97: 373–380.
13. Marchac D, de Olarte G. Reduction mammaplasty and correction of ptosis with a short inframammary scar. Plast Reconstruct Surg 1982; 69: 45–55.
14. Lejour M, Abboud M, Declety A, Kertesz P. Reduction des cicatrices de plastie mammaire: de l'ancre courte à la verticale. Ann Chir Plast Esthet 1990; 35: 369.
15. Lejour M, Abboud M. Vertical mammaplasty without inframammary scar and with breast liposuction. Perspect Plast Surg 1996; 4: 67–90.
16. Strombeck JO. Mammaplasty: report of a new technique based on the two-pedicle procedure. Br J Plast Surg 1960; 13: 79–90.
17. Skoog T. A technique of breast reduction – transposition of the nipple on a cutaneous vascular pedicle. Acta Chir Scand 1963; 126: 453–465.

18. Wiener DL, Aiache AE, SilverL, Tittiranonda T. A single dermal pedicle for nipple transposition in subcutaneous mastectomy, reduction mammaplasty or mastopexy. Plast Reconstruct Surg 1973; 51: 115.

19. Asplund O, Davies DM. Vertical scar breast reduction with medial flap or glandular transposition of the nipple-areola. Br J Plast Surg 1996; 49: 507–514.

20. Hammond DC. Short scar periareolar inferior pedicle reduction (SPAIR) mammaplasty. Plast Reconstruct Surg, 1999; 103: 890.

21. Hall-Findlay EJ. A simplified vertical reduction mammaplasty: shortening the learning curve. Plast Reconstruct Surg 1999; 104: 748.

22. Hall-Findlay EJ. Vertical breast reduction with a medially based pedicle. Operative strategies. Aesthet Surg J 2002; 22: 185–195.

23. Spear SL, Howard MA. Evolution of the vertical reduction mammaplasty. Plast Reconstruct Surg 2003; 112: 855–868.

24. Benelli L. A new periareolar mammaplasty: The 'round block' technique. Aesthet Plast Surg 1990; 14: 93.

25. Sampaio-Goes JC. Periareolar mammaplasty double skin technique. Breast Dis 1991; 4: 111.

26. Courtiss EH. Reduction mammaplasty by suction alone. Plast Reconstruct Surg 1993; 92: 1276–1284

27. Gray LN. Liposuction breast reduction. Aesthet Plast Surg 1998; 22: 159.

28. Mottura A. Circumvertical reduction mammaplasty. Aesthet Surg J 2000; 20: 199–204.

29. Graf R, Auersvald A, Bernardes A, Biggs TM. Reduction mammaplasty and mastopexy with shorter scar and better shape. Aesthet Surg J 2000; 20: 99–106.

30. Cooper A. On the anatomy of the breast and atlas. London: Longman, 1840.

31. Manchot C. Die Hautarterien des Menschlichen Korpers. Leipzig: Verlag von FCW Vogel, 1889.

32. Salmon M. Arteres de la peau, travaille du laboratoire d'anatomie de la Faculté de Marseille. Paris: Masson, 1936.

33. Palmer JH, Taylor GI. The vascular territories of the anterior chest wall. Br J Plast Surg 1986; 39: 287–299.

34. Schlenz I, Kuzbari R, Gruber H, Holle J. The sensitivity of the nipple–areola complex: An anatomic study. Plast Reconstruct Surg 2000; 105: 905–909.

35. Cruz-Korchin N, Korchin L. Breast-feeding after vertical mammaplasty with medial pedicle. Plast Reconstruct Surg 2004; 114: 890–894.

36. Schwartzmann E. Beitrag zur Vermeidung von Mammillennekrose bei einzeitiger Mammaplastik schwerer Fälle. (Avoidance of nipple necrosis by preservation of corium in one-stage plastic surgery of the breast.) Rev Chir Struct 1937; 7: 206–209.

37. Dufourmentel C, Mouly R. Plastie mammaire par la méthode oblique. Ann Chir Plast 1961; 6: 45.

38. Spector JA et al. The vertical reduction mammaplasty: a prospective analysis of patient outcomes. Plast Reconstruct Surg 2006; 117: 374–381.

39. Hall-Findlay EJ. Discussion: vertical reduction mammaplasty. Plast Reconstruct Surg 2006; 117: 382–383.

40. Berthe J-V, Massaut J, Greuse M, et al. The vertical mammaplasty: a reappraisal of the technique and its complications. Plast Reconstruct Surg 2003; 111: 2192–2199.

Breast Surgery in the Massive Weight-Loss Patient

13

author block
Dennis J. Hurwitz and Siamak Agha-Mohammadi

INTRODUCTION

After massive weight loss, obese women experience laxity of the skin proportional to the excess localized adiposity. The change in the breast is profound but unpredictable, owing to the variable gland to fat ratio, genetics, and prior pregnancies. Smaller breasts deflate; larger breasts flatten. For many, a singularly proud and voluptuous feature has been ruined. Further distorted by neighboring rolls of upper torso skin, these breasts conform poorly to brassieres. These women are resigned to concealing their breasts. Hence, among their many aesthetic concerns, breast reshaping is a priority. When given a choice, most weight-loss patients prefer mastopexy with autogenous tissue augmentation rather than augmentation with a silicone implant.

Nevertheless, skin reduction pattern mastopexy with silicone implant augmentation for volume is commonly presented in plastic surgery meetings. When the senior author became active in post-bariatric surgery body in the late 1990s, he favored that approach, and both authors still use it when there is inadequate neighboring discard tissue available for augmentation. Mastopexy with an implant is expeditious, resulting in dramatically improved breast contour, symmetry, and position of the nipple–areolar complex (NAC). Nevertheless, it is a complicated procedure that fails to address chest deformity and suffers from deteriorating aesthetics. The many solutions suggested for preventing recurrent ptosis after mastopexy or breast reduction in the general population attest to its high frequency and difficulty.[1-7]

Not only is there glandular ptosis, enhanced by the weight of the implants, but the breast loose skin conforms poorly to implants (Fig. 13.1). The upper pole of the breast empties and the lower pole fills excessively, resulting in descent of the inframammary fold (IMF), an excessive distance between the IMF and the NAC, and an upward rise to the NAC. This deformity is treated with an upper body lift and repositioning of the implant (Fig. 13.1). With mild skin laxity of the mid-torso one may pre-empt this unfavorable cascade of poor aesthetics with a secure permanent suture advancement of the IMF along the inferior implant space (Fig. 13.2). When there is adequate breast volume and minimal mid-torso laxity and breast descent, we advocate a mastopexy with dermal to rib suspension and internal shaping technique similar to that proposed by Rubin et al.[8] In addition we secure the IMF during the mastopexy.

Massive weight-loss patients usually accept increased risk and operative time of autogenous flaps for a more aesthetic, long-lasting outcome. Use of neighboring excess tissue for breast reshaping was proposed by Zook in the 1970s.[9] He placed de-epithelialized discard epigastric flaps beneath Pitanguy mastopexies. The inferior incision was carried around the trunk to correct undesirable rolls and bulk. Others used the Wise pattern and recruited skin folds below and lateral to the breasts to rebuild the breast.[9-13] Successful use of a lateral thoracic fasciocutaneous flap for breast reconstruction by Holstrom has ignited considerable interest in this trans-serratus perforator flap for post-mastectomy, cosmetic augmentation, and massive weight loss.[14-18]

Spiral flap breast reshaping with an upper body lift evolved to correct glandular ptosis (bottoming-out), poor breast projection, and inadequate lateral and superior pole fill with neighboring excess tissue.[19,20] The descended IMF is raised. The inferior pole of the breast is supported and augmented by the superior rotation of excess epigastric skin and fat. The lateral thoracic flap is tunneled under the superior breast to impart upper pole and lateral breast fullness and curvature. The operation combines well with the L brachioplasty[21] (Figs 13.3–13.5). Spiral flap refers to the invariable twisting and advancement under and around the breast of this compound superior epigastric and lateral thoracic flap. Previously presented in technical detail,[22] the

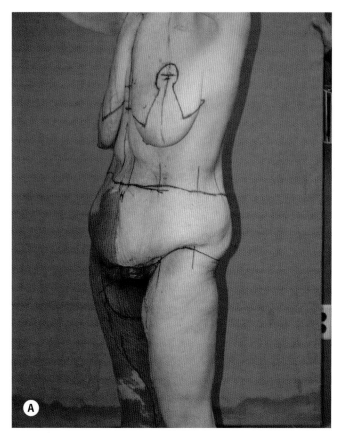

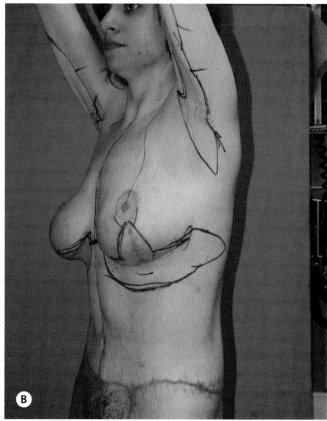

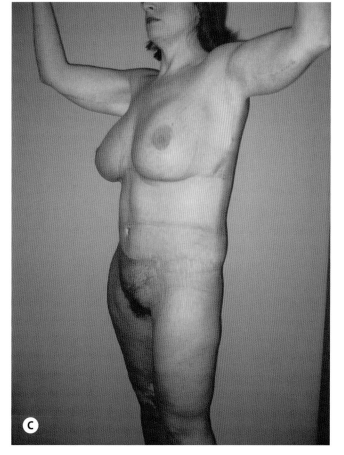

FIGURE 13.1 **A** Oblique anterior view show a 32-year-old 137-lb, 5 ft 4 in woman who lost 170 lb and is marked for total body lift surgery, including lower body lift, abdominoplasty, vertical thighplasty and Wise pattern mastopexy with 350 mL saline-filled silicone implant augmentation. **B** Six months later she is pleased with her lower body and thighs, but her breasts bottomed out with descent of her inframammary fold (IMF). Markings are drawn for revision of her mastopexy with a reverse abdominoplasty and an upper body lift, including raising her IMF. **C** The result 2 years after her breast revision with an upper body lift, showing an excellent breast shape, nipple position, and maintenance of her IMF suspension.

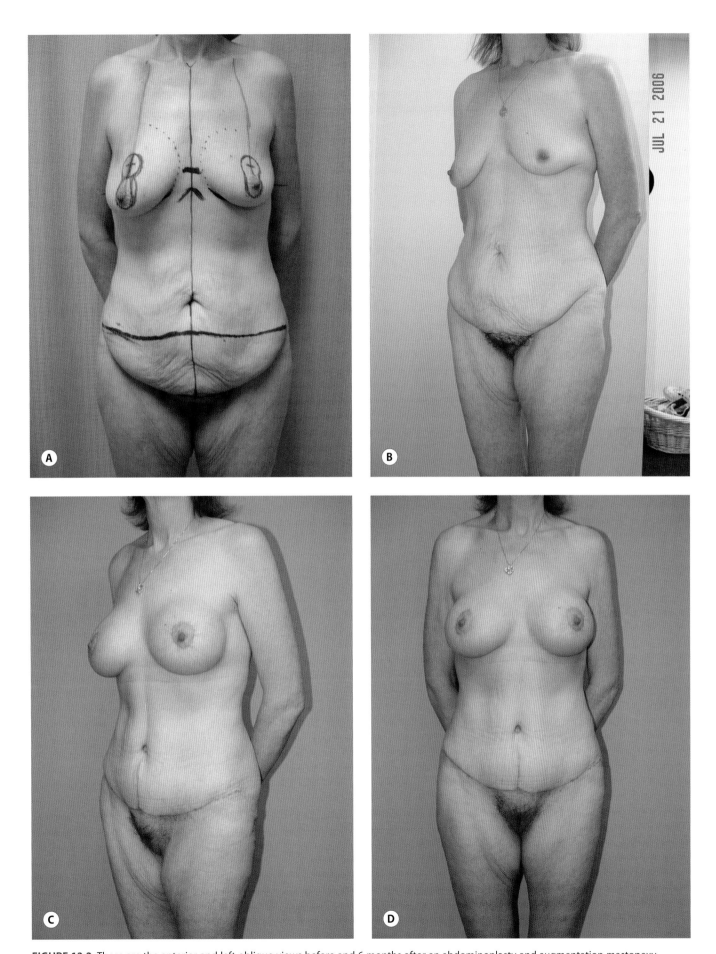

FIGURE 13.2 These are the anterior and left oblique views before and 6 months after an abdominoplasty and augmentation mastopexy with 325 mL on the right and 390 mL on the left. Suture stabilization of her inframammary folds (IMFs) was performed through the inferior portion of her implant dissection. She was 40 years old, 5 ft 6 in and 135 pounds, having lost 130 lb after gastric bypass surgery. Her breast shape and IMF have maintained position.

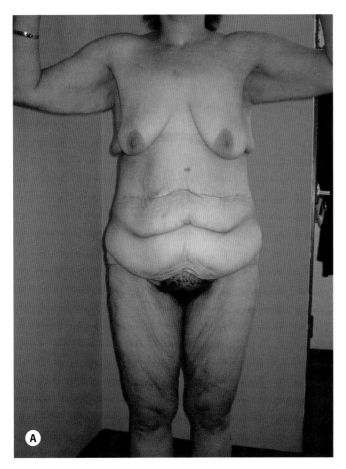

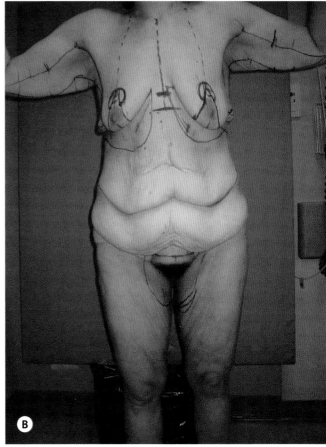

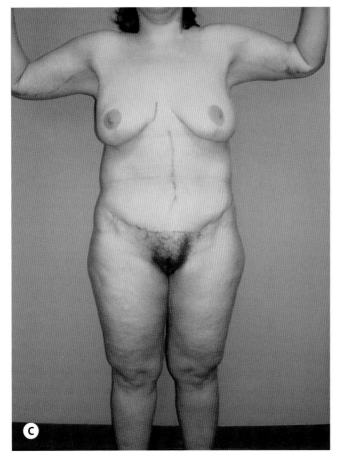

FIGURE 13.3–FIGURE 13.5 These are the preoperative and 1-year postoperative views of a 5 ft 4 in, 160 lb 42-year-old massive weight loss patient who had a single-stage total body lift followed by revisions of her right medial breast and central abdominal scars and vertical thighplasties. There is long-lasting correction of all her sagging skin and contour issues, with acceptably maturing scars. The considerable inferior extension of her breast flap onto the epigastrium is evident, as well as the lateral thoracic flaps. Both contributed volume and shaping to her breasts, which are symmetrical and firmly supported by inframammary folds (IMFs). Her convex lateral breast transitions into a concave but rounded anterior axillary fold. The hanging arm skin is corrected with reduction of the hyperaxilla and no constricting bands.

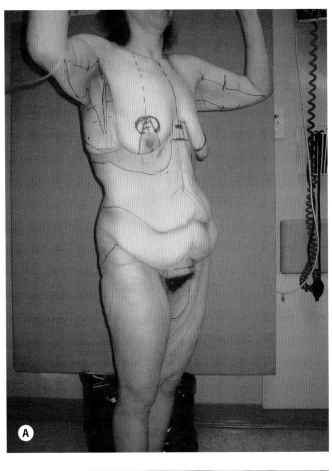

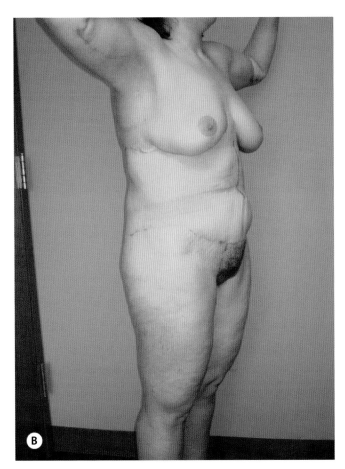

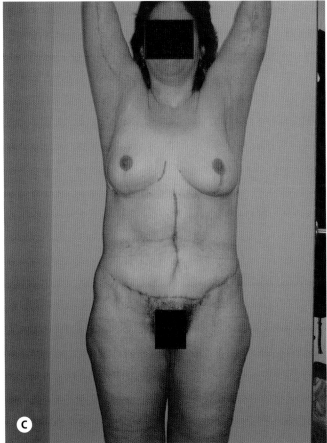

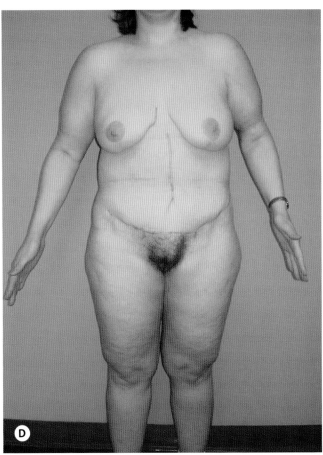

FIGURE 13.4

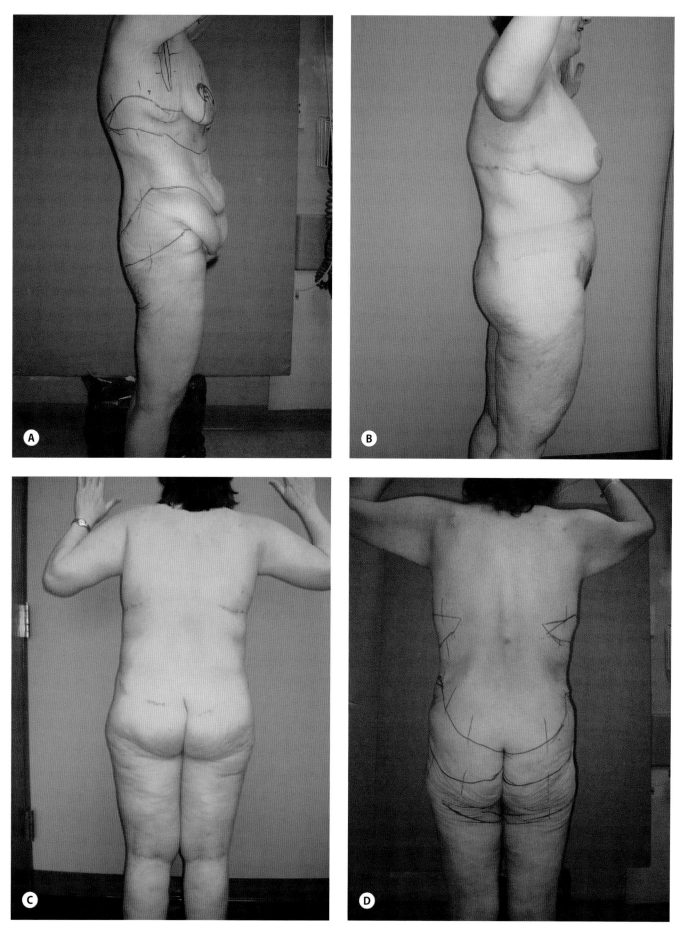

FIGURE 13.5

spiral flap description in this chapter focuses on the increasingly used modified sickle version harvested from a vertically oriented lateral thoracoplasty.

INDICATIONS AND CONTRAINDICATIONS FOR SPIRAL FLAP RESHAPING (Boxes 13.1–13.3)

Spiral flap breast reshaping with an upper body lift is indicated in patients with suitable torso anatomy who are in good health and have a good understanding of the procedure. We give our patient-oriented book, *Total Body Lift*, to facilitate their comprehension and preparation for surgery.[23] The patient needs to appreciate the value and difficulty of breast reshaping with upper body tissue discard. The patient accepts flap donor site and mastopexy scars that may extend around the back. Accompanying brachioplasty scars lie along the medial arm, across the axilla, and down the mid-lateral chest.

BOX 13.1 Indications

- Patient aversion to silicone implants
- Acceptance of risks and scars of flap reconstruction
- Severe excess skin and fat in the mid-torso
- Significant breast ptosis
- Inadequate breast volume

Obese patients with relatively poor vasculature and thick immobile flaps are generally poor candidates. Thin patients offer insufficient tissue. Patients who are medically and psychologically unstable, non-compliant, unreasonable, and using tobacco products are also generally poor candidates for these procedures.

BOX 13.2 Contraindications

- Smokers
- Unreasonable expectations
- Obese
- Underweight
- Minimal deformity

Spiral flap reshaping successfully treats the empty breast that is associated with extreme NAC ptosis and glandular descent following massive weight loss. A variety of breast shapes, ranging from broad and flat to constricted, are amenable to these operations. Patients who have had prior breast reduction and implant augmentation are also treatable. In women with excess skin and fat in the upper torso in which the lateral volume is greater than the medial volume, the operation can be accompanied by a simultaneous upper body lift. Upper body lift consists of a reverse abdominoplasty, excision of back skin excess, and creation of a raised IMF. The anticipated upper abdominal excess

tissue is left attached inferiorly to the breast mound to be de-epithelialized and flipped over the inferior pole. The roll of lateral chest and back tissue is left contiguous to the central breast mound as a transverse lateral thoracic extension. For lesser back laxity without rolls of skin, the lateral flap extension is modified to ascend superiorly along the mid-lateral chest to the axilla, which is the subject of the accompanying video demonstration.

OPERATIVE APPROACH

Spiral flap reshaping depends on an understanding of the above-described geometric interplay of upper body lift and breast anatomy and aesthetics. One must preserve blood supply to both the breast and this complex flap, and be technically facile in de-epithelialization, harvesting, moving, and shaping these flaps using an appropriate mastopexy technique.

Our clinical and cadaveric laboratory experience proves that the vasculature of the breast, axial pattern and perforators of the lateral thoracic, thoracoacromial, internal mammary and intercostal vessels emanates through suspending fascia from the third to the fifth ribs[24] (Fig. 13.6). Accordingly, the elevation of the descended breast from the eighth to the sixth ribs does not disrupt this critical mid-thoracic blood supply. Likewise, the creation of a lateral suprapectoral opening and superior tunnel over the third rib avoids critical axial vasculature. The mastopexy pattern varies from circumareolar to Wise. Because undermining is in the deep subcutaneous plane, the vascularity of the NAC and parenchyma is preserved. Our experience with limited skin necrosis is related to excessive tension at closure.

The spiral flap consists of both a broad-based inferior flap extension of the central breast mound and a narrow-based lateral thoracic fasciocutaneous flap supplied by trans-serratus fascial intercostal perforators. The patient with massive weight loss has large subcutaneous tissue vessels which are readily identified and supply these flaps to the tip of the scapula.

Finally, the breast reshaping depends on a complex interplay of mastopexy and autogenous tissue filling, with flip-up of an inferior flap of epigastric tissue and turning, twisting, and advancement of a large flap of lateral chest tissue tunneled under the upper pole of the breast. Persistent projection and natural contour without bottoming-out depend on secure suturing of the flaps and the reverse abdominoplasty to the costal cartilages and fascia.

Preoperative planning for the breast reshaping and upper body lift begins with a final assessment. Some patients lose or gain substantial amounts of weight, or may have altered their priorities and expectations. If a single-stage total body lift is planned, the lower body lift and abdominoplasty are drawn first, which is taken into consideration for the upper body lift.[25]

Severe skin laxity of the upper torso is optimally treated with a complete upper body lift, a transversely oriented de-epithelialized back flap, and a Wise pattern mastopexy (see Figs 13.3–13.5. The upper body lift combines a reverse abdominoplasty with removal of the back rolls, elevation

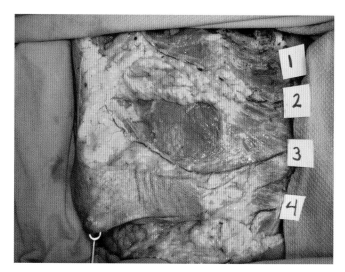

FIGURE 13.6 This right breast anatomical specimen was prepared with Microfil intravascular injections. Previous anatomical dissections have confirmed a mid-breast suspensory ligament containing a ring of dominant blood supply from internal mammary perforators to lateral intercostal and lateral thoracic vessels from the third to the fifth ribs. The NAC is being held with a hook. The spiral flap reshaping technique preserves these transverse dominant third to fifth rib vascular arcades.

and fixation of the inframammary fold, and breast reshaping. For severe deformity a Wise pattern mastopexy is needed for elevation of the NAC, removal of excess breast skin, and the inclusion of de-epithelialized discard from the mid-torso.

In patients with mild to moderate upper body skin laxity, the upper lift is modified to give fewer and less conspicuous scars. Moderate breast ptosis may only need a circumareolar or vertical pattern mastopexy. Isolated lateral IMF descent responds to elevation only along the lateral chest wall. The transverse back excision for the lateral thoracic flap harvest can be exchanged for a wide lateral chest de-epithelialized sickle shape. The back and lateral chest skin is then advanced to the mid-axillary line, with suture fixation to the serratus fascia. The sickle shape extends from the lateral breast to the short limb of the left brachioplasty.

For the following operation description refer to the accompanying video. Figures 13.6–13.8 show the preoperative surgical markings and the result at 4 months of the filmed patient.

Markings for the upper body lift begin with the patient standing, which allows the torso skin and breasts to descend. After the usual grid pattern is drawn, the ptotic breast is elevated off the chest wall to site and mark the current IMF along the nipple line. This level is registered across to the lower sternum. The low breast is pushed up to the sixth rib, and if the patient concurs that is the desired level this higher IMF level is sited and marked over the sternum. There will be a several but well-appreciated centimeter rise from the old IMF.

Because raising the IMF lowers the NAC, the new NAC is positioned several centimeters higher than the new IMF

along the nipple line. This point is also registered over the sternum. If there is excess skin and the breast needs to be narrowed, a Wise 'keyhole' pattern is drawn. To accommodate anticipated tissue fill, the descending vertical limbs are kept narrow and long.

The inferior incision line of the Wise pattern, which is usually placed about the current IMF, is positioned inferiorly onto the lower chest to include anticipated discard skin from the reverse abdominoplasty. To determine this additional area of skin, the patient should lift her breast mound to the anticipated higher level, then push the epigastric skin upward and laterally until the umbilicus moves slightly superior. The raised lower chest skin along the convergence of the nipple line and an imaginary horizontal extension of the new IMF are marked on the sternum with an ink dot. From the ink dot a rising line sweeps medially to the medial incision line of the Wise pattern near the sternum. From the nipple line inferior incision junction the line continues laterally and parallel to the lateral incision line of the Wise pattern. The advanced reverse abdominoplasty flap establishes the new IMF. Unless there is synmastia these upper reverse abdominoplasty incisions do not cross the anterior midline.

The next step involves determining the breadth and length of the transverse lateral chest and back skin roll to be removed, which was not performed in the patient in the video (Figs 13.1–13.3). This excess tissue provides fill and shape as a de-epithelialized, laterally based fasciocutaneous flap. The width of the tissue to be removed is determined by gathering the local redundant skin. The shape of flap resembles a hemiellipse rather than an equal-sided ellipse, with the longer inferior line advanced laterally during closure, which slightly reduces transverse width to narrow the waist. The placement of this excision pattern results in a closure along the brassiere line.

Alternatively, when there is only mild to moderate skin excess in the mid-torso and back, and the patient objects to a back scar, a sickle-shaped excision is drawn by pushing this excess skin superior and lateral to the breast and gathering the excess along the lateral chest, as seen in the video. The lateral chest excision continues into the axilla as the short limb of the L brachioplasty. For most patients, the upper body lift is completed with an L brachioplasty.[21] This complements the breast reshaping as it treats four intertwined deformities of the upper arm, axilla, and lateral chest. The brachioplasty corrects the canopy-like hanging skin, ptosis of the posterior axillary fold, oversized axilla, and lax lateral chest skin.

The L brachioplasty consists of a long-limbed hemielliptical excision of the inferior medial upper arm skin and a short-limbed vertical elliptical excision of the lateral chest connected by an inverted V excision through the axilla (see Figs 13.3, 13.4, 13.7 and 13.8, and video for details of the L brachioplasty markings). The superior incision line of the arm ellipse rises from the medial elbow along the bicipital groove to the deltopectoral groove. By gathering and pinching the excess skin of the arm, the inferior incision line extends from the medial elbow along the posterior margin of the arm to rise towards the deltopectoral groove. The

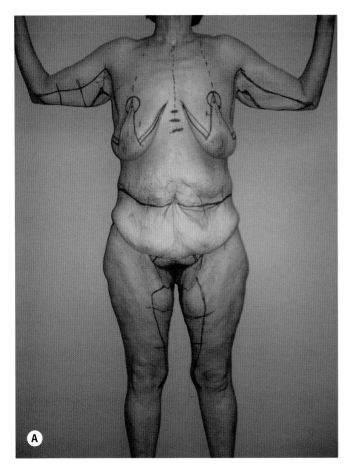

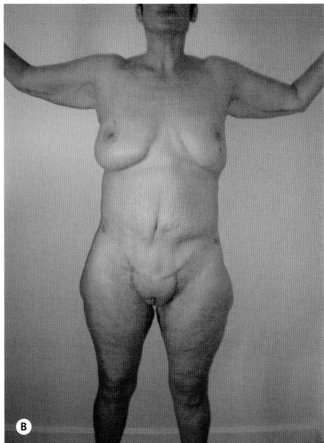

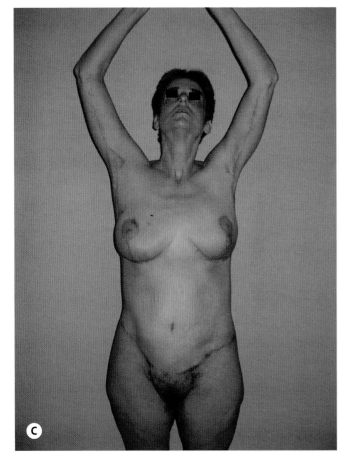

FIGURE 13.7–FIGURE 13.9 These are the preoperative and 27-month postoperative views of a 5 ft 6 in 175 lb, 37-year-old massive weight loss patient who had a single-stage total body lift. The upper body lift, spiral flap breast reshaping and L brachioplasty are demonstrated in the accompanying video. There is correction of all her sagging skin and contour issues, with acceptably maturing scars. Her breasts are symmetrical with adequate superior pole fullness and no glandular ptosis. Her convex lateral breast transitions into a concave but rounded anterior axillary fold. The hanging arm skin is corrected with reduction of the hyperaxilla and no constricting bands.

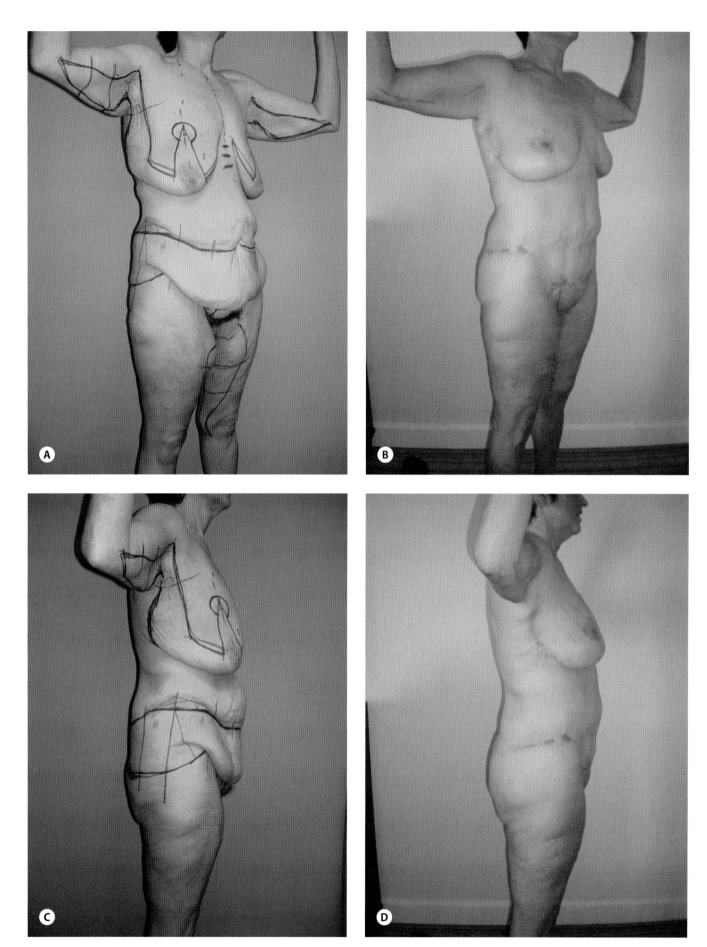

FIGURE 13.8

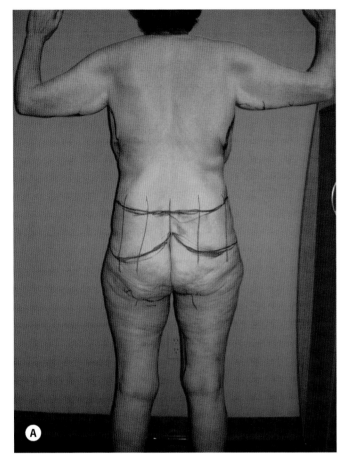

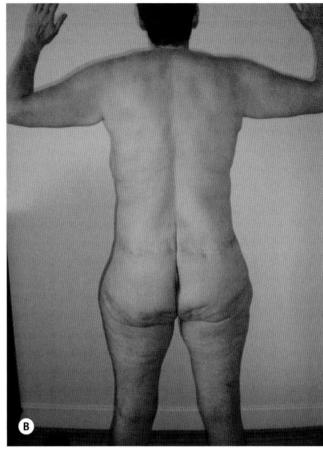

FIGURE 13.9

second ellipse drops vertically from the deltopectoral groove to include approximately the lateral half of the axilla and excess lateral chest wall skin. The chest portion of this ellipse is coordinated with the removal of a back roll performed during an upper body lift, and expansion of the breast by auto-augmentation.

An inferiorly based triangular flap is formed as the inferior arm incision meets the lateral incision of the vertically oriented lateral chest ellipse. The ability to advance this triangular flap to the deltopectoral groove is established by pinch approximation. This maneuver elevates the ptotic posterior axillary fold, tapering the arm into the axilla.

For the severe deformity, the upper body lift with spiral flap reshaping begins in the prone position with the harvesting of a lateral chest flap from mid-back excess. In mild to moderate situations the sickle flap modification is prepared in the supine position. In either case, the flap is de-epithelialized before elevation. As these flaps and the epigastric flaps are large areas, removal of thick, split-thickness grafts with an electric dermatome is preferred. A subsequent careful search for and removal of retained epithelium is essential to minimize cyst formation. The de-epithelialization commits the width of resection, so the surgeon must be accurate in preoperative marking. While the patient is prone in the severe cases, the perimeter inci-

sions are made through the subcutaneous fat to the latissimus dorsi muscle. After undermining for several centimeters, the flap is elevated from the muscular fascia extending medial to lateral. The muscular fascia is included with the flap near the lateral border of the latissimus dorsi, as when the serratus anterior muscle is reached the dissection stops. Prior infiltration with epinephrine-containing solutions is recommended to reduce blood loss. The edges of the excision are aligned with towel clips for the two-layer closure.

The patient is wrapped in a surgeon's gown and turned supine. The de-epithelialized lateral chest flaps remain attached to the serratus anterior and the central breast pedicle. When the width of the reverse abdominoplasty skin excision is confirmed, the extended Wise pattern is de-epithelialized. After marking the NAC with a 45 mm diameter cookie cutter, the Wise pattern mastopexy with its epigastric extension is de-epithelialized and extends to the previously raised lateral thoracic flap extension. This tedious process is expedited with the use of an electric dermatome set at 32 thousands of an inch. The medial, superior and lateral skin flaps of the Wise pattern are incised and undermined superficially as needed.

If the sickle-shaped modification of the spiral flap is chosen, the de-epithelialized flap perimeter incisions are made and the flap is raised from the serratus fascia, starting from the axilla. The flap's anterior limb incision is completed first. With identification of the lateral border of the pectoralis major muscle near the fourth rib, dissection of a tunnel for the flap continues across the muscle. Because the muscle is adherent to the skin, in thin patients it can be easily palpated along the anterior axillary line. The search for this junction is aided in heavier patients by incising to the anticipated level of the muscle and then retracting away. A dissection that is too deep tends to be associated with increased blood loss and may result in damage to major blood supply to the breast. Once the lateral border is identified, the dissection proceeds broadly over the anterior surface over the third and fourth ribs. A path from the base of the lateral thoracic flap to the window over the pectoralis muscle is created without injuring the large vessels overlying the serratus fascia. The pocket for the spiral flap is developed towards the parasternal region. The space is crescent-shaped, extending under the superior pole of the breast from lateral border of the pectoralis muscle near the fourth rib to the sixth sternochondral junction. The tunnel is widened enough to accept the lateral thoracic flap.

The next step includes the posterior incision and completion of flap elevation. The fifth, sixth, and perhaps the fourth intercostal trans-serratus perforators are protected by awareness of the lateral border of the latissimus dorsi muscle and the ribs. These vessels can be located by Doppler or direct visualization to the mid-axillary line. The lateral thoracic portion of the flap is nearly raised, but not until the entire breast is suspended, so the reverse abdominoplasty begins.

The long junction between the extended de-epithelialized flap and upper abdomen is incised from the parasternal region to the raised lateral thoracic flap. The breast with its epigastric flap extension is undercut along the rectus muscle fascia from the lower ribs to the sixth rib. The new IMF position, which has been registered over the sternum, guides this movement of the central breast pedicle. The termination of the tunnel for the lateral thoracic flap is completed under the medial flap of the Wise pattern parasternally about the sixth rib.

With the breast mobilized and the submammary tunnel completed, the lateral thoracic flap is prepared for augmentation by trimming back the distal tip until bright red bleeding is appreciated. A suture is placed through the distal end of the flap, followed by the insertion of a long clamp through the parasternal site. This is grasped and the back flap rotated along the lateral border of the pectoralis muscle, into the submammary space. This pulling suture is then stitched to the sixth costochondral junction, which holds the medial position of the flap. While in situ, the flap is tailored to optimally augment and reshape the breast. Generally the flap lies flat, but it may be rolled or further advanced on itself. The spiral flap is stitched to the lateral border entrance of the pectoralis major muscle. The breast usually slopes laterally with inadequate projection. Centralizing the breast requires suture suspension of the de-epithelialized flap, catching mid-epigastric flap dermis and pulling it medially by approximating it to the sixth rib cartilage.

The next step is to align the NAC and superior portion of the Wise pattern vertical flaps. The inferior epigastric extension is rotated upward and sutured to shape and project the mound.

Attention is again directed to the reverse abdominoplasty component. The inferior pedicle abdominal skin flap is directly undermined for several centimeters, and with the aid of graduated Brazilian dissector dilators the flap is discontinuously undermined over the rectus abdominis fascia beyond the costal margins. The breast pedicle is repositioned superiorly and the inferiorly based abdominal flap is advanced to the new IMF, which is usually at the fifth and sixth ribs. Approximately 12 interrupted 0 braided polyester sutures are placed in the subcutaneous fascial portion of the flap and along the sixth rib cartilage and periosteum. With the modified upper body lift and sickle flap, the advancement of the reverse abdominoplasty is in continuity with the lateral chest skin flap.

With the abdominal flap pushed firmly upwards, the sutures are sequentially tied. The closure of the reverse abdominoplasty forms the new inframammary fold, hidden under the breast.

The medial and lateral Wise pattern breast flaps are advanced over the breast mound and sutured together and along the IMF to complete the restoration of the breast. The added flap volume creates additional tension on the closure of the Wise pattern flaps. A high-tension closure of the lateral thoracic flap donor site from the axilla to the IMF appropriately flattens this area, emphasizing the newly created lateral breast fullness and projection. The lateral chest donor site closure is continuous with the advanced and stabilized new IMF. A firm fold also improves breast projection and eliminates bottoming-out. A matching procedure is performed on the contralateral breast.

The reverse abdominoplasty is closed in three layers. After the interrupted large braided permanent sutures, there are running absorbable sutures placed in the subdermal region and monofilament sutures placed in the dermis. During this closure, the L brachioplasty begins with thorough liposuction under the skin destined for resection. Ultrasound-assisted lipoplasty (UAL) with additional UAL of the arm is preferred and performed as needed. The posterior incision is followed by the anterior incision. The L-shaped strip of skin with very little fat is excised, leaving denuded vasculature and sensory nerves. Closure of the brachioplasty begins with deep suture advancement of the posterior axillary fold triangular flap across the axilla to the deltopectoral groove with 2/0 braided suture. Towel clips are used to align the skin closure. Closure is performed in two layers using an absorbable suture. Our experience with the speed, ease, and holding power of the Quill 0 double-armed barbed suture has been favorable. Quill 2/0 sutures can also be used for the dermal closure. The ipsilateral breast can be closed concurrently with the de-epithelialization on the contralateral breast.

The final intraoperative video and the results 2 weeks postoperatively are shown in the video. As the skin tension begins to equilibrate, the brachioplasty scar courses from the medial epicondyle along the medial arm, just inferior to the bicipital groove, coursing to the axillary dome before descending vertically and terminating on the chest, forming an inverted L. The inferior contour of the arm drops slightly at the mid-humerus and then rises distinctly to a superiorly positioned posterior axillary fold. The suspended posterior axillary fold skin conforms well to the axillary hollow. The brachioplasty scar zigzags through the axilla, descending and curving around the lateral breast, similar to the lateral brachiothoracoplasty of Pitanguy.[26] The mid-torso laxity has been corrected, and the breasts are raised, with improved fullness and shape.

COMPLICATIONS AND SIDE EFFECTS

Moderate incisional pain may linger for several weeks along the reconstructed IMF. Oral medication with narcotics is usually adequate. In cases where pain is protracted, an intercostal nerve block may be useful. Breasts in which the swelling and edema are moderate to severe generally relax and become ptotic, usually over the course of 1 month. Diffusely swollen upper extremities require higher elevation and more complete elastic wrapping.

The most common complication is distal flap necrosis of the lateral thoracic extension. Experience has demonstrated that some firmness may be palpable in about 20% of cases. This will generally resolve without treatment. From over 100 cases, inclusion cysts necessitating a biopsy or aspiration have been performed in only four. One patient suffered skin edge necrosis of the reverse abdominoplasty flap and cellulitis 1 week after an upper body lift. She had resumed cigarette smoking immediately after her surgery. Healing was by secondary intention. Scar revision restored an aesthetic result.

Some patients have experienced a diminution of superior pole fullness over time. Others have developed lateral breast fullness at the base of the lateral thoracic flap. In two patients the lateral breast was further advanced along the serratus fascia to correct this malposition. In the occasional case of breast size asymmetry, the fault lay in failing to consider the preoperative size discrepancies. Lateral IMF descent was significant in five breasts, probably owing to the large size of the flaps. This descent was corrected with readvancement of the lateral breast.

The L brachioplasty triangular flap across the axilla has a tenuous blood supply and may suffer necrosis, particularly if there is direct pressure. A small area of skin loss may lead to a large wound that may need to heal by secondary intention.

POSTOPERATIVE CARE

The incisions are usually covered with a skin glue together with a light gauze dressing and a surgical bra. No constricting binder is place across the mid-abdomen, although a long-leg elastic lower body garment is used. Patients are admitted for a single night's observation and care. The brachioplasty incisions are covered with large gauze pads and placed in an ACE wrap. These are replaced by elastic sleeves several days later. No direct pressure is placed on the triangular flap in the axilla as it is vulnerable to ischemic necrosis. As previously stated, considerable incisional pain may linger along the IMF, which may require and responds well to intercostal nerve blocks.

The scars may take years to mature, especially along the distal arm. Minor contour deformities of the breast are successfully treated with lipoaugmentation in the subcutaneous plane.

CONCLUSION

There are a variety of operations to reshape the breast after massive weight loss. It is the primary author's feeling that options using autologous tissue are preferable to those that use prosthetic devices, and therefore these flaps have become the treatment of choice A compound flap that includes an epigastric and a lateral thoracic extension to the central breast mound has been designed and termed a spiral flap based on the manner of usage. The spiral flap has been successfully combined with an upper body lift and L brachioplasty in over 100 patients. The sickle-shaped modification is demonstrated on video for this atlas.

REFERENCES

1. Regnault P. Breast ptosis. Clin Plast Surg 1976; 3: 193–203.
2. Spear SL, Majidian A. Mastopexy. In: Spear SL, ed. Breast surgery: principles and art. Philadelphia: Lippincott Williams & Wilkins, 1998: 673–684.
3. De Pina DP. Technical refinements in mammaplasty. Plast Reconstruct Surg 1983; 71: 50.
4. Exner K, Scheufler O. Dermal suspension flap in vertical-scar reduction mammoplasty. Plast Reconstruct Surg 2002; 109: 2289.

5. Frey M. A new technique of reduction mammoplasty: Dermis suspension and elimination of medial scars. Br J Plast Surg 1999; 52: 45.
6. Goes J. Periareolar mammoplasty with mixed mesh support: The double skin technique. Op Tech Plast Reconstruct Surg 1996; 3: 197.
7. Graf R, Biggs T. In search of better shape in mastopexy and reduction mammoplasty. Plast Reconstruct Surg 2002; 110: 309.
8. Rubin JP, O'Toole J, Agha-Mohammadi S. Approach to the breast after weight loss. In: Rubin JP, Matarasso A, eds. Aesthetic surgery after massive weight loss. Philadelphia: Saunders Elsevier, 2007; 37–38.
9. Zook EG. The massive weight loss patient. Clin Plast Surg 1975; 2: 457–466.
10. Wise RJ. A preliminary report on a method of planning the mammaplasty. Plast Reconstruct 1956; 17: 367–369.
11. Palmer B, Hallberg D, Backman L. Skin reduction plasties following intestinal shunt operations for treatment of obesity. Scand J Plast Reconstruct Surg 1975; 9: 47–52.
12. Shons AR. Plastic reconstruction after bypass surgery and massive weight loss. Surg Clin North Am 1979; 59: 1139–1152.
13. Holstrom H, Lossing C. The lateral thoracodorsal flap in breast reconstruction. Plast Reconstruct Surg 1986; 577: 933.
14. Heitmann C, Guerra A, Metzinger SW, et al. The thoracodorsal artery perforator flap: anatomical basis and clinical application. Ann Plast Surg 2003; 51: 23–29.
15. Levine JI, Soucid NE, Allen RJ. Algorithm for autologous breast reconstruction for partial mastectomy defects. Plast Reconstruct Surg 2005; 116: 762.
16. Van Landuyt K, Hamdi M, Blondeel P, Monstrey S. Autologous augmentation of pedicled perforator flaps. Ann Plast Surg 2004; 53: 322–327.
17. Pittet B, Mahajan AL, Alizadeh N, et al. The free serratus anterior flap and its cutaneous component. Plast Reconstruct Surg 2006; 117: 1277.
18. Kwei S, Borud LJ, Lee BT. Mastopexy with autologous augmentation after MWL: The intercostal artery perforator (ICAP) flap. Ann Plast Surg 2006; 57: 361.
19. Hurwitz DJ, Golla D. Breast reshaping after massive weight loss. In: Shenaq S, Spear SL, Davison S, eds. New trends in breast reduction and mastopexy. Semin Plast Surg 2004; 18: 179–187.
20. Hurwitz DJ, Agha-Mohammadi S. Post bariatric surgery breast reshaping: the spiral flap. Ann Plast Surg 2006; 56: 481–486.
21. Hurwitz DJ, Holland SW. The L brachioplasty: An innovative approach to correct excess tissue of the upper arm, axilla and lateral chest. Plast Reconstruct Surg 2006; 117: 403–411.
22. Hurwitz D. Breast reduction and mastopexy after massive weight loss. In: Spear S, ed. Surgery of the breast. Philadelphia: JB Lippincott, 2005; 1193–1209.
23. Hurwitz DJ. Total body lift: reshaping the breast, chest, arms, thighs, hips, waist, abdomen and knees after weight loss, aging and pregnancies. New York: MDPublish, 2005.
24. Wuringer E, Mader N, Posch E, et al. Nerve and vessel supplying ligamentous suspension of the mammary gland. Plast Reconstruct Surg 1998; 101: 1486.
25. Hurwitz DJ. Single stage total body lift after massive weight loss. Ann Plast Surg 2004; 52: 435–441.
26. Pitanguy I. Correction of lipodystrophy of the lateral thoracic aspect and inner side of the arm and elbow. Clin Plast Surg 1975; 2: 477.

14

Gynecomastia

Michael Zenn

INTRODUCTION

Gynecomastia is a benign enlargement of the male breasts. This may be due to proliferation of the glandular component or to an increase in the adipose component of the breast. Both etiologies are quite common. There is a bimodal distribution to the occurrence of gynecomastia. The first peak occurs during puberty, around the ages of 13 and 14 years; this trend declines through the late teenage years. The second peak is found in the adult population between 50 and 80 years. There is no racial difference in the prevalence of gynecomastia.[1,2]

Many medical conditions are associated with gynecomastia (Table 14.1), but it is beyond the scope of this chapter to go into each of these. The etiology should be diagnosed prior to treatment.[1–3]

INDICATIONS AND CONTRAINDICATIONS

Evaluation

Gynecomastia, due either to fatty enlargement or to glandular proliferation, can usually be discriminated by physical examination. Although some may consider gynecomastia due to fatty enlargement to be 'pseudogynecomastia,' both conditions are of concern to the patient and are treated by plastic surgery. The degree of fatty infiltration versus glandular breast tissue will ultimately dictate the course of action to be taken.

Any breast mass found on examination should not be assumed to be breast tissue, as other disorders, such as neurofibromas, lymphangiomas, lipomas, and dermoid cysts, can account for such masses. Breast cancer in men accounts for 1% of all breast cancers and should also always be in the differential diagnosis, especially if the mass has been enlarging and is asymmetric with the contralateral side.[1]

PREOPERATIVE HISTORY AND CONSIDERATIONS

Painful, tender gynecomastia appearing during puberty requires only history, physical examination, palpation, and examination of the testicles by palpation or ultrasound. If these are normal, reassurance and periodic follow-up are prescribed. In the majority of patients with this condition, spontaneous resolution will occur within 1–2 years. Evidence of feminization, such as small testicular size, lack of male hair distribution, or a eunuchoid body habitus, suggests a feminizing tumor and endocrine work-up is indicated, starting with serum testosterone, estradiol, luteinizing hormone, and dehydroepiandrosterone levels.[1,3,4]

Gynecomastia in men is quite common. Work-up should include a careful history, including medication use, social history, questions about hepatic dysfunction, testicular insufficiency, pulmonary symptoms, and hyperthyroidism. These questions will uncover most conditions associated with gynecomastia. If physical examination is normal, and if liver function, renal function, and thyroid function are all normal on laboratory examination, further examination is unwarranted. Drugs that may be causing gynecomastia (Table 14.2) should be discontinued if possible, and the patient should be re-evaluated in 1 month. If gynecomastia is progressive or new in onset and there are no abnormalities in physical examination or basic laboratory screening, measurements of chorionic gonadotropin, testosterone, estradiol, and luteinizing hormone are indicated.[1,3,4]

OPERATIVE APPROACH

Treatment

Treatment of the enlarged breast is indicated if gynecomastia causes pain, embarrassment, or emotional discomfort that interferes with the patient's daily life. The remainder **197**

TABLE 14.1 Conditions associated with gynecomastia

Neoplasms
Testicular (germ cell, Leydig cell or Sertoli cell)
Adrenal (adenoma or carcinoma)
Atopic production of HCG (lung, liver and kidney cancer)
Primary gonadal failure
Acquired (trauma, infection, torsion, radiation, chemotherapy)
Congenital
Secondary hypogonadism
Defects of testosterone production
Androgen-insensitivity syndromes
True hermaphroditism
Liver disease
Starvation
Renal disease
Hypothyroidism/thyrotoxicosis
Excessive extraglandular aromatase activity
Drugs (see Table 14.2)
Idiopathic gynecomastia

TABLE 14.2 Drugs associated with gynecomastia

Category	Drug
Hormones	Androgens
	Anabolic steroids
	Chorionic gonadotropin estrogens
Antiandrogens or inhibitors of androgen synthesis	Cyproterone
	Flutamide
Estrogen-binding blockers	Clomid
Antibiotics	Isoniazid
	Ketoconazole
	Metronidazole
Anti-ulcer medicines	Cimetidine
	Omeprazole
	Ranitidine
Cancer agents (anchorin agents)	
Cardiovascular	Amiodarone
	Captopril
	Digitoxin
	Enalapril
	Methyldopa
	Nifedipine
	Reserpine
	Verapamil
	Spironolactone
Psychoactive agents	Diazepam
	Haloperidol
	Phenothiazines
	Tricyclic antidepressants
Drugs of abuse	Alcohol
	Amphetamines
	Heroin/opiates
	Marijuana
Other	Phenytoin
	Penicillamine
	Auranofin
	Sulindac
	Theophylline

of this chapter will deal with the surgical treatment of gynecomastia when no other medical interventions are required for diagnosis or treatment.

Treatment will depend on the degree of gynecomastia and its composition. Patients who are smaller-breasted and have a large component of fatty tissue can be managed with liposuction alone. Patients with significant breast tissue which is not amenable to liposuction will require direct excision. Patients having a large breast with excessive skin as well as underlying breast tissue will require a procedure to reduce the volume of the breast as well as the skin envelope.

The ultimate goal of gynecomastia repair is a flat chest in line with the patient's body habitus, minimal scarring, and appropriately positioned and shaped nipple complexes. It is obvious to those of us who treat this condition commonly that patients may be treated in a variety of ways for a similar condition, and there are those who feel strongly that their way is the best. It is the goal of this chapter to lay out all possible treatments for gynecomastia and leave it to the clinician to decide which would be the most appropriate in any particular case. It is helpful, when deciding which procedure should be performed, to involve the patient as much as possible and help him make decisions regarding scar placement, morbidity, and downtime from the different surgical procedures, and ultimately, the final outcome.

Liposuction

In cases of minor gynecomastia with minimal skin excess and a majority of fatty tissue excess, liposuction alone can

be successful.[5,6] This can be done through a remote-access incision in the axillae, or in the periareolar area. Some cases can be done in a stepwise fashion, performing liposuction first and determining whether any direction excision is required secondarily. Some people advocate performing gynecomastia in two separate stages when there is skin excess.[2] In such cases liposuction is performed to removed the fatty component and allow the skin to retract. Secondary resection of skin and breast is then performed when the requirements for resection have diminished. This may limit the ultimate quantity of scar, but the patient must agree to a two-stage procedure. Most recently, ultrasonic liposuction has been championed as the treatment for the majority of cases of gynecomastia, even where there is significant glandular tissue.[4,7]

Direct excision

Before liposuction, the gold standard for gynecomastia repair was direct excision. In minimal and some moderate cases, reduction can be carried out through a periareolar excision only, excising both skin and fatty tissue. The more modern version of this procedure involves central resection of breast tissue only and peripheral liposuction at the same time. Most cases can be managed by this technique.[8] The disadvantages of this procedure include insensitivity of the nipple, as direct breast tissue excision will, by definition, divide the innervation to the nipple–areolar complex. Spontaneous reinnervation may occur to varying degrees, but this cannot be guaranteed.

There is also an art to the excision procedure to ensure that enough tissue remains under the nipple so that the contour with the surrounding skin and subcutaneous tissue is seamless. One must remember in these cases that removal of all breast tissue is not the goal. This is a contouring procedure, and thinking about it as such will avoid contour-related problems later.

Limited skin resection procedures

In cases of moderate to severe gynecomastia where excess skin, breast ptosis, and an enlarged areola are characteristically seen, limited procedures will not suffice. In addition to removing volume via liposuction or direct excision, skin must also be removed. The most common mistake made in skin removal procedures is to treat the male breast like the female breast and perform skin resection with an inverted T or 'Wise pattern' excision. Performance of a T excision in the male shows a lack of understanding of its design. In a female breast, T excision is largely hidden by the breast mound itself. In a male gynecomastia repair, where the goal is a flat chest and limited scar, a T incision becomes quite conspicuous.

The goal of limiting scarring from skin excision in gynecomastia would be best met if it were possible to hide the scar in the periareolar area only. This is possible if only moderate ptosis exists.[9,10] Examples of significant skin reduction in cases of significant ptosis using only a periareolar scar have been reported, but have limited applicability.[11] The final skin contour must be smooth without wrinkling, and this is the limiting factor in using the periareolar approach.

Historically, many limited skin incision designs have been performed[12–20] (Fig. 14.1). Common to many of these procedures is the maintenance of a periareolar scar and limiting the length and locations of any additional scars. The optimal skin incision design used would be patient-dependent and based on clinical judgment at the time of the procedure. In general, scars that extend laterally and inferiorly from the periareolar area are perhaps best hidden. One should try to avoid medial or superior extension when possible.

Maximal skin removal procedures

Many patients presenting with gynecomastia, especially those presenting after bariatric surgery, have large skin envelopes which are essentially empty. Nipples can be mal-positioned quite distant from their normal location. Large skin excisions need to be performed in these cases and, as with much post-bariatric surgery, contour is the primary concern and the length of the scars secondary. Patients will accept large scars so that they may wear clothes comfortably and not have any hanging skin. Although small nipple movements can retain a nipple on a small dermal pedicle and still maintain its viability, larger nipple movements are best treated with free nipple grafting.[21] The goal in these procedures is to maximally remove skin symmetrically so that a flat contour is left. In most cases of skin excision, whether maintaining the nipple on a pedicle or free grafting it, nipple sensation will probably be absent and there is the added increase risk of necrosis or graft loss.

Nipple positioning

Important considerations in gynecomastia repair is the ultimate location, size, and shape of the nipple–areolar complex once the reduction is performed.[22–24] In cases of volume reduction without skin excision, one can expect a larger areola to contract significantly once there is no volume underneath it. The degree of reduction is variable but should be symmetric. Although the final areola may still be large, it is desirable to avoid complete periareolar scars when possible. A slightly enlarged areola has a more natural appearance out of clothes than one with a concentric scar.

In cases where skin excision is planned, one must pay close attention to locating the nipple–areolar complex and making it the appropriate size. Although there is natural variation, the appropriate-size nipple–areolar complex in a male is smaller than that of a female. Whereas the female nipple–areolar complex tends to be round, with an average diameter of 40 mm, the male complex is oval in shape, with an average horizontal diameter of 27 mm and an average vertical diameter of 20 mm. Many papers have been written on localization of the nipple–areolar complex.[22–24] In general, most nipples are located in the fourth or fifth intercostal space over the inferior margin of the pectoralis muscle. Although some publications recommend reliance on anatomic and soft tissue landmarks such as the acromioclavicular joint and the anterior superior iliac spine, others use more sophisticated calculations. One such method reported by Beer et al.[24] uses measurements of the circumference of the chest and length of the sternum to help localize the new nipple–areolar complex. Clinically, it is helpful to compare clinical judgment to these formulas for placement as a check prior to final nipple placement. Bear in mind that in all techniques some settling may occur. This will vary depending on the patient's anatomy and tissue characteristics.

Complications

As with other breast procedures, common complications of gynecomastia repair include bleeding, infection, seroma, asymmetry, bad scarring, pain, and a poor cosmetic result. The most common reasons for patient dissatisfaction include the appearance of scars, persisting fullness in the chest, irregularity of the skin, nipple and skin insensitivity, and chronic pain.

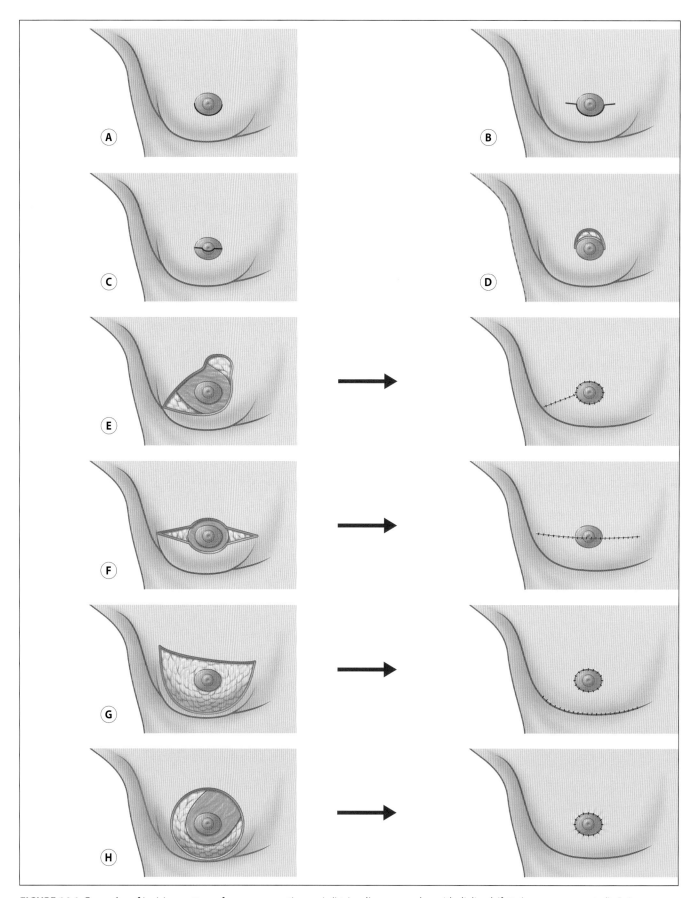

FIGURE 14.1 Examples of incision patterns for gynecomastia repair ('striped' areas are de-epithelialized; 'fatty' areas are resected). **A.** Lower periareolar (Webster[12]) **B** Omega (Barsky[13]). **C** Transareolar (Pitanguy[14]). **D** Superior areolar (Letterman and Schurter[15]). **E** Nipple transposition with lateral excision (Letterman and Schurter[16]). **F** Bipedicle (Pers[17], Peters[18]). **G** Mastectomy with free nipple graft (Wray[19]). **H** Periareolar excision with purse-string closure (Huang[20], Colic[11], Persichette[10]).

CASE EXAMPLES

Case 1 A 58-year-old man with gynecomastia which is largely adipose. He underwent ultrasound-assisted liposuction of 300 mL on each side. This is his 4-month follow-up (Fig. 14.2).

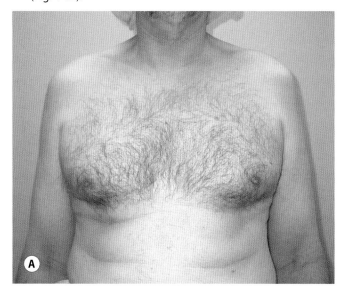

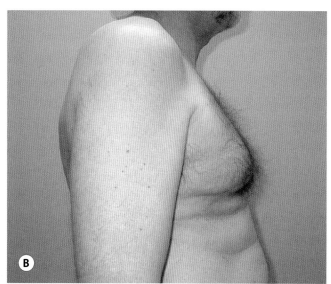

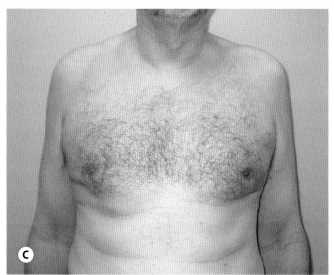

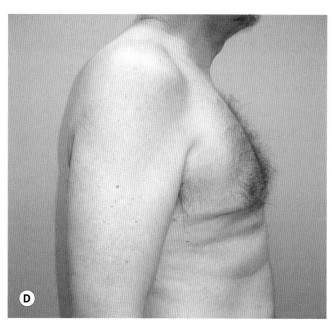

Case 2 A 48-year-old man with palpable breast tissue and adiposity who underwent direct excision via a lower peri-areolar approach (left 100 g, right 80 g) and tumescent liposuction (225 mL total). This is his 5-month follow-up (Fig. 14.3).

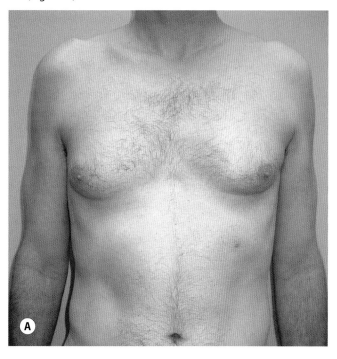

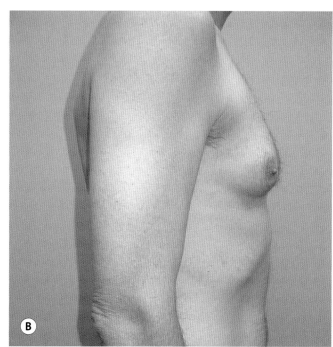

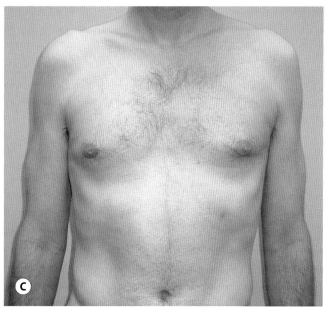

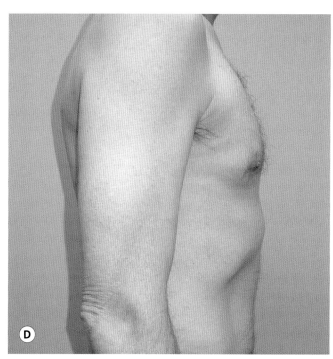

Case 3 A 15-year-old male with palpable breast tissue and some skin excess with an enlarged areola. He underwent periareolar skin excision, direct excision of breast tissue (left 70 g, right 90 g), and chest tumescent liposuction (200 mL total). This is his 4-month follow-up (Fig. 14.4).

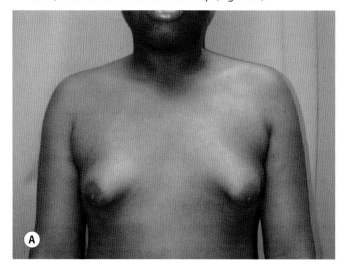

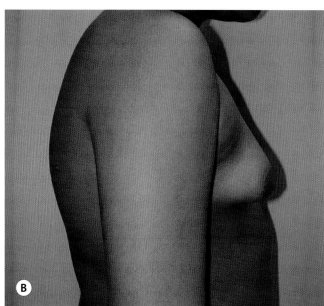

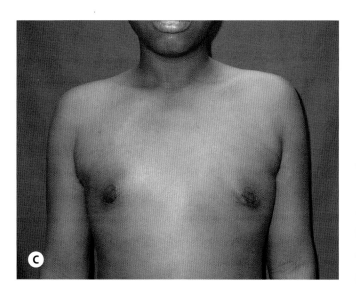

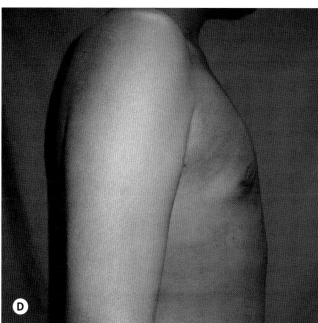

Case 4 A 50-year-old man who underwent previous gynecomastia repair via an inframammary incision. He continued to have skin and volume excess and just wanted to be flat. He underwent a direct excision of skin to incorporate the inframammary scar (512 g on right, 446 g on left) and free nipple grafting. This is his 9-month follow-up. (Fig. 14.5). Nipple hypopigmentation has nearly resolved and usually does so by 1 year postoperatively.

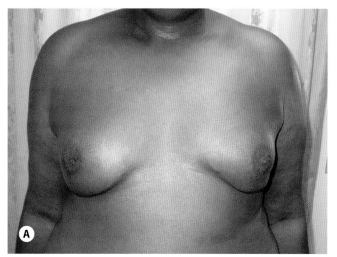

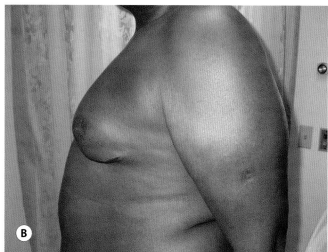

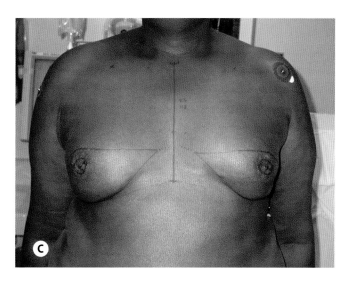

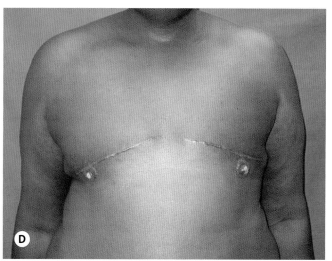

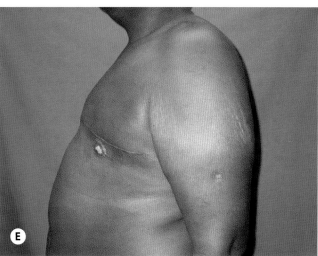

CONCLUSIONS

Gynecomastia repair incorporates basic plastic surgery principles to achieve successful results. Unlike female breast reduction, the goal of gynecomastia repair is a flat chest which is in proportion to the patient's overall body habitus. A gynecomastia patient must be willing to accept the possibility of noticeable skin irregularity in the simplest cases, to noticeable scars, nipple insensitivity, and asymmetry in more complex cases. Despite this, with proper patient selection and preoperative counseling, a successful result can be achieved.

REFERENCES

1. Braunstein GD. Gynecomastia. N Engl J Med 1993; 328: 490–495.
2. Bostwick J. Gynecomastia. In: Bostwick J III (ed) Plastic and reconstructive breast surgery. St Louis: Quality Medical Publishing, 2000.
3. Daniels IR, Layer GT. Gynaecomastia. Eur J Surg 2001; 167: 885–892.
4. Rohrich RJ, Ha RY, Kenkel JM, Adams WP. Classification and management of gynecomastia: defining the role of ultrasound-assisted liposuction. Plast Reconstruct Surg 2003; 111: 909–923.
5. Rosenberg GJ. Gynecomastia. In: Spear SL (ed) Surgery of the breast: principles and art. Philadelphia: Lippincott Williams & Wilkins, 2006.
6. Rosenberg GJ. Gynecomastia: suction lipectomy as a contemporary solution. Plast Reconstruct Surg 1987; 80: 379–386.
7. Hodgson ELB, Fruhstorfer BH, Malata CM. Ultrasonic liposuction in the treatment of gynecomastia. Plast Reconstruct Surg 116: 646–653.
8. Mladick RA. Gynecomastia. Clin Plast Surg 1991; 18: 815–822.
9. Smoot EC. Eccentric skin resection and purse-string closure for skin reduction with mastectomy for gynecomastia. Ann Plast Surg 1998; 41: 378–383.
10. Persichette P, Berloco M. Gynecomastia and the complete circumareolar approach in the surgical management of skin redundancy. Plast Reconstruct Surg 2001; 107: 948–954.
11. Colic MM, Colic MM. Circumareolar mastectomy in the female-to-male transsexuals and large gynecomastias: a personal approach. Aesthet Plast Surg 2000; 24: 450–454.
12. Webster JP. Mastectomy for gynecomastia through a semi-circular intra-areolar incision. Ann Surg 1946; 124: 557.
13. Barsky AJ, Kahn S, Simon BE. Principles and practice of surgery. New York: McGraw Hill, 1964.
14. Pitanguy I. Transareolar incision for gynecomastia. Plast Reconstruct Surg 1966; 38: 414–419.
15. Letterman G, Schurter M. The surgical correction of gynecomastia. Am Surg 1969; 35: 322–325.
16. Letterman G, Schurter M. Surgical correction of massive gynecomastia. Plast Reconstruct Surg 1972; 49: 259–262.
17. Pers M, Bretteville-Jensen G. Reduction mammaplasty based on the vertical vascular bipedicle and 'tennis ball' assembly. Scand J Plast Reconstruct Surg 1972; 6: 61.
18. Peters HM, Vastine V, Knox L, Morgan RF. Treatment of adolescent gynecomastia using a bipedicle technique. Ann Plast Surg 1998; 40: 241.
19. Wray RC, Hoopes JE, Davis GM. Correction of exreme gynaecomastia. Br J Plast Surg 1974; 27: 39–41.
20. Huang TT, Hidalgo JE, Lewis SR. A circumareolar approach in surgical management of gynecomastia. Plast Reconstruct Surg 1982; 69: 35–40.
21. Murphy TP, Ehrlichman RJ, Seckel BR. Nipple placement in simple mastectomy with free nipple grafting for severe gynecomastia. Plast Reconstruct Surg 1994; 94: 818–823.
22. Beckstein MS, Windle BH, Stroup RT. Anatomical parameters for nipple position and areolar diameter in males. Ann Plast Surg 1996; 36: 33–36.
23. Shulman O, Badani E, Wolf Y, Hauben DJ. Appropriate location of the nipple–areola complex in males. Plast Reconstruct Surg 2001; 108: 348–351.
24. Beer GM, Budi S, Seifert B, et al. Configuration and localization of the nipple–areolar complex in men. Plast Reconstruct Surg 2001; 108: 1947–1952.

Nipple–Areola Reconstruction

15

Kenneth C. Shestak

The nipple is an essential aesthetic feature of the breast and is the visual center around which the rest of the gland emanates. The nipple is surrounded by areolar tissue, which is a darkly pigmented epithelium that has a small number of ducts opening into it. The areolar skin is visually darker than the surrounding breast skin but slightly lighter in pigmentation than the nipple[1] (Fig. 15.1).

The nipple is most aesthetically positioned at the point of maximal projection on the breast mound.[1,2] It can be located by the transposition of the inframammary fold (done routinely when planning a breast reduction) or by measurements from fixed points of reference on the anterior chest (done in most nipple reconstructions following a previous breast reconstruction). The distance from the nipple to the suprasternal notch and the inframammary fold varies from patient to patient (Fig. 15.2B). In the absence of previous surgery or an obvious developmental asymmetry, the nipple positions are most often roughly symmetric.

GUIDELINES FOR NIPPLE RECONSTRUCTION

When performing nipple–areola reconstruction the optimal visual appearance of the reconstructed nipple is achieved by simulating the best possible position, projection, and pigmentation relative to the nipple features on the opposite breast. The author has come to recognize that perhaps the most important feature is the color patch symmetry of the areola with the opposite areola. Visual symmetry between the color and location of the nipple–areola complex on the opposite breast and its position on the reconstructed breast mound is paramount for the optimal visual appearance of the reconstructed nipple. In the past this was accomplished by the transplantation of a darkly pigmented full-thickness skin graft (vulva or proximal medial thigh skin). Currently,

however, it is best done with an intradermal tattoo, which can produce the most predictable symmetry with the opposite areola over a wide variety of colors.[1,2] This characteristic of the color of the areola around the reconstructed nipple is more important than either position or projection. Indeed, good color patch symmetry can often compensate for partial or even significant loss of nipple projection or slight abnormalities in position. This is illustrated in the patient in Figure 15.3 (A–D), who sustained a significant loss of nipple projection marring what was otherwise a good left breast reconstruction with a transverse rectus abdominis musculocutaneous (TRAM) flap. This situation was 'rescued' by a well-done intradermal tattoo[2] which produced an excellent aesthetic outcome.

In terms of timing, the author believes that nipple–areola reconstruction is best done at a second stage rather than at the primary breast reconstruction. This allows the breast mound to evolve in terms of shape and gravitational settling. In my practice, nipple reconstruction is most often combined with a procedure to revise the reconstructed breast and reshape the opposite breast. At this time adjustments in nipple position on both breasts contribute to symmetry and overall aesthetic appearance. Nipple reconstructions performed at the time of breast reconstruction carry a high probability of subsequent asymmetry unless they are done following an ultimate skin-sparing mastectomy where the nipple and areola alone are removed. In this case, replacement of the skin with a simultaneous nipple reconstruction on this skin paddle (as described by Hammond) may yield a good result. Similarly, performing a simultaneous nipple reconstruction at the time of exchanging the expander for an implant carries with it a small but definite increased risk of losing the implant owing to problems with wound healing and subsequent exposure and/or infection at the site of nipple reconstruction.[3,4] For this reason I have not adopted this procedure in my practice.

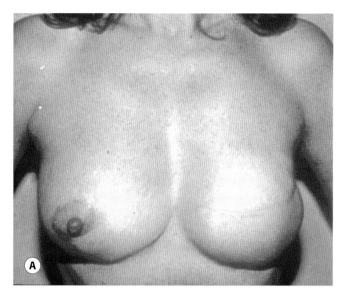
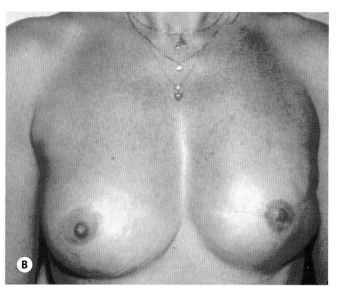

FIGURE 15.1 **A** Preoperative AP view of a patient who has undergone a left breast reconstruction with an implant. **B** Postoperative appearance of same breast reconstruction following nipple reconstruction and areolar tattoo. Note vivid dimension of realism.

NIPPLE RECONSTRUCTION OPTIONS

Historically, the options for nipple–areola reconstruction have included tattoo alone, the use of composite grafts such as toe pulp,[5] earlobe,[6] labia minora,[7] or most commonly a composite graft of a portion of the contralateral nipple[8] from the opposite breast (in patients with extremely large nipples). Over the past 20 years, 'pullout' skin flaps raised at the desired nipple position have represented the 'state of the art' in nipple reconstruction.[9–14] The most commonly used flaps are listed below. Formerly the areolar region was reconstructed using a full-thickness graft of darkly pigmented skin.[15] Most recently, however, the areola is replicated by an intradermal tattoo,[16,17] which is the best way to create symmetry of areolar color.

The most recent addition to this lineup of 'pullout flap' procedures is the double opposing periareolar flap reconstruction, introduced by us.[13] A similar procedure has been popularized by Hammond.[14]

An intradermal tattoo alone for nipple reconstruction may be sufficient in the elderly, high-risk patient who desires a semblance of visual symmetry[17] but in whom it may not be wise to have a formal reconstruction because of local tissue conditions (scarring of skin, atrophy of dermis, and subcutaneous adipose tissue), advanced age, or senescence.

I believe that there is still a place, albeit in the very rare situation, for 'nipple sharing.'[8] This technique is applicable in special circumstances of primary reconstruction where there are extremely thin and attenuated tissues or scars in the desired position of nipple reconstruction, in the patient who has a large opposite nipple which might serve as donor tissue for reconstruction (Fig. 15.4A–D).

Nipple sharing involves removal of either the distal or the most anterior aspect of the nipple (Fig. 15.4A), or the excision of a pie-shaped portion of the nipple including the most anterior aspect and the core shaft of the nipple,

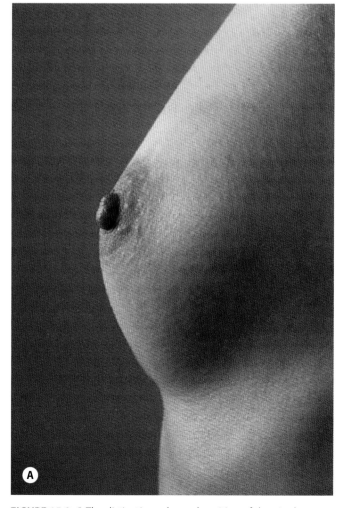

FIGURE 15.2 **A** The distinctive color and position of the nipple–areolar complex, which ideally is located at the highest point of the breast mound.

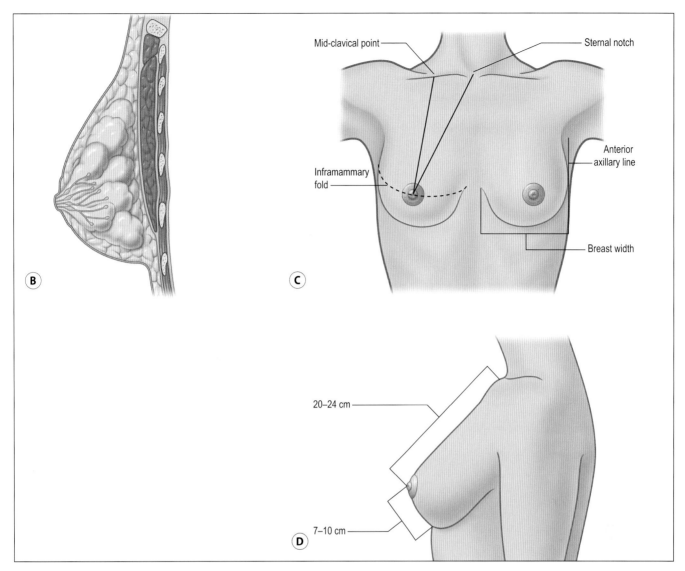

FIGURE 15.2, cont'd **B** Schematic illustrating ducts draining the lobules and emanating through the nipple. **C, D** Typical position of nipple relative to topographical landmarks on the chest wall.

harvested both on its anterior and under surfaces (Fig. 15.4B). This obviously reduces the size of the new nipple, which in some cases may be a benefit. It does also result in a scar on the donor nipple, and obviously a reduction in size. However, when such composite grafts are placed in the appropriate location and surrounded by an intradermal tattoo they can produce a good simulation of the patient's opposite nipple (Fig. 15.4D).

Currently the most popular technique for nipple reconstruction involves the use of a 'pullout flap'[9–14] of skin and subcutaneous adipose tissue at the ideal site on the reconstructed breast mound, with the application of intradermal tattoo for the areolar reconstruction. Many designs are possible, and these are outlined in Figure 15.5. There are varying degrees of success with pullout flap reconstructions, based on their design. That is to say, the design of the specific nipple flap may indeed play a role in the ultimate projection. I believe that some flap designs are inherently better than others. For example, I have found that the quadrapod design[18] (Fig. 15.6), which employs a direct elevation of the tissue with closure of flaps at the base of the nipple, is unreliable in terms of producing and maintaining long-term nipple projection. This technique often produces a nipple which looks excellent on the operating table but loses most of its projection with time (by 1 year postoperatively). When studying this design and analyzing the technique of elevation, the loss of nipple projection would seem to be almost intuitive. This is because the forces of wound contraction act to pull this tissue directly back down to the plane of the breast surface, thereby predisposing it to loss of projection.

In contrast, the flap techniques that elevate skin and adipose tissue off the reconstructed breast, detaching it at all areas but the base of the flap and then reconfiguring it into the desired nipple shape, are more successful in terms of maintaining their projection.[9–14,19–26] The elements in the

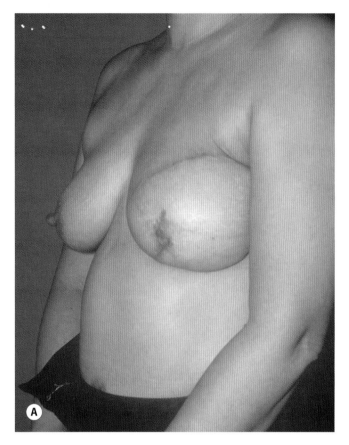

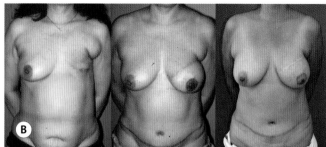

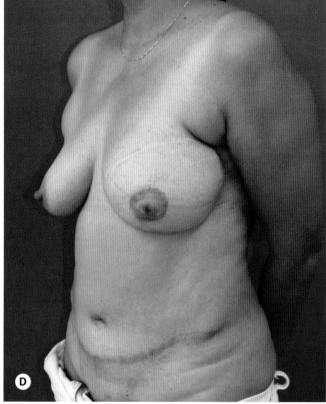

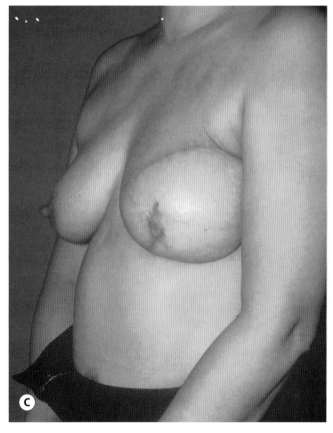

FIGURE 15.3 A Suboptimal nipple reconstruction with significant loss of projection resulting in major asymmetry. **B** The areolar tattoo transforms this suboptimally projecting nipple into an aesthetically pleasing appearance. **C, D** The oblique views of the same patient before and after the tattoo. This is a 7-year postoperative view.

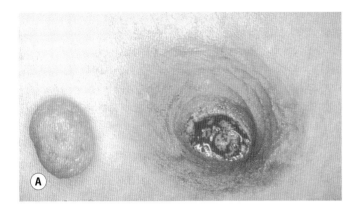

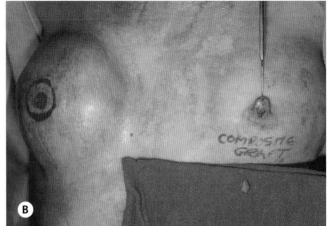

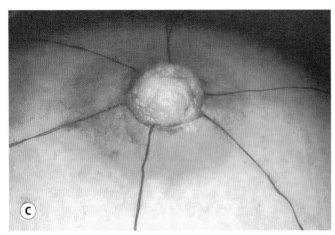

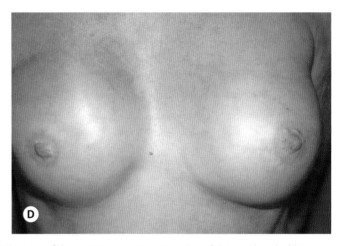

FIGURE 15.4 A 'Nipple-sharing' technique of nipple reconstruction, with harvest of the anteriormost aspect wedge of the nipple, which is ready for transfer as a composite graft. **B** Alternatively, a wedge of the inferior aspect of the opposite nipple can be harvested for transfer as a composite graft. **C** Composite graft of nipple placed on recipient bed. **D** Healed appearance of composite nipple graft.

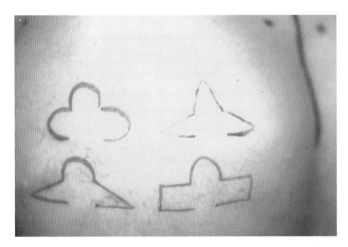

FIGURE 15.5 Pullout flaps. These are the most commonly used skin designs of skin and subcutaneous adipose flaps for nipple reconstruction.

flap responsible for nipple projection are adipose tissue and the thickness of the dermis. These more reliable designs are those in which the flap tissue used for reconstruction of the new nipple is elevated or 'pulled out' to at least a 90° angle from the surface of the breast mound. Such proce-

dures are variations of the skate design originally proposed by Hartrampf,[11] subsequently modified and refined by Little and Spear[12,20] (Fig. 15.7).

It has been my observation that the modified star design[21] can reliably produce small to moderately projecting nipples (less than or equal to 5 mm) (Fig. 15.8). For the reconstruction of larger nipples, my choice is the skate design[12,20] (Fig. 15.7). The fishtail flap developed by McCraw[22] (Fig. 15.9) also has the ability to produce a nipple with very marked projection. Such designs may allow the maintenance of greater long-term projection. Of particular advantage is a modification of the fishtail flap design which is used when there is a transversely oriented scar slightly above or below the desired nipple position[13] (Fig. 15.10). This design makes it possible to reconstruct the nipple without creating any new scars on the reconstructed breast. It may be based either superiorly or inferiorly, depending on the desired nipple position.

Most recently we further modified the skate flap by a design that closes the donor area primarily by virtue of employing a second flap directly juxtaposed to the nipple reconstruction and its 'parent' flap. We have called this modification the double opposing periareolar or DOPA flap

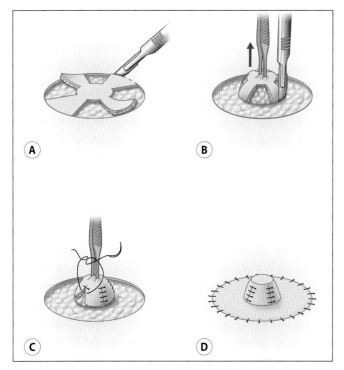

FIGURE 15.6 A–D The quadrapod flap. This is a type of pullout flap that does not involve separation and reconfiguring of the nipple. Inherently it allows the forces of wound contraction to pull the nipple back down to the base.

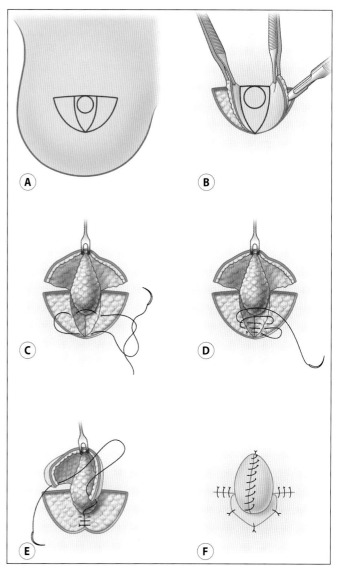

FIGURE 15.7 A–F The skate flap is the classic 'pullout' flap. It entails elevating a composite of skin and fat out of the breast to a 90° angle and configuring the nipple, with closure of the donor site in a way so as to support nipple projection.

(Fig. 15.11A–D).[13] A very similar procedure was simultaneously introduced by Hammond.[14]

To learn more about the natural history of nipple reconstruction, we have recently completed a prospective analysis of projection loss studied every 3 months for 1 year following nipple reconstruction. Our data indicate a loss of projection of 40% with all types of flap, and the majority of this loss occurs within the first 6 months.[10]

PRIMARY NIPPLE RECONSTRUCTION: PLANNING AND PATIENT MARKING

In planning nipple reconstruction the surgeon must study the opposite breast carefully. It is important to note the position of the nipple relative to the breast mound on the contralateral breast. This must be visually assessed and then careful measurements from a fixed point, most often the suprasternal notch, are taken. The next reference point is the distance from the midline on the horizontal plane to the position from the suprasternal notch, and this is also an important parameter. These measurements are then cross-referenced with the patient's opinion as to where the nipple should be created (Fig. 15.2B).

In this regard I will ask the patient to use a removable EKG lead as a simulated nipple–areola complex and place it on her reconstructed breast. I will ask her to do this while standing in front of a full-length mirror as I leave the room.

This affords the best visual scenario for her to check the position. I then return to the room and will either agree with the position or make appropriate suggestions for modification. At this time the aesthetic judgment of the surgeon comes very much into play. This relates to changing the position relative to the shape and projection of the opposite breast and considerations imposed by any scars that may fall directly near or in the selected position for nipple placement. Once the position of the nipple is established, measurements from the suprasternal notch and the midline are recorded, and reviewed the evening before surgery.

The projection of the opposite nipple, its base width, and the shape and position of the areola all need to be carefully assessed and considered in the preoperative plan

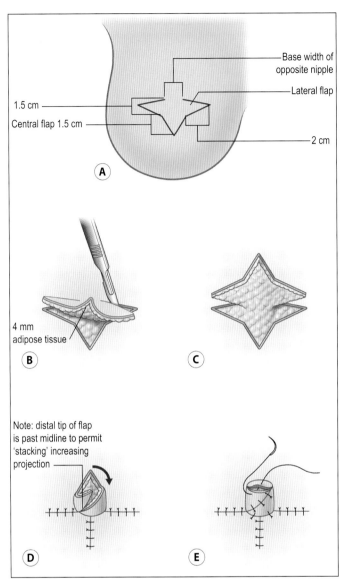

FIGURE 15.8 A–E The modified star flap. This is very useful in primary and secondary reconstruction of the nipple. It is a derivative of the skate flap.

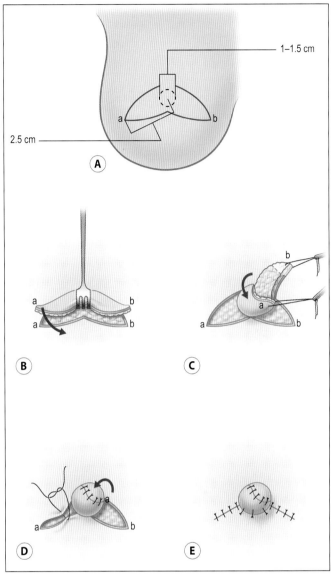

FIGURE 15.9 A–E The design and elevation of the fishtail flap.

for nipple reconstruction, in conjunction with its planned position relative to existing scars on the reconstructed breast (Fig. 15.12A–C). Occasionally the patient will request that the nipple be positioned well away from the most projecting point of the breast mound so as to simulate the position on the opposite breast. Such requests generally result from significant breast ptosis, as in the patient in Figure 15.12D, who had significant ptosis of her contralateral breast and specifically requested that no modification of that breast be done, and that the nipple be reconstructed in a position to match that on her native breast mound.

The base width and the projection of the normal nipple on the contralateral breast determine the base dimension and width of the lateral wings of the flap used for the new

nipple. These are important guides no matter which technique is selected. These features are taken into account during the preoperative planning and are highlighted in Figures 15.7, 15.8 and 15.11: the skate flap, the modified star, and the DOPA flap.

The essential steps in reconstruction of the nipple are:
- Establish the best possible position for the nipple to be reconstructed.
- Verify the patient's acceptance of the nipple position.
- Plan to match the base width of the opposite nipple.
- Select the best technique to match the projection of the opposite nipple.
- Maintain all of the scars for the nipple reconstruction within the area of the intended areola (the area that will be tattooed).

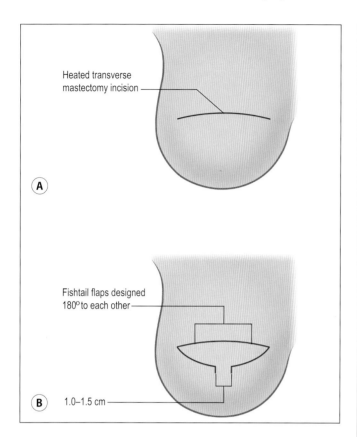

FIGURE 15.10 A, B Alternative and very useful design of the fishtail flap which can be used when there is a transverse scar on the breast.

- Review the procedure with the patient using photographs to illustrate average outcomes, emphasizing that a medical tattoo is the finishing touch that will confer the maximum possible realism to the reconstructed nipple.

SURGICAL TECHNIQUE

This procedure is routinely performed under local anesthesia in the outpatient setting unless the patient is having additional procedures necessitating general anesthesia. I will generally use local anesthesia containing epinephrine for all areas of the procedure, except for the very base of the nipple flap, where I will use xylocaine without epinephrine. The nipple reconstruction need not be performed in the hospital operating environment as it can be safely done in an office operating room or even in a treatment room. However, in cases where an implant breast reconstruction has been performed I believe that maximizing an environment of sterility by performing the procedure in an operating room environment is essential. Therefore, in my opinion, a nipple reconstruction procedure following an implant-based breast reconstruction requires the use of an operating room where sterility can be maximally preserved.

In performing nipple reconstruction the surgeon must realize that, no matter which technique is used, these are

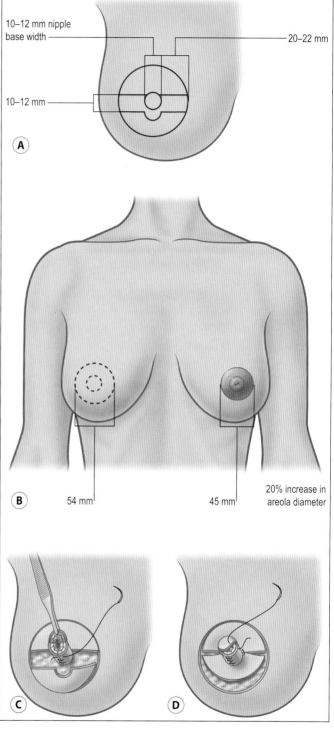

FIGURE 15.11 A Plan for positioning of the nipple on the reconstructed breast. Ideally the nipple is placed at the highest point of the breast mound. It can be positioned according to dimensions derived from fixed points on the torso, including the suprasternal notch, and distance from the midline. The base (here lateral) of the new nipple should not be encroached upon by existing scars on the breast. **B** Outline for modified star flap reconstruction with 15 mm base width. **C** Nipple placed in dependent position on left breast reconstruction to match right nipple, which was in a dependent position.

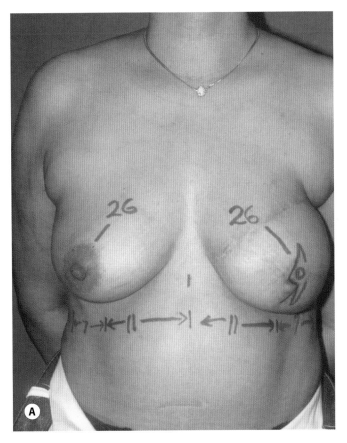

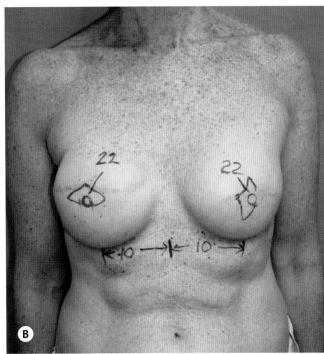

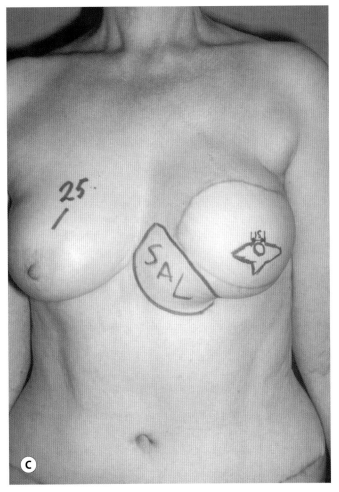

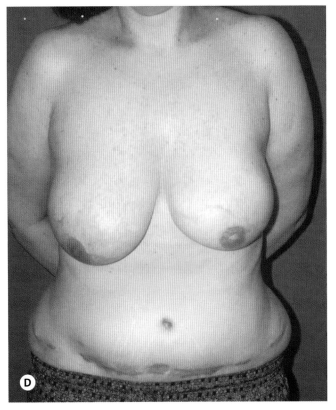

FIGURE 15.12 A–D Planning for a combination of lipocontouring of the breast and modified star flap reconstruction.

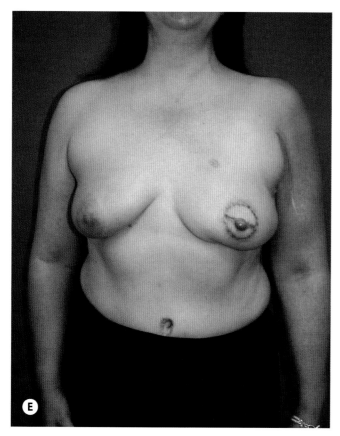

FIGURE 15.12, cont'd

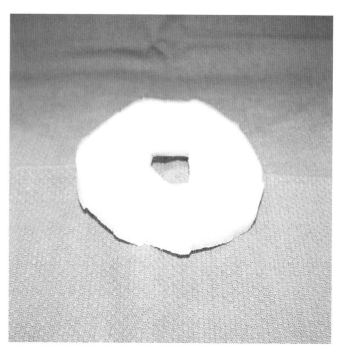

FIGURE 15.13 Sterile foam rubber 'doughnut' to be placed around the reconstructed nipple at the time of surgery to protect it from compression over the first 3 weeks of healing.

delicate flaps. They must be handled with extreme care using skin hooks or fine forceps employed primarily with sharp dissection with the scalpel or sharp scissors for flap elevation. In configuring and suturing the flaps, the surgeon must be careful not to twist or bend the flaps excessively. Flap loss due to ischemia may result from 'overtightening' the skin, excessive bending of the flap(s), or usng too many sutures. Any element of flap compromise must be recognized at the time of the nipple reconstruction and necessary sutures removed or flap transpositions altered so as to immediately reverse any flap ischemia during folding and configuring the nipple. Generally only one or two sutures need to be removed to avoid such a problem.

Achieving primary wound healing is a key concept. As already mentioned, the surgeon must avoid ischemia of these delicate flaps, which most often will lead to flap separation and open wounds. This condition results in increased wound contraction, often dramatically reducing nipple projection or altering the shape, inclination, and even the position of the reconstructed nipple.

Following nipple–areola reconstruction, I feel it is necessary to protect the nipple from external compressive forces. To do this I use a 'foam rubber doughnut' placed around the nipple, which I ask patients to wear inside their bra for approximately 1 month. I believe that such a device may help prevent the loss of projection due to early mechanical compression (Fig. 15.13).

If a skin graft is used for the areolar reconstruction a 'bolster-type' dressing is placed to ensure maximal contact of the graft with the underlying graft bed. This is left in place for a minimum of 5 days. When skin grafts are needed, full-thickness grafts are my preference. I do not feel it necessary or advisable to harvest pigmented skin from the area of the proximal inner thigh or labial region, as these donor sites can be uncomfortable and/or painful. Almost all full-thickness skin grafts undergo hypopigmentation with the passage of time. It has been my experience that an intra-dermal tattoo is the best way to optimize the color match between the normal areola and areolar tissue around the new nipple.

A skate flap requires a small or large skin graft to close the donor area. The traditional skate involved a doughnut or 'washer-shaped' skin graft, whereas more recent designs have employed smaller rectangular skin grafts at the base of the nipple. It is important to oppose the edges of the dermis to close the donor area of the fat component on the deep surface of the skate flap (Fig. 15.7D,E).

The use of the star flap (Fig. 15.8A–E) includes primary closure of the donor area and does not require a skin graft. The donor area in this technique is closed directly by edge-to-edge skin approximation (Fig. 15.8D) in two layers. It is important to realize that for this technique the sutures which have been used to configure the nipple must be left in for at least 2 weeks (Fig. 15.8E). A subsequent areolar tattoo can camouflage the scars from the donor closure areas which extend radially away from the nipple base (Fig. 15.8D,E). Direct closure of the donor area slightly flattens the contour of the reconstructed breast.

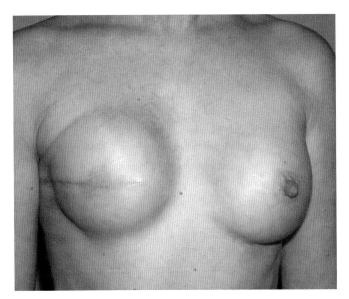

FIGURE 15.14 Patient with significant scar and atrophy of subcutaneous tissue following a right breast reconstruction with tissue expander and implant.

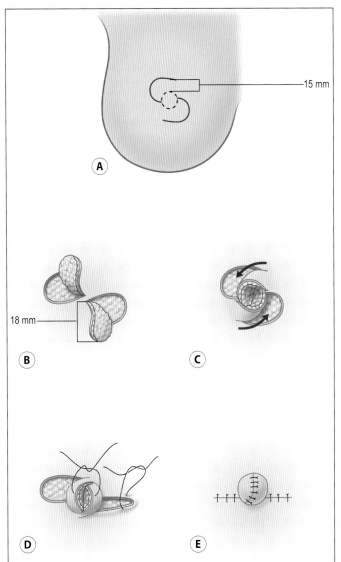

FIGURE 15.15 The double opposing tab flap. This is a nipple reconstruction based on flaps which are elevated and wrapped around each other. It is useful when the scar from the mastectomy runs directly through the site of intended nipple reconstruction. It is important to make the base of these flaps sufficiently wide (18 mm) to ensure vascularity to the reconstructed nipple.

When assessing a patient for nipple reconstruction the surgeon must be especially wary of tissues that are excessively thin, and this situation is common following the use of tissue expansion for breast reconstruction (Fig. 15.14). Because tissue expansion definitely results in thinning of subcutaneous fat layer and dermis, at the time of exchange of the expander for the chosen implant I will always make special note of the thickness of the muscle layer, subcutaneous adipose tissue, and dermis, specifically noting any significant atrophy in the subcutaneous adipose layer. As previously mentioned, I believe that it is helpful to perform the nipple reconstruction at a third stage in individuals who are undergoing implant reconstruction following the placement of a tissue expander.

The presence of scars (Fig. 15.14) on the breast is often a significant factor in selecting the type of nipple reconstruction. Their position, width, and the quality of the surrounding skin and deep tissue must be carefully assessed and a plan developed to minimize any negative impact they might have on the nipple reconstruction.

Scars from previous biopsies or the mastectomy can be very problematic. They do influence the choice of technique, and especially if the scar runs right through the area of the planned base of a new nipple reconstruction. In this situation it is often advisable to use a technique that 'straddles'[22–27] the scar (Fig. 15.15). The technique that best accomplishes this is the double opposing tab flap described by Knoll.[23,27] Scars can be particularly important when they lie right where the nipple is to be centered. Previous radiation therapy causes fibrosis of the skin and dermis, and confers to the skin flaps a stiff quality which makes folding and configuring difficult. There is also decreased circulation in such flaps. A history of smoking further complicates these conditions and poses special problems. Therefore I urge all patients who smoke to quit completely for at least 4 weeks prior to surgery.[28]

In summary, I believe that it is essential to alter the design of the nipple reconstruction procedure so that the blood supply to the flaps is minimally affected by existing scar tissue. Radiation therapy poses its own set of difficulties, especially if multiple skin scars are also present. Patients who smoke also appear to have more in the way of circulatory problems in the breast skin. As mentioned above, this must be pointed out to the patient preoperatively and a plea made for temporary cessation of smoking.[28]

Finally, primary nipple reconstruction must be carefully planned and executed in a precise manner, as secondary reconstructions are more difficult. For this reason, a few comments about the planning and technique of primary nipple reconstruction are in order.

NIPPLE RECONSTRUCTION TECHNIQUES

My choice of nipple reconstruction technique depends on the projection of the nipple I am attempting to match on the contralateral breast. For nipples with 5 mm or less of projection I favor the modified star flap (Fig. 15.8A–E). For nipples with greater projection I will sometimes use a skate flap (Fig. 15.7A–F). Another indication for the skate flap is the situation where no flattening of the anterior contour of the breast is desired. Here, a skate flap and a skin graft may be preferable. Finally, I will consider the use of a double opposing tab flap (Fig. 15.15A–E) when the mastectomy scar runs directly through the site where the base of the nipple would be ideally located. The following section outlines how I perform each of these techniques.

The modified star flap

The design of the flap in a particular case is dependent on the base width and projection of the opposite nipple: the base width of the new nipple is created to match that of the opposite nipple. The width of the lateral limbs determines the ultimate nipple projection. When planning this dimension it is important to realize that there will be an approximately 30–40% loss of projection with time. Therefore, I usually make the lateral limbs a minimum of 1.5 cm wide and 2 cm long (Fig. 15.8A). The total height of the nipple is planned for at least 1 cm. By making the distance from the base of the lateral flap to the tip 2 cm, the flap will fold around the central core of the nipple, allowing skin closure without tension. These flaps are elevated with 2–4 mm of adipose tissue (Fig. 15.8B) on their deep surface (deep to the dermis), which allows folding of the flaps without tension.

After the injection of 1% xylocaine without epinephrine, the lateral flaps or 'wings' are elevated first, followed by the central flap. The dissection proceeds toward the central portion of the design. As the central core of the nipple is approached it is important to access a deeper plane in the adipose layer. In a primary nipple reconstruction the dissection proceeds unencumbered. In secondary cases the surgeon will be elevating scarred elements of the previous unsuccessful nipple, and so it is important to preserve the maximal amount of blood supply to the adipose tissue and skin arising deep within the flap. For this reason I elevate the most proximal portion of the flap at its base, delicately with blunt dissection, using either a tenotomy scissors or, in some cases, the handle of the scalpel. This tends to optimally preserve the blood supply to the central core of adipose tissue and skin of the new nipple. The donor area is closed primarily and in layers, with the deep dermis closed first (with coated polyglycolic acid suture Maxxon or PDS 3/0) followed by a skin closure with interrupted 5/0 nylon. The nipple elements are then assembled, starting with the lateral flaps. These flaps are advanced past the midline to achieve a 'stacking' in the portion of the nipple

opposite the base so as to maximally increase the projection (Fig. 15.8D).

The 5/0 nylon sutures used for configuration of the nipple are left in place for 3 weeks to ensure good healing and to prevent the folded flaps 'unfurling'. Removing these sutures before the end of the 3-week period has resulted in wound separation in several cases. Finally, the newly reconstructed nipple is protected from direct compression by a foam rubber 'doughnut' (Fig. 15.13), which can be inserted into a bra during the first month of healing.

The skate flap

The skate flap (Fig. 15.7A–F) can produce a large nipple with significant projection and is my choice when the contralateral nipple has a projection of 7 mm or more. The nipple is located according to patient wishes and aesthetic concerns. It is optimally positioned at the highest point of the breast mound.

I will often give the patient an EKG lead which she can place on her reconstructed breast, so as to choose her preferred position for the new nipple. The design of the skate flap is variable, and the dimensions are dependent on the projection of the opposite nipple. The base width is planned to match that of the opposite nipple, with an approximately equal distance of skin on either side to comprise the 'lateral wing.' The distance from the base of the nipple to the portion of the areola furthest from it is approximately twice the projection of the opposite nipple (Fig. 15.7A). This 2 : 1 dimension of the central axis of the nipple allows for loss of projection due to the normal processes of contraction and wound healing. The patient should be informed preoperatively of the discrepancy in nipple height that will be present immediately after surgery, the reconstructed nipple being much larger. This central axis is also the region from which the core of fat comprising the main substance of the nipple will be elevated. The central core of the flap is adjoined on either side by extensions of skin which, elevated together, leave a circular outline (Fig. 15.7D,E). The position of the nipple and design of the flap are checked just prior to taking the patient to surgery.

The skin markings of the flap are injected with local anesthetic without epinephrine (1% xylocaine). The outline of the design is incised peripherally on all sides. Next the lateral flaps are elevated from peripheral to central at the deepest dermal level. Yellow adipose tissue should not be visible at this point. As the point of transition between the lateral elements and the central core of the flap is reached, the dissection is deepened by incising completely through the dermis into the adipose tissue, thereby raising a core or 'finger-like projection' of adipose tissue in continuity with the skin in the central portion of the flap. This core is gently raised with a scalpel, leaving behind a deep V-shaped trough defect in the subcutaneous adipose tissue. The width of this core progressively increases as the dissection moves toward the base of the flap. As the base of the flap is reached it is important to preserve as much blood flow to the fat as possible. This blood flow is derived from vertically oriented blood vessels running in the fat, and to spare them I will gently spread or stretch this tissue with either the dissecting scissors or the handle of the scalpel. The dermis on either side is incised to the nipple base to permit a full 90° elevation of the flap. When the elevated flap is held perpendicular to the plane of the breast it resembles a sunfish or skate – hence its name, the skate flap.

The V-shaped donor area in the center (Fig. 15.7D) is then closed with 4/0 chromic sutures which bring dermis edge to dermis edge, taking care to bury the knots. This closed wound will create a platform on which to assemble the new nipple. The nipple is reconstructed by configuring the lateral wings around the central core, by starting at its base and working towards the apex. The most lateral tip of each lateral wing is sewn to its counterpart with interrupted 5/0 chromic sutures. The flaps are closed without excessive tension.

The donor area of the skate flap is most often closed with a full-thickness skin graft, harvested from any area of skin excess. It need not be taken from an area of skin with increased pigmentation, such as the inner thigh or labia. The graft is thoroughly defatted and sutured to the periphery of the defect. It is preferable to raise a skin graft rather than to close the wounds under excess tension. Closure under tension will almost invariably produce a spread scar, which will be unsightly and which does not take tattoo pigment well.

A tie-over bolster dressing is used to maximize contact between graft and recipient bed, and is usually left in place for a minimum of 5 days. The reconstructed nipple is again protected from compression by clothing with a foam rubber doughnut, which is worn for 1 month.

The optimal time for areolar reconstruction with an intradermal tattoo is approximately 3–4 months after healing of the skin graft. The skate flap method permits the reconstruction of a nipple of virtually any size, and it is my technique of choice when the projection of the contralateral nipple exceeds 6 mm.

The double opposing periareolar flap

My current flap of choice for nipple reconstruction in most circumstances is a derivative of the skate flap. This is a pullout flap which involves the construction of two flaps within a circular construct of a new areola. The site of the nipple is located as with the other techniques just described. The nipple itself is derived from the larger of two flaps. The base width of the flap is determined by the base dimension of the nipple on the opposite breast. The width of the lateral wings determines the eventual projection of the nipple, and this dimension is determined by assessing the projection of the opposite nipple. It typically varies in width between 10 and 12 mm (Fig. 15.11A). The nipple is elevated by raising the 'lateral wings' and the central aspect of the nipple flap. The lateral wings are raised with 1 mm or 2 mm of adipose thickness until the central aspect of the nipple is reached. Here it is necessary to include a plug of additional adipose tissue that will vary from 4 to 8 mm in thickness. This adipose tissue is raised in contiguity with the flap, as in the development of both the skate and modified star flaps. The

dissection of the wings is complete when the nipple stands upright without sutures. Care is taken to maintain as much blood supply as possible to the nipple flap. A small additional 'cap' of skin is included with the elevation of the lateral wings (Fig. 15.11C), creating a central donor area. The nipple is then reconstructed using 5/0 nylon sutures. The 'cap' closes over the most projecting aspect of the nipple.

The central donor area thus created is closed by mobilizing both the parent flap for the nipple and the 'opposing flap' designed opposite to it. These flaps are mobilized by releasing the dermis peripherally. This is done by placing the flaps on tension with a double skin hook and incising through the dermis only with a sharp scalpel. There will be a definite 'give' when the dermis is divided. The dissection stops at that point so as to preserve the subdermal plexus of blood vessels. This maneuver creates considerable ability of the flaps to 'slide' toward each other on their subcutaneous pedicles. There is no undermining of either the parent flap or the opposing flap. This maneuver allows easy approximation of the flap edges, permitting closure of the central donor area. The nipple flap itself is sutured to the edge of the smaller flap or to a small de-epithelialized surface on this smaller flap. This flap surface provides a solid foundation for the nipple flap and this may minimize subsequent loss of nipple projection

A peripheral donor area is produced by this maneuver. The peripheral donor area is then closed with a 'purse-string' suture of 2/0 or 3/0 Maxon to create the appearance of an areola. The skin is closed with interrupted sutures of 5/0 nylon. A protective dressing using Adaptic non-adherent layer, gauze, and a sterile foam doughnut is then applied, and the patient placed in a surgical bra. The sutures are removed no sooner than 2 weeks after surgery.

The double opposing periareolar flap has become our technique of choice for nipple reconstruction in primary cases. It avoids the use of skin grafts and seems to have the advantage of maximizing nipple projection in the long term. The appearance of the peripheral and central scars following surgery simulates the appearance of the visual lines of a nipple (Fig. 15.12E), even prior to intradermal tattooing. This technique is similar to that described by Hammond.[14] It is different in that, apart from the nipple flap itself, there is no undermining of the parent or opposing flaps.

Caution is needed when using this technique in patients who have undergone previous irradiation of the breast skin flaps, and in those who have very thin flaps following previous tissue expansion and implant placement. In the former situation there may be concern about the blood supply of the flaps, and it may be advisable to design the parent flap of the nipple and the corresponding 'opposing' flap as large as possible so as to maximize the area of the subcutaneous pedicles. In the latter case care must be taken when the flaps are very thin following previous surgery and tissue expansion. Preservation of the subcutaneous plexus is essential, as is allowing sufficient time to elapse from the implant placement procedure so that the mobility and the elasticity of the tissues at the site of nipple reconstruction will have returned as close to normal as possible. This

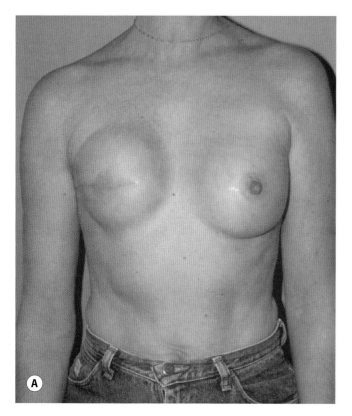

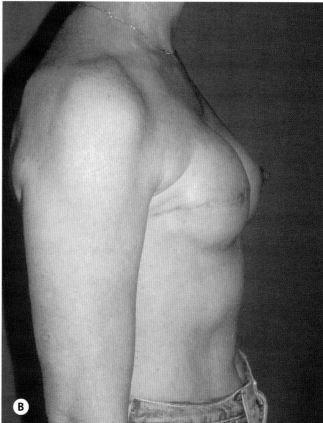

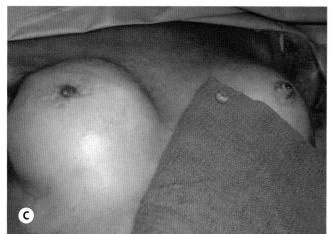

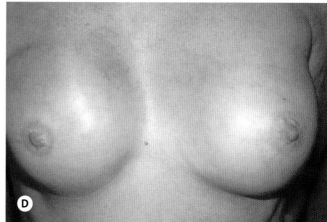

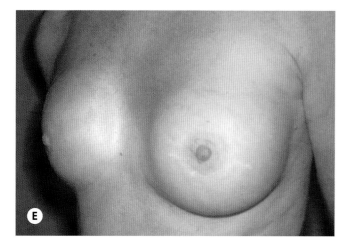

FIGURE 15.16 A Partial loss of previous left nipple reconstruction following tissue expander and implant noted on AP view. **B** Lateral view of same patient. Note lack of projection in the reconstructed nipple. **C** Composite nipple graft harvested from opposite nipple. **D** Postoperative result of redo nipple reconstruction 9 months after surgery on AP view. **E** Lateral view of composite nipple reconstruction 9 months following surgery.

usually means that the interval between implant placement and nipple reconstruction is 4–6 months.

The double opposing tab flap

As previously mentioned, a potential problem situation for nipple reconstruction results when the scar from the mastectomy runs directly through the intended site of reconstruction. This scar can cause problems with the vascularity of the flap(s) used for the nipple reconstruction, and reduces the amount of subcutaneous adipose tissue available on the deep surface of the skin flaps. The situation can be addressed with the use of flaps raised on either side of the scar. Such a technique is that of the double opposing tab flap as proposed by Kroll[23,27] (Fig. 15.15A,E).

If this double opposing design is used it is essential to make the base width of the flaps a minimum of 15 mm. This will help ensure an adequate blood supply to the flaps as they are elevated. Unfortunately, closure of the created donor defect does confer a definite 'flatness' to the reconstructed breast mound at this point. This remains an unsolved problem. Nevertheless, the double opposing tab flap remains a useful technique when the mastectomy scar runs directly though the ideal position for nipple creation.

It is important to realize that, no matter which technique is selected, contraction will occur as part of the healing process, and therefore the nipple needs to be made larger than the opposite nipple at the time of reconstruction. Prior to the study noted above we had the strong clinical impression that the 'shrinkage' rate was somewhere between 40% and 60% when projection is seen as a function of time from surgery and the projection is carefully studied for 1 year. As corroborated in our study, most of the projection is lost within the first 6 months, loss continuing for up to a year but being apparently stable after that. This is an important concept for the surgeon to be aware of when trying to achieve long-term nipple symmetry from the standpoint of projection.

REVISING THE SUBOPTIMAL NIPPLE RECONSTRUCTION

Cases of minor projection loss may be compensated for by an intradermal tattoo (Fig. 15.3A–C). This tends to produce color patch symmetry, giving the visual appearance of a normal breast and nipple symmetry on casual glance. I believe that a well-done tattoo can 'rescue' or salvage a suboptimal nipple reconstruction in many cases (Fig. 15.3D).

Major loss of projection following nipple reconstruction is disappointing for both the patient and the surgeon. This result is an asymmetry which detracts from the overall appearance of the reconstruction. This situation can be addressed in several ways.

An uncommon but helpful method is to use a composite graft of nipple from the opposite breast – if the nipple is sufficiently large and the patient is willing to permit a surgical procedure on it with the placement of incisions.

The utility of this technique is illustrated by the following case.

The patient in question had undergone a previous nipple reconstruction following breast reconstruction with a tissue expander and subsequent implant. The reconstructed nipple had suboptimal projection (Fig. 15.16A,B). Because the patient had a wide thin scar at the intended site of nipple reconstruction only, with attrition of the skin and subcutaneous fat from the tissue expansion process, and a very large contralateral nipple, we addressed this problem by de-epithelialization of the skin overlying the suboptimal nipple reconstruction and placing a composite graft from the opposite nipple (Fig. 15.16C). This remedied the deficient projection and enhanced symmetry between the nipples (Fig. 15.16D,E).

More commonly a modified star flap[21] is very helpful as a source of 'booster' tissue (Fig. 15.17) for the suboptimal nipple reconstruction. This flap can be elevated at the site of the original nipple reconstruction as long as it is oriented such that the base is not encroached upon or compromised by existing scar tissue. The use of this flap to augment nipple projection in a patient who had previously undergone nipple reconstruction with a modified star procedure is illustrated in Figure 15.18(A–F). This was a young woman who had had an immediate left breast reconstruction with a TRAM flap. Eight months after surgery she underwent

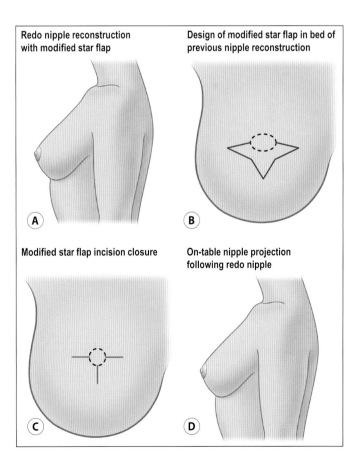

Redo nipple reconstruction with modified star flap

Design of modified star flap in bed of previous nipple reconstruction

(A) (B)

Modified star flap incision closure

On-table nipple projection following redo nipple

(C) (D)

FIGURE 15.17 Outline of redo nipple reconstructed with a modified star flap. The flap is designed such that the base (blood supply) is oriented in the same direction as the previous reconstruction.

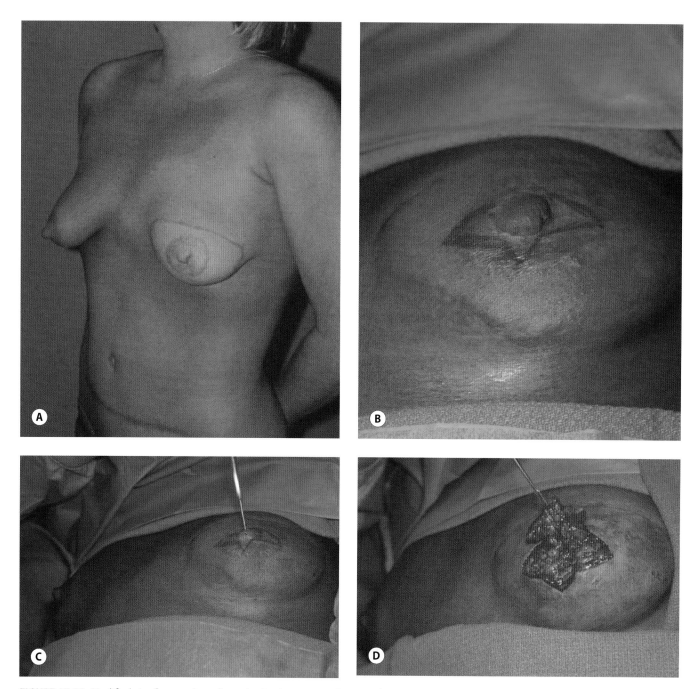

FIGURE 15.18 Modified star flap used as a 'boost' to inadequate previous nipple reconstruction. **A** Inadequate projection of reconstructed nipple compared to significant projection of the nipple on the patient's opposite breast. **B** Design of redo nipple reconstruction with the modified star flap used as a 'boost' to address the inadequate projection of the previous reconstruction. **C, D** Surgical elevation of the flap. Gentle handling of the tissue is accomplished with a skin hook.

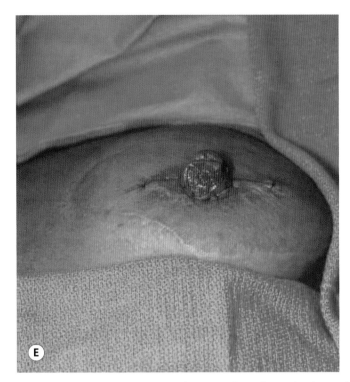

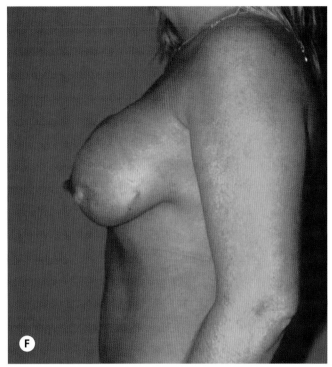

FIGURE 15.18, cont'd E Flap tissue being 'configured' into the shape of a nipple. **F** Enhanced projection noted postoperatively on the lateral view.

nipple reconstruction with a superiorly based modified star flap. She sustained wound separation at the site of flap inset, which resulted in excessive wound contraction and a 70% loss of nipple projection. Five months after complete healing we performed another modified star flap to increase her nipple projection (Fig. 15.18B,C). This was done by orienting the flap in the exact same direction as the original flap, elevating most of the previous flap with the new modified star flap (Fig. 15.18D). This produced a very satisfactory outcome from the standpoint of symmetry with the contralateral nipple (Fig. 15.18E,F).

REFERENCES

1. Bostwick J 3rd. Plastic and reconstructive breast surgery. St Louis: Quality Medical Publishing, 1990; 1174.
2. Shestak KC. Re-operative plastic surgery of the breast. Philadelphia: Lippincott Williams & Wilkins, 2006.
3. Slavin SA, Colen SR. Sixty consecutive breast reconstructions with the inflatable expander: a critical appraisal. Plast Reconstruct Surg 1990; 86: 910–919.
4. Maxwell GP, Falcone PA. Eighty-four consecutive breast reconstructions using a textured silicone tissue expander. Plast Reconstruct Surg 1992; 89: 1022–1034; discussion 1035–1036.
5. Klatsky SA, Manson PN. Toe pulp free grafts in nipple reconstruction. Plast Reconstruct Surg 1981; 68: 245.
6. Brent B, Bostwick J 3rd. Nipple–areola reconstruction with auricular tissues. Plast Reconstruct Surg 1977; 60: 353.
7. Adams WM. Labial transplant for correction of loss of the nipple. Plast Reconstruct Surg 1949; 4: 295.
8. Bhatty MA, Berry RB. Nipple–areola reconstruction by tattooing and nipple sharing. Br J Plast Surg 1997; 50: 331–334.
9. Little JW. Nipple–areolar reconstruction. In: Cohen, Mimis (ed.) Mastery of surgery: plastic and reconstructive surgery. Vol. II. Boston: Little, Brown, 1994.
10. Shestak KC, Gabriel A, Landecker A, et al. Assessment of long-term nipple projection: a comparison of three techniques. Plast Reconstruct Surg 2002; 110: 780–786.
11. Hartrampf CR Jr, Culbertson JH. A dermal-fat flap for nipple reconstruction. Plast Reconstruct Surg 1984; 73: 982.
12. Little JW 3rd. Nipple–areola reconstruction. Clin Plast Surg 1984; 11: 351.
13. Shestak KC, Nguyen TD. The double opposing peri-areolar flap: a novel concept for nipple–areola reconstruction. Plast Reconstruct Surg 2007; 119: 473–480.
14. Hammond DC. Nipple reconstruction with a variation of the skate flap. Plast Reconstruct Surg (in press).
15. Broadbent TR, Woolf RM, Metz PS. Restoring the mammary areola by a skin graft from the upper inner thigh. Br J Plast Surg 1977; 30: 220.
16. Spear SL, Convit R, Little JW 3rd. Intradermal tattoo as an adjunct to nipple–areola reconstruction. Plast Reconstruct Surg 1989; 83: 907.
17. Becker H. The use of intradermal tattoo to enhance the final result of nipple–areola reconstruction. Plast Reconstruct Surg 1986; 77: 673.
18. Little JW 3rd, Munasifi T, McCulloch DT. One-stage reconstruction of a projecting nipple: the quadripod flap. Plast Reconstruct Surg 1983; 71: 126.
19. Little JW. Nipple–areolar reconstruction. In: Cohen, Mimis ed. Mastery of surgery: plastic and reconstructive surgery. Vol. II. Boston: Little, Brown, 1994.
20. Little JW. Nipple–areola reconstruction. In: Spear SL, Little JW, Lippman ME, Wood WC, eds. Surgery of the breast: principles and art. Philadelphia: Lippincott-Raven, 1998.

21. Eskenazi L. A one-stage nipple reconstruction with the 'modified star' flap and immediate tattoo: a review of 100 cases. Plast Reconstruct Surg 1993; 92: 671–680.

22. McCraw JB, Colen L. The fish-tail flap in nipple reconstruction. Personal communication.

23. Kroll SS, Hamilton S. Nipple reconstruction with the double-opposing-tab flap. Plast Reconstruct Surg 1989; 84: 520.

24. Hugo NE, Sultan MR, Hardy SP. Nipple–areola reconstruction with intradermal tattoo and double-opposing pennant flaps. Ann Plast Surg 1993; 30: 510–513.

25. Weiss J, Herman O, Rosenberg L, Shafir R. The S nipple–areola reconstruction. Plast Reconstruct Surg 1989; 83: 904–906.

26. Lossing C, Brongo S, Holmstrom H. Nipple reconstruction with a modified S-flap technique. Scand J Plast Reconstruct Hand Surg 1998; 32: 275–279.

27. Kroll SS, Reece GP, Miller MJ, et al. Comparison of nipple projection with the modified double-opposing tab and star flaps. Plast Reconstruct Surg 1997; 99: 1602–1605.

28. Rohrich RJ, Coberly DM, Krueger JK, Brown SA. Planning elective operations on patients who smoke: survey of North American plastic surgeons. Plast Reconstruct Surg 2002; 109: 350–355; discussion 356–357.

Index

Page numbers relating only to illustrations are in *italics*.